T0226665

Standing Surgery

Editor

JEREMIAH T. EASLEY

VETERINARY CLINICS OF NORTH AMERICA: EQUINE PRACTICE

www.vetequine.theclinics.com

Consulting Editor
A. SIMON TURNER

April 2014 • Volume 30 • Number 1

ELSEVIER

1600 John F. Kennedy Boulevard • Suite 1800 • Philadelphia, Pennsylvania, 19103-2899

http://www.vetequine.theclinics.com

VETERINARY CLINICS OF NORTH AMERICA: EQUINE PRACTICE Volume 30, Number 1
April 2014 ISSN 0749-0739, ISBN-13: 978-0-323-29022-7

Editor: Patrick Manley; p.manley@elsevier.com
Developmental Editor: Donald Mumford

© 2014 Elsevier Inc. All rights reserved.

This periodical and the individual contributions contained in it are protected under copyright by Elsevier, and the following terms and conditions apply to their use:

Photocopying

Single photocopies of single articles may be made for personal use as allowed by national copyright laws. Permission of the Publisher and payment of a fee is required for all other photocopying, including multiple or systematic copying, copying for advertising or promotional purposes, resale, and all forms of document delivery. Special rates are available for educational institutions that wish to make photocopies for non-profit educational classroom use. For information on how to seek permission visit www.elsevier.com/permissions or call: (+44) 1865 843830 (UK)/(+1) 215 239 3804 (USA).

Derivative Works

Subscribers may reproduce tables of contents or prepare lists of articles including abstracts for internal circulation within their institutions. Permission of the Publisher is required for resale or distribution outside the institution. Permission of the Publisher is required for all other derivative works, including compilations and translations (please consult www.elsevier.com/permissions).

Electronic Storage or Usage

Permission of the Publisher is required to store or use electronically any material contained in this periodical, including any article or part of an article (please consult www.elsevier.com/permissions). Except as outlined above, no part of this publication may be reproduced, stored in a retrieval system or transmitted in any form or by any means, electronic, mechanical, photocopying, recording or otherwise, without prior written permission of the Publisher.

Notice

No responsibility is assumed by the Publisher for any injury and/or damage to persons or property as a matter of products liability, negligence or otherwise, or from any use or operation of any methods, products, instructions or ideas contained in the material herein. Because of rapid advances in the medical sciences, in particular, independent verification of diagnoses and drug dosages should be made.

Although all advertising material is expected to conform to ethical (medical) standards, inclusion in this publication does not constitute a guarantee or endorsement of the quality or value of such product or of the claims made of it by its manufacturer.

Veterinary Clinics of North America: Equine Practice (ISSN 0749-0739) is published in April, August, and December by Elsevier Inc., 360 Park Avenue South, New York, NY 10010-1710. Business and Editorial Offices: 1600 John F. Kennedy Blvd., Suite 1800, Philadelphia, PA 19103-2899. Subscription prices are $270.00 per year (domestic individuals), $431.00 per year (domestic institutions), $130.00 per year (domestic students/residents), $315.00 per year (Canadian individuals), $543.00 per year (Canadian institutions), $365.00 per year (international individuals), $543.00 per year (international institutions), and $180.00 per year (international and Canadian students/residents). To receive student/resident rate, orders must be accompanied by name of affiliated institution, date of term, and the signature of program/residency coordinator on institution letterhead. Orders will be billed at individual rate until proof of status is received. Foreign air speed delivery is included in all *Clinics* subscription prices. All prices are subject to change without notice. **POSTMASTER:** Send address changes to *Veterinary Clinics of North America: Equine Practice*, 3251 Riverport Lane, Maryland Heights, MO 63043. Customer Service (orders, claims, online, change of address): Elsevier Health Sciences Division, Subscription Customer Service, 3251 Riverport Lane, Maryland Heights, MO 63043. Tel: 1-800-654-2452 (U.S. and Canada); 314-447-8871 (outside U.S. and Canada). Fax: 314-447-8029. E-mail: journalscustomerservice-usa@elsevier.com (for print support); E-mail: journalsonlinesupport-usa@elsevier.com (for online support).

Reprints. For copies of 100 or more of articles in this publication, please contact the Commercial Reprints Department, Elsevier Inc., 360 Park Avenue South, New York, NY 10010-1710. Tel.: 212-633-3874; Fax: 212-633-3820; E-mail: reprints@elsevier.com.

Veterinary Clinics of North America: Equine Practice is covered in *MEDLINE/PubMed (Index Medicus), Excerpta Medica, Current Contents/Agriculture, Biology and Environmental Sciences,* and *ISI.*

Contributors

CONSULTING EDITOR

A. SIMON TURNER, BVSc, MS, DVSc
Diplomate, American College of Veterinary Surgeons; Professor Emeritus, Department of Clinical Sciences, College of Veterinary Medicine and Biomedical Sciences, Colorado State University, Fort Collins, Colorado

EDITOR

JEREMIAH T. EASLEY, DVM
Diplomate, American College of Veterinary Surgeons; Assistant Director, Surgical Research Laboratory; Assistant Professor, Department of Clinical Sciences, College of Veterinary Medicine and Biological Sciences, Colorado State University, Fort Collins, Colorado

AUTHORS

ARIC ADAMS, DVM
Diplomate, American College of Veterinary Surgeons; Associate Surgeon, Equine Medical Center of Ocala, Ocala, Florida

SAFIA Z. BARAKZAI, BVSc, MSc, DESTS, MRCVS
Diplomate, European College of Veterinary Surgeon; Equine Surgeon, Chine House Veterinary Hospital, Sileby, Leicestershire, United Kingdom

DENNIS E. BROOKS, DVM, PhD
Diplomate of the American College of Veterinary Ophthalmologists; Comparative Ophthalmology Service, Department of Large Animal Sciences; Comparative Ophthalmology Service, Department of Small Animal Sciences, College of Veterinary Medicine, University of Florida, Gainesville, Florida

PHIL A. CRAMP, BSc, BVM&S, MS, MRCVS
Diplomate, American College of Veterinary Surgeons; Diplomate, European College of Veterinary Surgeon; Hambleton Equine Clinic, Hutton Rudby, North Yorkshire, England

PADRAIC M. DIXON, MVB, PhD, MRCVS
Professor of Equine Surgery, Dick Vet Equine Hospital, Easter Bush Vet Centre, University of Edinburgh, Roslin, Midlothian, United Kingdom

JACK EASLEY, DVM
Diplomate, American Board of Veterinary Practitioners; Equine Veterinary Practice, Easley Equine Dentistry, Shelbyville, Kentucky

JEREMIAH T. EASLEY, DVM
Diplomate, American College of Veterinary Surgeons; Assistant Director, Surgical Research Laboratory; Assistant Professor, Department of Clinical Sciences, College of Veterinary Medicine and Biological Sciences, Colorado State University, Fort Collins, Colorado

DAVID FREEMAN, MVB, PhD
Diplomate, American College of Veterinary Surgeons; Large Animal Clinical Sciences, University of Florida, College of Veterinary Medicine, Gainesville, Florida

FERNANDO L. GARCIA-PEREIRA, DVM, MS
Diplomate, American College of Veterinary Anesthesia and Analgesia; Assistant Professor in Veterinary Anesthesia, Department of Large Animal Clinical Science, College of Veterinary Medicine, University of Florida, Gainesville, Florida

JANIK C. GASIOROWSKI, VMD
Diplomate, American College of Veterinary Surgeons; Associate Surgeon, Department of Surgery, Mid-Atlantic Equine Medical Center, Ringoes, New Jersey

SARAH GRAHAM, DVM
Diplomate, American College of Veterinary Surgeons; Diplomate, American College of Veterinary Sports Medicine and Rehabilitation; Clinical Assistant Professor, Large Animal Clinical Sciences, University of Florida, Gainesville, Florida

DEAN A. HENDRICKSON, DVM, MS
Diplomate, American College of Veterinary Surgeons; Associate Dean, Professional Veterinary Medicine, Colorado State University, Fort Collins, Colorado

MICHALA DE LINDE HENRIKSEN, DVM, PhD
Comparative Ophthalmology Service, Department of Veterinary Clinical Sciences, College of Veterinary Medicine, University of Minnesota, Saint Paul, Minnesota

ROBERT J. HUNT, DVM, MS
Diplomate, American College of Veterinary Surgeons; Davidson Surgery Center, Hagyard Equine Medical Institute, Lexington, Kentucky

ROBERT A. MENZIES, BVSc
Diplomate, American Veterinary Dental College; Dentistry & Oral Surgery Service, Faculty of Veterinary Medicine, Veterinary Teaching Hospital, University of Helsinki, Helsinki, Finland

FRANK A. NICKELS, MS, DVM
Diplomate, American College of Veterinary Surgeons; A203 Veterinary Medical Center, College of Veterinary Medicine, Michigan State University, East Lansing, Michigan

THOMAS O'BRIEN, MVB
Diplomate, American College of Veterinary Surgeons; Fethard Equine Hospital, Fethard, Tipperary, Ireland

ERIN G. PORTER, DVM
Diplomate of the American College of Veterinary Radiology; Clinical Assistant Professor, Diagnostic Imaging, Department of Small Animal Clinical Sciences, University of Florida, Gainesville, Florida

TIMO PRANGE, DVetMed, MS
Diplomate, American College of Veterinary Surgeons; Equine and Farm Animal Veterinary Center, NC State College of Veterinary Medicine Veterinary Health Complex, Raleigh, North California

DEAN W. RICHARDSON, DVM
Diplomate, American College of Veterinary Surgeons; Charles W. Raker Professor of Equine Surgery, Chief, Large Animal Surgery, Section of Surgery, New Bolton Center, University of Pennsylvania, Kennett Square, Pennsylvania

JIM SCHUMACHER, DVM, MS, MRCVS
Diplomate, American College of Veterinary Surgeons; Department of Large Animal
Clinical Sciences, University of Tennessee, Knoxville, Tennessee

KATHRYN A. SEABAUGH, DVM, MS
Diplomate, American College of Veterinary Surgeons; Department of Large Animal
Medicine, College of Veterinary Medicine, University of Georgia, Athens, Georgia

ALESSIO VIGANI, DVM, PhD
Diplomate, American College of Veterinary Anesthesia and Analgesia; Resident in Small
Animal Emergency and Critical Care, Department of Small Animal Clinical Science,
College of Veterinary Medicine, University of Florida, Gainesville, Florida

NATASHA M. WERPY, DVM
Diplomate of the American College of Veterinary Radiology; Clinical Associate Professor,
Diagnostic Imaging, Department of Small Animal Clinical Sciences, University of Florida,
Gainesville, Florida

Contents

The advantages of performing standing male urogenital surgeries are numerous when compared with performing the same surgery in the anesthetized animal. Some traditional standing male urogenital surgeries, such as castrations, may be faster and cheaper to perform. Laparoscopic standing male urogenital surgeries may allow for improved visualization of the surgical field, decreased hemorrhage, and decreased morbidity and convalescence. Limitations of standing procedures may include increased danger to the surgeon because of fractious behavior of the patient, and increased expense and training associated with instrumentation for specialized procedures such as laparoscopy.

Many urogenital procedures of the mare are commonly performed with the mare standing. Ovariectomy via colpotomy was described as early as 1903, and the Caslick vulvoplasty was first described in 1937. As knowledge expands and instruments become more specialized, techniques will improve. With the introduction of laparoscopy, clinicians have not only been able to improve the previously described urogenital procedures but also to devise new procedures. This article describes multiple surgeries of the female urogenital tract, all of which can be performed with the mare standing, and describes a variety of approaches to some portions of the female urogenital tract.

This article describes diagnostic arthroscopy and arthroscopic management of selected lesions in the standing equine patient. Details on case selection, patient and operating room preparation, and surgical technique are presented. This information will add techniques that avoid general anesthesia to the equine surgeon's armamentarium.

In all surgeries with the patient standing under chemical and physical restraint, patient compliance is of the utmost importance. All fractures of the third metacarpal or metatarsal condyles and sagittal fracture of the first phalanx are not amenable to internal fixation with the horse standing, and young unhandled horses may not have a suitable disposition for standing surgical treatment of septic pedal osteitis, or implantation and removal of transphyseal screws. Previous operator experience in performing the procedure or technique under general anesthesia is beneficial. Appreciation of appropriate topographic anatomic landmarks is important, and intraoperative radiographic control is useful.

This article addresses the clinical application of magnetic resonance imaging (MRI) and computed tomography (CT) as applied to the standing equine patient. This discussion includes the logistics, advantages, disadvantages, and limitations of imaging a standing horse. In addition, a brief review is given of the physics of these modalities as applied in clinical practice, and the currently available hardware and software required by these techniques for image acquisition and artifact reduction. The appropriate selection of clinical cases for standing MRI and CT is reviewed, focusing on cases that are capable of undergoing standing surgeries following lesion diagnosis.

VETERINARY CLINICS OF
NORTH AMERICA: EQUINE PRACTICE

THE CLINICS ARE NOW AVAILABLE ONLINE!
Access your subscription at:
www.theclinics.com

Preface

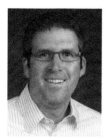

Jeremiah T. Easley, DVM
Editor

It has been an honor and pleasure to be the editor of the *Veterinary Clinics of North America: Equine Practice* on standing surgery. This issue is meant to summarize extensive advancements made over the past 20 years since the last *Veterinary Clinics* issue on standing surgery was published in 1991. The many advancements can be attributed to improvements made in minimally invasive equine surgery. Other advancements can be attributed to innovative and original thinking surgeons who realized a need and pursued a new surgical technique in the standing horse to avoid the complications involved with general anesthesia related to a particular procedure. The authors contributing to this issue have strived to present the most recent and up-to-date standing equine procedures with the goal of improving veterinarians' understanding of this rapidly growing topic.

For each article, I recruited authors with diverse experiences in each topic. My goal was to pair newer veterinary scientists establishing their early careers with experienced and highly accomplished experts in various fields of study. This edition will not only present the most current literature, but will also include previous experiences that may benefit a surgeon performing a specific surgery for the very first time in the standing horse. I would like to personally thank the authors for their contributions. I hope the reader finds the articles complete and all encompassing.

In my opinion, standing surgery is always advantageous to the horse, owner, and often the surgeon as long as the surgery can be performed safely, as effectively, and with equivalent outcomes as the procedure performed under general anesthesia. This will vary tremendously between cases based on surgical experience and patient cooperation. However, there are obvious cases where general anesthesia is required or warranted to ensure safety to the patient and the personnel. Standing surgery cannot be performed in all scenarios, and many of the standing procedures described in this text should be reserved for qualified surgeons who are comfortable and experienced performing these surgeries in the recumbent horse as well.

While my career as a surgeon may be short to date, I have been fortunate to learn from very gifted professionals in such a brief time. I am very grateful for my experiences at the Equine Medical Center of Ocala, the University of Florida, and Colorado State University. My internship, surgical residency, and current position have afforded me

Vet Clin Equine 30 (2014) xiii–xiv
http://dx.doi.org/10.1016/j.cveq.2013.11.013
0749-0739/14/$ – see front matter © 2014 Elsevier Inc. All rights reserved.

opportunities to learn from and work alongside highly talented veterinarians who have guided my career and opened doors I never knew existed. I would like to thank those clinicians for the amazing experiences I have had under their leadership. I would also like to thank Dr. A. Simon Turner for the opportunity to be the guest editor for this exciting issue of *Veterinary Clinics of North America: Equine Practice*. Drs Simon Turner and Howard B. Seim, III, are extraordinary mentors and friends, who never stop teaching or helping young professionals establish their careers. Lastly, I want to thank my father, Jack Easley, and my wife, Jennifer Hatzel (both equine veterinarians), for being daily role models in this wonderful career path I have chosen.

Jeremiah T. Easley, DVM
Surgical Research Laboratory
Department of Clinical Sciences
College of Veterinary Medicine and Biological Sciences
Colorado State University
300 West Drake Road
Fort Collins, CO 80523, USA

E-mail address:
jeremiah.easley@colostate.edu

Anesthesia and Analgesia for Standing Equine Surgery

Alessio Vigani, DVM, PhD[a],*, Fernando L. Garcia-Pereira, DVM, MS[b]

KEYWORDS

- Standing equine surgery • Equine Anesthesia • Standing sedation
- Epidural equine analgesia • Epidural catheterization

KEY POINTS

- Standing sedation represents a safe and effective alternative to general anesthesia for many diagnostic and surgical procedures in horses.
- Patient selection and preparation are critical aspects for a successful standing sedation procedure.
- α2-Agonists represent the main-stem class of sedatives for standing sedation.
- The use of drug combinations and continuous rate infusions are recommended to provide a balanced and steady-state level of sedation and analgesia during the procedure. The use of short-acting agents favors rapid titration to effect and recovery.
- Single-injection or continuous epidural anesthesia/analgesia provides significant advantages for selected procedures to abdominal cavity and perineal region.

INTRODUCTION

The risks associated with equine anesthesia are well known to any professional involved in equine medical care. It has been repeatedly shown that general anesthesia in horses has the highest complication rate of any other domestic species. An anesthetic-related mortality of up to 1% for elective procedures, and 10% for emergency procedures, has been reported.[1–3] These worrisome data should always be kept in mind when contemplating whether the benefit of general anesthesia for a specific patient and procedure outweighs the risks. However, considering mortality alone significantly underestimates the overall morbidity of equine anesthesia in terms of nonlethal injuries occurring during recovery.[4] The astronomically high complication rate seems to be mainly due to the cardiovascular and respiratory alterations caused

Funding Sources: None.

Conflict of Interest: None.

[a] Department of Small Animal Clinical Science, College of Veterinary Medicine, University of Florida, 2015 Southwest 16th Avenue, Gainesville, FL 32608, USA; [b] Department of Large Animal Clinical Science, College of Veterinary Medicine, University of Florida, 2015 Southwest 16th Avenue, Gainesville, FL 32608, USA

* Corresponding author.

E-mail address: alessio.vigani@gmail.com

http://dx.doi.org/10.1016/j.cveq.2013.11.008

0749-0739/14/$ – see front matter © 2014 Elsevier Inc. All rights reserved.

by anesthesia and recumbency.[1] Decreased tissue perfusion and oxygenation to the muscles and visceral organs are also responsible for the development of myopathy and gastrointestinal dysfunction.[3,4]

The development and practice of sedative protocols that would allow the practitioner to perform diagnostic and surgical procedures with the patient remaining standing would therefore be ideal in certain circumstances. Sedation maintains the physiologic cardiovascular compensatory mechanisms that are commonly depressed during general anesthesia. Maintaining the horse in a standing position also has the absolute advantage over general anesthesia of eliminating the detrimental effect of recumbency on gas exchange and muscle perfusion.

However, the physiologic advantages of standing sedation are counterbalanced by the inherent difficulties of maintaining appropriate patient restraint for the surgical procedure. Excessive sedation and muscle relaxation would induce tremors, ataxia, or worse, causing the animal to fall. A plane of sedation that is too superficial instead would potentially induce delirium and hypersensitivity to stimulation. In this regard, the use of short-acting sedatives because titrated continuous infusion seems to be preferable over bolus dosing of longer-acting agents. Infusion of short-acting agents allows the achievement of the wanted effect and the titration to a steady state of sedation in a more rapid fashion. Bolus dosing alone instead will likely produce intermittent peaks and troughs of levels of sedation and possibly higher risk of over- or undersedation. The use of continuous infusions would likely provide a more constant sedative effect once the initial loading bolus has been administered.

The combination of drugs with different pharmacologic action allows for reduced doses of individual drugs, thereby decreasing their side effects. A balanced approach by supplementing sedatives and tranquilizers with systemic analgesic or regional anesthetic techniques facilitates standing procedures. Multimodal analgesia would also provide superior analgesia with potentially fewer side effects than a single-agent approach.[5]

Although standing sedation is widely recognized to be associated with a lower risk of severe complications compared with general anesthesia, the current literature is lacking in precise indications in regard to the complication rate and mortality. Due to the lack of definitive evidence of superiority of one sedative protocol over another, the management of standing sedation in horses is still based on tradition, personal bias, and institutional preference rather than on scientific approaches.

Nevertheless, a critical consideration is related to the safety of the staff. The safety of the personnel involved in the procedure represents the most important factor to consider when approaching a procedure under standing sedation in horses. In this regard, the margin of error becomes much narrower than during general anesthesia and the anesthetist has the responsibility, not only to ensure the highest level of anesthetic care to the patient but also to provide a safe and protected working condition for the operators involved.

PATIENT ASSESSMENT AND PREPARATION

Dr Robert Moors Smith, an icon of human pediatric anesthesiology, when asked an opinion about what is the role of his profession in modern medicine, briefly answered: "There are no safe anesthetic agents, there are no safe anesthetic procedures, there are only safe anesthetists." This statement brilliantly summarizes the critical importance of the appropriate selection and direct supervision of any sedated or anesthetized patient. Preliminary examination, appropriate patient stabilization, and intraprocedural monitoring by the anesthetist are compulsory to performing a safe and uneventful standing sedation.

Patient selection is the first step for a successful standing procedure. Fractious or highly stressed horses are unlikely to tolerate any manual restraining and handling. It is notorious that highly sympathetically driven animals appear to be resistant to standard doses of sedatives. However, unpredictable oversedation may result with the use of higher dosages. Therefore for these reasons and because of the potential risk for the personnel involved, these patients should be considered poor candidates for standing sedation.

"Plan for the worst!" is a general rule for any sedation or anesthesia in horses. When planning for a standing procedure, it is critical to anticipate the possible occurrence of complications to be prepared for a prompt intervention. For example, a major risk of standing sedation is the falling of the patient on the ground. In this unfortunate scenario, the recommended intervention is a rapid induction of general anesthesia and placement of the patient in an appropriately padded stall for recovery. Therefore, it is indicated to always calculate and have available appropriate doses of induction agents (ie, ketamine and diazepam). In addition, endotracheal tubes of different sizes and oxygen supply should be available in case of a need for rapid intubation after induction of anesthesia. All equipment and emergency medications should be prepared in advance to ensure appropriate intervention under emergency conditions.

As part of the patient's preparation, an intravenous catheter should be placed for drugs and fluid administration, and the horse's mouth should be washed in case there is a need for endotracheal intubation. For prolonged procedures (>1 hour), the placement of a urinary catheter is recommended for urine collection, especially when $\alpha2$-agonists are used. The aim is to prevent the spread of urine on the floor that could increase the risk of accidental fall of the animal.

A quiet location, devoid of stimulating factors such as bright light, noise, and other horses, should be chosen for the procedure. Use of blinders and placing swabs in the ears once the patient is sedated help to reduce stimulation. For prolonged procedures, the use of a dedicated room, equipped with specific stocks to confine the horse, is highly recommended. Fully walled stocks should be avoided. The stocks should be constructed of metal bars only to leave free access to the animal from all sides.

Indications for standing sedation must consider the complexity and duration of the procedure. Complexity of the surgical procedure has been associated with the risk of anesthetic-related complications.[1,4] Increasing duration also, independently from the type of surgical procedure, was associated with increased risk.[1] These principles would likely also apply to standing sedation. Prolonged procedures expose the patient to drug accumulation, increased risk of undesired effects, and prolonged recovery. Therefore, the practitioner's familiarity with the procedure and the experience of the personnel involved in the procedure play an important role at decreasing the risk of complications.[2]

With appropriate sedation and analgesia, there are several procedures that can be performed in the standing conscious horse. Diagnostic procedures, such as magnetic resonance imaging, scintigraphy, and endoscopy, usually require minimal or no analgesia, whereas invasive surgical interventions may require a multimodal approach to control pain.

Minor surgical procedures, which are often considered for standing sedation, include tracheostomy, placement of a subpalpebral lavage system, tarsorrhaphy, removal of the nictitating membrane, and cryosurgery for removal of small cutaneous masses.

Sinus surgery, excision of large cutaneous masses, thoracoscopy, and laparascopy are examples of more invasive indications for standing sedation in which appropriate analgesia is critical for successful results. Standing laparoscopy is commonly used for diagnostic biopsy, ovariectomy, cryptorchidectomy, and colopexy. Perineal surgery and urethral surgery are other common indications for standing sedation. The standing position in these cases maintains the symmetry of the anatomic landmarks, hence facilitating the surgical approach. Profound analgesia for perineal surgery can be successfully provided with regional techniques such as epidural analgesia and a pudendal nerve block. The combination of these analgesic techniques with the sedation protocol would significantly reduce nociceptive stimulation and the risk of unwanted reactions of the patient. Other procedures performed in the standing position are included in later articles within this issue.

PHARMACOLOGY

Ideal drug combinations for standing procedures should provide reliable sedation, cause minimal ataxia, and provide adequate analgesia. Virtually all of these combinations include α2-agonists along with another agent with synergistic effect. Following is a description of some recommended protocols with relative duration of effect and practical indications for use.

Acepromazine

Acepromazine is commonly used for premedication. It is very effective as an anxiolytic; however, it provides only a mild to moderate degree of sedation. Acepromazine at the dose of 0.02 to 0.04 mg/kg can provide sufficient restraint for clipping and placement of an intravenous catheter. The intramuscular route of administration is associated with a delay in the peak sedative effect of about 30 to 45 minutes. With intravenous injection, the sedative effect is achieved usually within 15 minutes.[6] The duration of sedation is 3 to 4 hours. Acepromazine does not provide any analgesic effect.[7] Occasionally paradoxic excitement may occur. Acepromazine provides a good calming effect, and it significantly decreases the requirements of other sedatives used in combination. In horses it also has antiarrhythmogenic properties.[8] If profound sedation is needed, acepromazine alone is likely to be insufficient even at high doses. Increasing the dose will only increase the duration of action, without further increasing the intensity of sedation. For this reason, it should always be used in combination with other drugs, such as α2-agonists and opioids.[6]

Acepromazine can cause sudden collapse in excited horses, although this occurrence is extremely rare. The suggested mechanism for this overresponse is that sympathetically driven animals have high circulating levels of catecholamines. Circulating epinephrine preferentially acts at β-adrenergic receptors, causing skeletal muscle vasodilation and, as peripheral α1-receptors are blocked by acepromazine, this will unmask the vasodilation, with secondary profound hypotension and possible collapse. Acepromazine is not suitable for use in hypovolemic or septic patients, because drug-induced vasodilatation will worsen the preexisting cardiovascular instability. Acepromazine is contraindicated in breeding stallions, because it has been associated with priapism and paraphimosis, although this has been proven to be extremely rare.[9]

α2-Agonists

α2-Adrenoreceptor agonists are undoubtedly the main-stem component of any standing sedation in horses. It is realistically impossible to provide a reliable, stable, and profound degree of sedation without using an α2-adrenoreceptor agonist. Xylazine, romifidine, detomidine, and dexmedetomidine are available for use in horses.[10] Their peak effect occurs approximately 2 to 5 and 15 to 30 minutes after intravenous and intramuscular administration, respectively.[11] The intramuscular dose required to produce similar intensity of sedation is approximately double the intravenous dose for all of the agents belonging to this class.

Recently, the pharmacokinetics and pharmacodynamics of a detomidine gel administered sublingually have been investigated. At the dose of 0.04 mg/kg, mild to moderate sedation was observed. The time of onset of sedation was about 40 minutes, and duration was approximately 2 hours. Large interindividual variability of effect was observed.[12]

All α2-agonists produce reliable, sedative, visceral, and somatic analgesic, and muscle-relaxant effects.[13] α2-Agonists are characterized by a "ceiling" sedative effect, whereby increasing the dose extends the duration but does not increase the intensity of sedation.[14] After the initial bolus, there are 2 options to maintain sedation for prolonged procedures. Supplemental intravenous doses can be given as needed when the sedative effects start decreasing, at approximately one-quarter to one-half of the initial dose. Alternatively, many authors recommend the administration as continuous intravenous infusions, avoiding the "peaks and troughs" seen with repeat bolus injections.

Common side effects of all α2-agonists include bradycardia, second-degree atrioventricular block, biphasic hypertension followed by hypotension, increased urine production, moderate hyperglycemia, sweating, and decreased gastrointestinal motility.[10] Ataxia appears more profound with xylazine compared with romifidine or detomidine.[15] Increased myometrial contractility and intrauterine pressure have been shown to occur with xylazine; therefore, it should not be used during the last trimester of pregnancy. Conversely, detomidine has been shown to reduce intrauterine pressure, and therefore, it represents the sedative of choice in pregnant mares at late stages of pregnancy.[16]

The intravenous administration of detomidine was also shown to decrease intraocular pressure in clinically normal horses and may represent a safe sedative when performing ocular procedures.[17]

α2-Agonists given as a bolus cause a temporary increase in afterload with secondary depression of ventricular function and cause myocardial hypoxia due to coronary vasoconstriction. The magnitude of these effects appears to be largely dose independent and is demonstrated by the near-maximal magnitude of cardiovascular changes occurring even at microdoses of these agents. Therefore the use of "low doses" should not be considered safer than high doses. Instead, the preliminary evaluation and appropriate patient selection are the most important factors in determining the safety of the use of any α2-agonist.[18]

The solution for a continuous infusion can be prepared by adding the selected α2-agonist agent to a bag of isotonic crystalloid fluids. This solution is initially administered at a calculated drip rate and then titrated to effect on a case-by-case basis. Bolus doses and infusion rates for many α2-agonists have been investigated for standing sedation in horses. The duration of sedation is longest with romifidine, followed by detomidine, dexmedetomidine, and xylazine, when equipotent intravenous doses are used.[19] The recommended infusion rates should be adjusted based on the patient response and the level of sedation required. The combination of any α2-agonist with butorphanol also allows the reduction of the infusion rate to up to one-half of the rate of the drug used alone.[20,21]

Recommended bolus doses and infusion rates are listed below and reported in **Table 1**:

- Xylazine: The recommended bolus is 0.8 to 1 mg/kg followed by an infusion rate of 0.65 mg/kg/h. Significant ataxia has been shown at high doses and with prolonged infusions.[20]

Table 1	
Recommended intravenous boluses and CRI for α2-agonists	
Drug	**Recommended Intravenous Bolus and Infusion Rate**
Xylazine	Bolus: 0.8–1 mg/kg CRI: 0.65 mg/kg/h
Romifidine	Bolus: 0.1 mg/kg CRI: 0.03 mg/kg/h
Detomidine	Bolus: 0.01 mg/kg CRI: 0.01–0.04 mg/kg/h
Dexmedetomidine	Bolus: 0.003–0.005 mg/kg CRI: 0.005 mg/kg/h

- Romifidine: The initial recommended dose is 0.1 mg/kg followed by 0.03 mg/kg/h.[21] The time to maximal sedation and complete recovery is longer with romifidine than with other α2-agonists. The onset of sedation is 5 to 10 minutes after intravenous bolus and the duration of effect is about 60 minutes.[22]
- Detomidine: An initial bolus of 0.01 mg/kg intravenously can be followed by an infusion of 0.01 to 0.04 mg/kg/h.[23,24] At the high-dose range, ataxia is a common occurrence. When higher infusion rates are required for extended periods of time to maintain an adequate level of sedation, combination with other agents is recommended. The authors commonly use a standard bolus of 0.01 mg/kg followed by an infusion at 0.03 mg/kg/h. If the degree of sedation achieved at this rate does not meet the requirement for the procedure, the addition of butorphanol is then indicated. The combination of butorphanol with detomidine produces a potent synergistic effect. Individual constant rate infusion (CRI) doses should be halved to avoid oversedation.[25]
- Dexmedetomidine is the most potent agent among the commercially available α2-agonists. A bolus of 0.003 to 0.005 mg/kg intravenously has been used by the authors for standing sedation of brief duration (<30 minutes). For longer procedures, an infusion at 0.005 mg/kg/h is indicated. After bolus administration, dexmedetomidine has been shown to produce cardiopulmonary changes similar to other α2-agonists, but of very short duration. Pharmacokinetic studies of dexmedetomidine in horses showed rapid distribution and rapid clearance. These pharmacokinetic characteristics favor its use as a CRI.[26] The cost of the drug, however, still represents the major obstacle to the routine use of dexmedetomodine in equine sedation.

The intravenous solutions of α2-agonists for infusion for a 450-kg horse can be prepared by the following:

- 400 mg xylazine added to a 500-mL bag of saline (0.8 mg/mL), administered at a rate of 1 drop/s (10 drops/mL infusion set). This solution provides 80 minutes of infusion at approximately 0.65 mg/kg/h. When combined with opioids, the infusion rate should be decreased to 1 drop/2 s (0.3g/kg/h)
- 20 mg romifidine added to a 500-mL bag of saline (0.04 mg/mL), administered at a rate of 1 drop/s (10 drops/mL infusion set). This solution provides 80 minutes of infusion at approximately 0.03 mg/kg/h. When combined with opioids, the infusion rate should be decreased to 1 drop/2 s (0.015 mg/kg/h)
- 25 mg of detomidine added to a 500-mL bag of saline (0.05 mg/mL), administered at a rate of 1 drop/s (10 drops/mL infusion set). This solution provides

approximately 80 minutes of infusion at 0.04 mg/kg/h. When combined with opioids, the infusion rate should be decreased to 1 drop/2 s (0.02 mg/kg/h)
- 3.5 mg of dexmedetomidine added to a 500-mL bag of saline (0.007 mg/mL), administered at a rate of 1 drop/s (10 drops/mL infusion set). This solution provides 80 minutes of infusion at approximately 0.005 mg/kg/h. When combined with opioids, the infusion rate should be decreased to 1 drop/2 s (0.002 mg/kg/h)

α2-ANTAGONISTS

The α2-antagonist atipamezole (0.05–0.15 mg/kg IM) has been used successfully to reverse sedation from detomidine, xylazine, romifidine, and medetomidine. Atipamezole completely reverses the sedation, but recurrence of sedation can occur if high doses of α2-agonist are used, mainly due to the short duration of action of atipamezole.[27]

Opioids

The analgesic effect of opiates in horses still represents a major topic of discussion and current investigation. The effect of opioids on somatic and visceral pain has been largely investigated in horses.[28–32] Opioids have also been shown to provide a significant synergistic effect on sedation produced by α2-agonists. The combination of an α2-agonist with an opioid allows a significant reduction of the effective dose of either agent to about half of the dose of each drug used alone (see **Table 4**).[33–36]

The potential side effects of opioids have limited their widespread use in the past. Signs of excitement, such as head shaking and continuous pacing and gastrointestinal hypomotility, are the most feared adverse effects. These complications are rare at analgesic doses, but they can occur at much higher doses (0.5–1 mg/kg morphine) than those used clinically.[37–39] However, the debate on the safety of these agents is still open. Morphine has been implicated in postanesthetic colic in one institution,[40] although results from other studies showed no such risk.[41,42] A reduction in fecal output has been reported in horses given morphine. However, general anesthesia, pain, stress, and changes in diet have all been shown to produce a significant effect on gastrointestinal motility.[43–46] Fecal output is also easily monitored and adding oil to feed may be considered if there is any concern about gastrointestinal motility. The authors encourage the use of opioid analgesics in horses whenever invasive surgical procedures are performed, given that the benefits of their use largely outweigh the risks.[47]

Opioid-induced histamine release, causing urticaria and hypotension, is possible after rapid intravenous injection. This occurrence is particularly rare; however, opioids should be given by slow injection when administered intravenously. Histamine release is more commonly seen after meperidine administration, so this drug, if ever used in horses, should only be administered by the intramuscular route.[48]

Recommended bolus doses and infusion rates are listed below and reported in **Table 2**.

Butorphanol

A single intravenous bolus has a short duration of action, between 30 and 60 minutes. CRIs of butorphanol, used to maintain a steady level of sedation and decrease possible behavioral side effects, have been described.[49] A loading dose of 0.02 mg/kg intravenously, followed by an infusion rate of 0.024 mg/kg/h, was shown to produce both sedative and analgesic effects, without causing behavioral changes, whereas a single dose of butorphanol (0.1 mg/kg, IV) resulted in a significant increase in locomotor activity and ataxia. The use of butorphanol has been associated with increased head

| Table 2 | |
| Recommended intravenous boluses and CRI for opioids | |
Drug	Recommended Intravenous Bolus and Infusion Rate
Butorphanol	Bolus: 0.02 mg/kg CRI: 0.024 mg/kg/h
Morphine	Bolus: 0.1–0.2 mg/kg CRI: 0.03 mg/kg/h
Methadone	Bolus: 0.15 mg/kg CRI: 0.05 mg/kg/h
Buprenorphine	Bolus: 0.005–0.01 mg/kg

shaking and twitching, so it is not ideal for procedures requiring the head to be static (ie, ocular procedures). When combined with α2-agonists, butorphanol produces a potent synergistic effect. Individual CRI doses should be halved to avoid oversedation.[35,50]

Morphine and methadone
Morphine at 0.1 to 0.2 mg/kg intravenously produces sedation and analgesia of longer duration than butorphanol. The effect after bolus administration lasts 4 to 6 hours. Morphine has been used successfully as an infusion at 0.03 mg/kg/h, following an initial bolus of 0.05 mg/kg intravenously, in combination with an α2-agonist for standing surgery.[51] Methadone at 0.15 mg/kg intravenously produces a similar degree of sedation to morphine, but the rate for constant infusion has not been determined at present.[37] The authors have used methadone as a CRI at 0.05 mg/kg/h combined with α2-agonists for standing sinus surgery with successful results.

Buprenorphine
Buprenorphine has recently been studied in horses and appears to provide satisfactory analgesia for 8 to 12 hours.[52,53] Buprenorphine at 0.005 to 0.01 mg/kg intravenously has been shown to provide adequate analgesia in combination with α2-agonists for standing laparoscopy.[54] The onset of analgesia is slow and the peak effect occurs at 45 to 60 minutes after bolus administration.[55,56] Given the long duration of action of buprenorphine, no constant infusion for this agent has been investigated.

The intravenous solutions of opioids for infusion for a 450-kg horse can be prepared by adding the following:

- 15 mg butorphanol to a 500-mL bag of saline (0.03 mg/mL), administered at a rate of 1 drop/s (10 drops/mL infusion set). This solution provides 80 minutes of infusion at approximately 0.024 mg/kg/h. When combined with α2-agonists, the infusion rate should be decreased to 1 drop/2 s (0.012 mg/kg/h)
- 20 mg morphine to a 500-mL bag of saline (0.04 mg/mL), administered at a rate of 1 drop/s (10 drops/mL infusion set). This solution provides 80 minutes of infusion at approximately 0.03 mg/kg/h. When combined with α2-agonists, the infusion rate should be decreased to 1 drop/2 s (0.015 mg/kg/h)
- 30 mg methadone to a 500-mL bag of saline (0.06 mg/mL), administered at a rate of 1 drop/s (10 drops/mL infusion set). This solution provides 80 minutes of infusion at approximately 0.05 mg/kg/h. When combined with α2-agonists, the infusion rate should be decreased to 1 drop/2 s (0.025 mg/kg/h)

Ketamine

Ketamine, besides its common use as an induction agent, can be administered at sub-anesthetic doses in standing horses to provide analgesia, particularly in cases of inflammatory diseases. Ketamine is effective in cases whereby adjunctive analgesia is required. The duration of action of a subanesthetic ketamine bolus (0.1–0.5 mg/kg) is short (30 minutes). At these doses, ketamine appears to provide somatic analgesia and rapid onset of sedation. An infusion of ketamine may then be beneficial for a prolonged procedure when the analgesia provided by α2-agonists or opioids appears insufficient. Ketamine can be infused at 0.3 to 0.6 mg/kg/h intravenously, with minimal side effects (**Table 3**).[57] Ketamine can be used in combination with α2-agonists, opioids, and/or lidocaine for extended infusion.[58] When using combinations, the individual infusion rates should be maintained at the lower end of the dose range to avoid oversedation.

Ketamine is also useful in cases of insufficient sedation from α2-agonists. A bolus of 0.1 to 0.2 mg/kg intravenously is effective as rescue intervention in the case of intra-procedural sudden lightening of the level of sedation. A 50-mg (0.1 mg/kg) intravenous bolus in an average adult horse would provide rapid onset of profound sedation with the horse remaining still for about 15 minutes. This intervention, referred to as the "ketamine stun," should only be used while the sedation from another agent is still effective to avoid excitation.

In recent years, ketamine has been shown to possess several properties beyond its anesthetic and analgesic activity. Most interestingly, ketamine has a substantial anti-inflammatory effect by down-regulating the production of pro-inflammatory cytokines.[59] In virtue of this action, ketamine has been gaining interest for use in the course of laminitis and other severe inflammatory processes in horses.

The intravenous solutions of ketamine for infusion for a 450-kg horse can be prepared as follows:

- 200 mg ketamine added to a 500-mL bag of saline (0.4 mg/mL), administered at a rate of 1 drop/s (10 drops/mL infusion set). This solution provides 80 minutes of infusion at approximately 0.3 mg/kg/h.

Lidocaine

Lidocaine can be administered systemically in horses to provide analgesia, sedation along with anti-inflammatory, prokinetic, and anti-endotoxaemic effects.[60,61] The mechanisms whereby systemic lidocaine exerts analgesic and nonanalgesic actions have not been fully elucidated, but activity on specific peripheral and central sodium channels has been hypothesized.[62] Following a loading dose of 1 to 2 mg/kg given intravenously over 5 to 10 minutes, lidocaine is usually infused at 0.025 to 0.05 mg/kg/min (see **Table 3**).[63]

One important consideration when using lidocaine is the relatively low therapeutic index of this drug. Noticeably, the high end of the effective dose approximates closely

Table 3	
Recommended intravenous boluses and CRI for ketamine and lidocaine	
Drug	**Recommended Intravenous Bolus and Infusion Rate**
Ketamine	Bolus: 0.1–0.2 mg/kg CRI: 0.3–0.6 mg/kg/h
Lidocaine	Bolus: 1–2 mg/kg CRI: 0.025–0.05 mg/kg/min

the dose at which adverse effects may start to occur. The plasma concentration for central nervous system (CNS) side effects in horses is 2 to 3 times the target therapeutic level achieved using the rate of 50 μg/kg/min. Toxic plasma levels can therefore be easily achieved by accumulation of lidocaine with prolonged infusions.[64] The first signs of toxicity are CNS effects, which can present as muscle facsiculations, anxiety, and incoordination. This can progress to loss of consciousness, seizures, and respiratory arrest if severe overdosing occurs. If muscle facsiculations are seen, then the rate should be halved or stopped. Because lidocaine is rapidly metabolized, cessation of therapy or reduction of infusion rate may be all that is required to relieve minor symptoms. Seizures or excitement should be treated with induction of general anesthesia rather than diazepam alone. This recommendation is based on the risk of worsening the incoordination and delirium by using diazepam alone.

If cardiovascular collapse occurs, it should be treated with aggressive fluid resuscitation and vasopressor agents. Rarely, collapse occurs before the onset of muscle fasciculations; this is because there is large variation between individuals. Cardiovascular effects usually occur at a much higher plasma concentration than the one causing CNS signs. Cardiovascular side effects include bradycardia, hypotension, ventricular arrhythmias, and cardiac arrest.[65]

The accumulation of lidocaine and its metabolites during a prolonged infusion (>2 hours) would likely produce ataxia. As a preventive measure, even in the absence of signs of toxicity, after 2 hours of infusion at the high-dose rate (0.0 5 mg/kg/min), it is then recommended to halve the rate (0.025 mg/kg/min).

The intravenous solutions of lidocaine for infusion for a 450-kg horse can be prepared by adding the following:

- 2000 mg lidocaine to a 500-mL bag of saline (4 mg/mL), administered at a rate of 1 drop/s (10 drops/mL infusion set). This solution provides 80 minutes of infusion at approximately 0.05 mg/kg/h. The infusion rate should be halved after 2 hours of infusion.

SEDATIVE COMBINATIONS

When sedative combinations are used, possible chemical interactions between different agents mixed in the same solution can cause precipitation and affect drug stability. To avoid this possible occurrence and to better titrate the effect of each sedative or analgesic drug of the combination, the authors recommend using separate infusion bags for each drug. Infusion rates for sedative combinations commonly used for standing sedation are listed in **Table 4**.

EPIDURAL ANESTHESIA/ANALGESIA

Caudal or intercoccygeal epidural anesthesia and analgesia provide desensitization of the tail, anus, rectum, perineum, vulva, vagina, urethra, and bladder in conscious standing horses.[66] Local anesthetics, α2-agonists, ketamine, and opioids have been administered by caudal epidural injection, providing long-lasting pain relief in standing horses.[67–78] The aim is to produce sensory desensitization without losing the motor function of the hind limbs. Numerous drug combinations have been described. A local anesthetic agent combined with an α2-agonist or an opioid is commonly used.[68,70,71,73]

Epidural α2-agonists provide a direct analgesic effect and a synergistic action with local anesthetics, prolonging their duration of action. Epidural ketamine produces analgesia by a noncompetitive antagonist effect on spinal N-methyl-D-aspartate

Table 4
Recommended intravenous CRI for common sedative combinations (See the text for details on how to prepare infusion bags of each agent of the sedative combination. The solutions for infusion of each sedative or analgesic drug should be prepared in separate bags. It is not recommended to mix multiple drugs in the same infusion bag, due to the risk of possible chemical interactions.)

Drug Combinations	Recommended Intravenous Infusion Rate
Detomidine	0.02 mg/kg/h
Butorphanol	0.012 mg/kg/h
Xylazine	0.03 mg/kg/h
Butorphanol	0.012 mg/kg/h
Romifidine	0.015 mg/kg/h
Butorphanol	0.012 mg/kg/h
Dexmedetomidine	0.002 mg/kg/h
Butorphanol	0.012 mg/kg/h
Detomidine	0.02 mg/kg/h
Morphine	0.015 mg/kg/h
Dexmedetomidine	0.002 mg/kg/h
Morphine	0.015 mg/kg/h
Detomidine	0.02 mg/kg/h
Morphine	0.015 mg/kg/h
Ketamine	0.3 mg/kg/h
Xylazine	0.03 mg/kg/h
Ketamine	0.3 mg/kg/h
Lidocaine	0.025 mg/kg/h

receptors. Analgesia following epidural injection of opioids is mainly due to the local action on opioid receptors in the spinal cord.[79,80] Epidural morphine, by virtue of its hydrophilic nature, produces profound analgesia with no detectable drug in the plasma.[81] Lipid solubility of opioids injected epidurally affects the onset and duration of analgesia. Onset of analgesia is slower but the duration of analgesia is longer with hydrophilic agents such as morphine.[79] Interestingly, highly lipophilic opioids, such as methadone, hydromorphone, and fentanyl, produce analgesia primarily by systemic absorption; hence, no advantage exists in injecting these agents epidurally.[79]

The volume of anesthetic/analgesic injected epidurally depends on the size of the horse and type of agent used. If local anesthetics are used, no more than a total volume of 10 mL per adult horse should be injected, to avoid hind limb paralysis.[82] Opioids, ketamine, and α2-agonists can be administered epidurally in adult horses, as diluted solution, at total volumes up to 20 mL. The commercially available solutions of these agents are usually highly concentrated and can be diluted with sterile saline to obtain the desired volume to be injected. A total volume of 20 mL per adult horse produces cranial migration of the solution for up to 10 vertebral spaces.[66]

For single epidural injections, the authors recommend the use of an 18-G 7.5-cm spinal needle placed in the first intercoccygeal space (Co1-Co2) in standing horses held in stocks. Epidural catheterization is performed using an epidural Huber point (Tuohy) needle instead of a spinal needle. For a detailed description of the techniques for epidural injection and catheterization in horses, the reader is referred to a recent review article on the topic.[83]

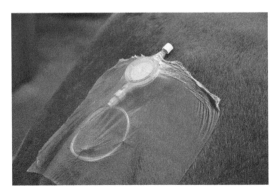

Fig. 1. Epidural catheter inserted between first and second coccygeal vertebrae for long-term use. The catheter must be secured to the skin using a tape butterfly sutured to the skin. A bacterial filter may be attached to the catheter connector. The site of catheter penetration should be maintained sterile and the region should be covered with sterile gauze sponges and an adhesive plastic dressing.

Epidural catheterization can be used for repeated epidural delivery of analgesics and anesthetics in horses (**Fig. 1**). Continuous epidural drug administration in horses has been repeatedly shown to produce profound analgesia in various clinical conditions. Long-term epidural drug administration is not associated with apparent adverse

Table 5
Common single agents and drug combinations for epidural analgesia/anesthesia in standing adult horses (If local anesthetic is used, no more than a total volume of 10 mL per adult horse is injected. Opioids, ketamine, and α2-agonists can be administered epidurally in adult horses, as diluted solution at total volumes up to 20 mL. The commercial solutions of these agents are usually highly concentrated and can be diluted with sterile saline to obtain the desired volume to be injected.)

Recommended Agents for Epidural Use	Recommended Volume of Solution per Adult Horse (mL)
Local anesthetics	
Lidocaine 2%	5
Mepivacaine 2%	5
Bupivacaine 0.25%	10
Ropivacaine 0.2%	10
α2-agonists	
Xylazine (0.17 mg/kg)	10
Detomidine (0.02 mg/kg)	10
Opioids	
Morphine (0.1 mg/kg)	20
Other agents	
Ketamine (1 mg/kg)	20
Drug combinations	
Lidocaine 2% + Xylazine (0.17 mg/kg)	5–8
Lidocaine 2% + Morphine (0.1 mg/kg)	5–8
Xylazine (0.17 mg/kg) + Morphine (0.1 mg/kg)	20
Bupivacaine 0.25% + Morphine (0.1 mg/kg)	10
Detomidine (0.02 mg/kg) + Morphine (0.1 mg/kg)	20

systemic effects in horses. Minor complications associated with epidural catheters are mainly related to catheter malfunction rather than to injury to the patient.[69,84,85]

Single agents and drug combinations for epidural injection, with relative dosages and volume of injection in adult horses, are shown in **Table 5**.

REFERENCES

1. Johnston GM, Eastment JK, Wood JL. The confidential enquiry into periopera-tive equine fatalities (CEPEF): mortality results of phases 1 and 2. Vet Anaesth Analg 2002;29:159–70.
2. Bidwell LA, Bramlage LR, Rood WA. Equine perioperative fatalities associated with general anaesthesia at a private practice – a retrospective case series. Vet Anaesth Analg 2007;34:23–30.
3. Senior JM. Morbidity, mortality, and risk of general anesthesia in horses. Vet Clin North Am Equine Pract 2013;29(1):1–18.
4. Wagner AE. Complications in equine anesthesia. Vet Clin North Am Equine Pract 2008;24(3):735–52.
5. Dutton DW, Lashnits KJ, Wegner K. Managing severe hoof pain in a horse using multimodal analgesia and a modified composite pain score. Equine Vet Ed 2009;21(1):37–43.
6. Marroum PJ, Webb AI, Aeschbacher G, et al. Pharmacokinetics and pharmaco-dynamics of acepromazine in horses. Am J Vet Res 1994;55(10):1428–33.
7. Love EJ, Taylor PM, Murrell J, et al. Effects of acepromazine, butorphanol and buprenorphine on thermal and mechanical nociceptive thresholds in horses. Equine Vet J 2012;44(2):221–5.
8. Dyson DH, Pettifer GR. Evaluation of the arrhythmogenicity of a low dose of ace-promazine: comparison with xylazine. Can J Vet Res 1997;61:241–5.
9. Driessen B, Zarucco L, Kalir B, et al. Contemporary use of acepromazine in the anaesthetic management of male horses and ponies: a retrospective study and opinion poll. Equine Vet J 2011;43:88–98.
10. England GC, Clarke KW. Alpha 2 adrenoceptor agonists in the horse - a review. Br Vet J 1996;152(6):641–57.
11. Grimsrud KN, Mama KR, Thomasy SM, et al. Pharmacokinetics of detomidine and its metabolites following intravenous and intramuscular administration in horses. Equine Vet J 2009;41(4):361–5.
12. Dimaio Knych HK, Stanley SD. Pharmacokinetics and pharmacodynamics of detomidine following sublingual administration to horses. Am J Vet Res 2011; 72(10):1378–85.
13. Rohrbach H, Korpivaara T, Schatzmann U, et al. Comparison of the effects of the alpha-2 agonists detomidine, romifidine and xylazine on nociceptive withdrawal reflex and temporal summation in horses. Vet Anaesth Analg 2009;36(4): 384–95.
14. Valverde A. Alpha-2 agonists as pain therapy in horses. Vet Clin North Am Equine Pract 2010;26(3):515–32.
15. Ringer SK, Portier K, Torgerson PR, et al. The effects of a loading dose fol-lowed by constant rate infusion of xylazine compared with romifidine on seda-tion, ataxia and response to stimuli in horses. Vet Anaesth Analg 2013;40(2): 157–65.
16. Schatzmann U, Jossfck H, Stauffer JL, et al. Effects of alpha 2-agonists on intra-uterine pressure and sedation in horses: comparison between detomidine, romi-fidine and xylazine. Zentralbl Veterinarmed A 1994;41(7):523–9.

17. Holve DL. Effect of sedation with detomidine on intraocular pressure with and without topical anesthesia in clinically normal horses. J Am Vet Med Assoc 2012;240(3):308–11.
18. Yamashita K, Tsubakishita S, Futaok S, et al. Cardiovascular effects of medetomidine, detomidine and xylazine in horses. J Vet Med Sci 2000;62(10): 1025–32.
19. England GC, Clarke KW, Goossens L. A comparison of the sedative effects of three alpha 2-adrenoceptor agonists (romifidine, detomidine and xylazine) in the horse. J Vet Pharmacol Ther 1992;15:194–201.
20. Ringer SK, Portier KG, Fourel I, et al. Development of a xylazine constant rate infusion with or without butorphanol for standing sedation of horses. Vet Anaesth Analg 2012;39:1–11.
21. Ringer SK, Portier KG, Fourel I, et al. Development of a romifidine constant rate infusion with or without butorphanol for standing sedation of horses. Vet Anaesth Analg 2012;39:12–20.
22. Freeman SL, England GC. Comparison of sedative effects of romifidine following intravenous, intramuscular, and sublingual administration to horses. Am J Vet Res 1999;60(8):954–9.
23. van Dijk P, Lankveld DP, Rijkenhuizen AB, et al. Hormonal, metabolic and physiological effects of laparoscopic surgery using a detomidine buprenorphine combination in standing horses. Vet Anaesth Analg 2003;30:72–80.
24. Mama KR, Grimsrud K, Snell T, et al. Plasma concentrations, behavioural and physiological effects following intravenous and intramuscular detomidine in horses. Equine Vet J 2009;41(8):772–7.
25. Taylor PM, Browning AP, Harris CP. Detomidine-butorphanol sedation in equine clinical practice. Vet Rec 1988;123:388–90.
26. Bettschart-Wolfensberger R, Freeman SL, Bowen IM, et al. Cardiopulmonary effects and pharmacokinetics of i.v. dexmedetomidine in ponies. Equine Vet J 2005;37(1):60–4.
27. Hubbell JA, Muir WW. Antagonism of detomidine sedation in the horse using intravenous tolazoline or atipamezole. Equine Vet J 2006;38(3):238–41.
28. Stout RC, Priest GT. Clinical experience using butorphanol tartrate for relief of abdominal pain in the horse. In: Moore JN, White NA, Becht JL, editors. Equine colic research. Proceedings of the second symposium at the University of Georgia. vol. 2. Lawrenceville (NJ): Veterinary Learning Systems; 1986. p. 68–70.
29. Walker AF. Sublingual administration of buprenorphine for long-term analgesia in the horse. Vet Rec 2007;160:808–9.
30. Corletto F, Raisis AA, Brearley JC. Comparison of morphine and butorphanol as pre-anaesthetic agents in combination with romifidine for field castration in ponies. Vet Anaesth Analg 2005;32(1):16–22.
31. Love EJ, Taylor PM, Clark C, et al. Analgesic effect of butorphanol in ponies following castration. Equine Vet J 2009;41:552–6.
32. Sanz MG, Sellon DC, Cary JA, et al. Analgesic effects of butorphanol tartrate and phenylbutazone administered alone and in combination in young horses undergoing routine castration. J Am Vet Med Assoc 2009;235:1194–203.
33. Clarke KW, England GC, Goossens L. Sedative and cardiovascular effects of romifidine alone and in combination with butorphanol in the horse. J Vet Anaesth 1991;18:25–9.
34. Dyson DH, Pascoe PJ, Viel L, et al. Comparison of detomidine hydrochloride, xylazine, and xylazine plus morphine in horses: a double blind study. J Equine Vet Sci 1987;7:211–6.

35. Clarke KW, Paton BS. Combined use of detomidine with opiates in the horse. Equine Vet J 1988;20:331–4.

36. Schatzman U, Armbruster S, Stucki F, et al. Analgesic effect of butorphanol and levomethadone in detomidine sedated horses. J Vet Med A Physiol Pathol Clin Med 2001;48:337–42.

37. Combie J, Dougherty J, Nugent E, et al. The pharmacology of narcotic analgesics in the horse. IV. Dose and time response relationships for behavioral responses to morphine. Meperidine, pentazocine, anileridine, methadone, and hydromorphone. J Equine Med Surg 1979;3:377–85.

38. Amadon RS, Craigie AH. The actions of morphine on the horse. Preliminary studies: diacetylmorphine (heroin), dihydrodesoxymorphine-D (desomorphine) and dihydroheterocodeine. J Am Vet Med Assoc 1937;91:674–8.

39. Carregaro AB, Luna SP, Mataqueiro MI, et al. Effects of buprenorphine on nociception and spontaneous locomotor activity in horses. Am J Vet Res 2007;68: 246–50.

40. Senior JM, Pinchbeck GL, Dugdale AH, et al. Retrospective study of the risk factors and prevalence of colic in horses after orthopaedic surgery. Vet Rec 2004; 155(11):321–5.

41. Andersen MS, Clark L, Dyson SJ, et al. Risk factors for colic in horses after general anaesthesia for MRI or nonabdominal surgery: absence of evidence of effect from perianaesthetic morphine. Equine Vet J 2006;38:368–74.

42. Love EJ, Lane JG, Murison PJ. Morphine administration in horses anaesthetized for upper respiratory tract surgery. Vet Anaesth Analg 2006;33:179–88.

43. Tinkler MK, White NA, Lessard P, et al. Prospective study of equine colic risk factors. Equine Vet J 1997;29:454–8.

44. Cohen ND, Gibbs PG, Woods AM. Dietary and other management factors associated with colic in horses. J Am Vet Med Assoc 1999;215:53–60.

45. Hillyer MH, Taylor FG, Proudman CJ, et al. A case control study of simple colonic obstruction and distension colic in the horse. Equine Vet J 2002;34:455–63.

46. Jones RS, Edwards GB, Brearley JC. Commentary on prolonged starvation as a factor associated with post operative colic. Equine Vet Educ 1991;3:16–8.

47. Clutton RE. Opioid analgesia in horses. Vet Clin North Am Equine Pract 2010; 26(3):493–514.

48. Flacke JW, Flacke WE, Bloor BC, et al. Histamine release by four narcotics: a double-blind study in humans. Anesth Analg 1987;66(8):723–30.

49. Sellon DC, Roberts MC, Blikslager AT, et al. Effects of continuous rate intravenous infusion of butorphanol on physiologic and outcome variables in horses after celiotomy. J Vet Intern Med 2004;18:555–63.

50. Spadavecchia C, Arendt-Nielsen L, Spadavecchia L, et al. Effects of butorphanol on the withdrawal reflex using threshold, suprathreshold and repeated subthreshold electrical stimuli in conscious horses. Vet Anaesth Analg 2007;34(1): 48–58.

51. Solano AM, Valverde A, Desrochers A, et al. Behavioural and cardiorespiratory effects of a constant rate infusion of medetomidine and morphine for sedation during standing laparoscopy in horses. Equine Vet J 2009;41:153–9.

52. Love EJ, Murrell J, Whay HR, et al. Antinociceptive effects of buprenorphine in horses: a dose finding study. Proceedings of the American College of Veterinary Anesthesiologists. Phoenix (AZ): 2008. p. 14.

53. Taylor PM, Love EJ, McCluskey L, et al. Analgesic effects of buprenorphine following castration in ponies. Proceedings of the American College of Veterinary Anesthesiologists. Phoenix (AZ): 2008. p. 15.

54. Taylor P, Coumbe K, Henson F, et al. Evaluation of sedation for standing clinical procedures in horses using detomidine combined with buprenorphine. Vet Anaesth Analg 2013. [Epub ahead of print]. http://dx.doi.org/10.1111/vaa.12055.

55. Love EJ, Taylor PM, Murrell J, et al. Assessment of the sedative effects of buprenorphine administered with 20 microg/kg detomidine in horses. Vet Rec 2011; 168(15):409.

56. Love EJ, Taylor PM, Murrell J, et al. Assessment of the sedative effects of buprenorphine administered with 10 µg/kg detomidine in horses. Vet Rec 2011; 168(14):379.

57. Larenza MP, Peterbauer C, Landoni MF, et al. Stereoselective pharmacokinetics of ketamine and norketamine after constant rate infusion of a subanesthetic dose of racemic ketamine or S-ketamine in Shetland ponies. Am J Vet Res 2009;70:831–9.

58. Wagner AE, Mama KR, Contino EK, et al. Evaluation of sedation and analgesia in standing horses after administration of xylazine, butorphanol, and subanesthetic doses of ketamine. J Am Vet Med Assoc 2011;238(12):1629–33.

59. Hirota K, Lambert DG. Ketamine: new uses for an old drug? Br J Anaesth 2011; 107(2):123–6.

60. Cook VL, Shults JJ, McDowell MR, et al. Anti-inflammatory effects of intravenously administered lidocaine hydrochloride on ischemia-injured jejunum in horses. Am J Vet Res 2009;70(10):1259–68.

61. Cook VL, Shults JJ, McDowell MR, et al. Attenuation of ischaemic injury in the equine jejunum by administration of systemic lidocaine. Equine Vet J 2008;40(4):353–7.

62. Thomas J, Doherty TJ, Seddighi MR. Local anesthetics as pain therapy in horses. Vet Clin North Am Equine 2010;26:533–49.

63. Robertson SA, Sanchez LC, Merritt AM, et al. Effect of systemic lidocaine on visceral and somatic nociception in conscious horses. Equine Vet J 2005;37: 122–7.

64. Dickey EJ, Mckenzie HC III, Brown JA, et al. Serum concentrations of lidocaine and its metabolites after prolonged infusion in healthy horses. Equine Vet J 2008;40(4):348–52.

65. Meyer GA, Lin HC, Hanson RR, et al. Effects of intravenous lidocaine overdose on cardiac electrical activity and blood pressure in the horse. Equine Vet J 2001; 33(5):434–7.

66. Skarda RT, Tranquilli WJ. Local and regional anesthetic and analgesic techniques: horses. In: Tranquilli WJ, Thurmon JC, Grimm KA, editors. Lumb and Jones' veterinary anesthesia. 4th edition. Ames (IA): Blackwell Publishing; 2007. p. 605–43.

67. Scheling CG, Klein LV. Comparison of carbonate lidocaine and lidocaine hydrochloride for caudal epidural anesthesia in horses. Am J Vet Res 1985;46: 1375–7.

68. Grubb TL, Riebold TW, Huber MJ. Comparison of lidocaine, xylazine, and xylazine/lidocaine for caudal epidural analgesia in horses. J Am Vet Med Assoc 1992;20:1187–90.

69. Martin CA, Kerr CL, Pearce SG, et al. Outcome of epidural catheterization for delivery of analgesics in horses: 43 cases (1998–2001). J Am Vet Med Assoc 2003;222(10):1394–8.

70. Chopin JB, Wright JD. Complications after the use of a combination of lignocaine and xylazine for epidural anaesthesia in a mare. Aust Vet J 1995;72:354–5.

71. Robinson EP, Natalini CC. Epidural anesthesia and analgesia in horses. Vet Clin North Am Equine Pract 2002;18:61–82.

72. Skarda RT, Muir WW. Comparison of antinociceptive, cardiovascular, and respiratory effects, head ptosis, and position of pelvic limbs in mares after caudal epidural administration of xylazine and detomidine hydrochloride solution. Am J Vet Res 1996;57:1338–45.
73. Sysel AM, Pleasant SR, Jacobson JD. Efficacy of an epidural combination of morphine and detomidine in alleviating experimentally induced hindlimb lameness in horses. Vet Surg 1996;25:511–8.
74. Skarda RT, Muir WW. Caudal analgesia induced by epidural or subarachnoid administration of detomidine hydrochloride solution in mares. Am J Vet Res 1994;55:670–80.
75. Skarda RT, Muir WW. Analgesic, hemodynamic and respiratory effects of caudal epidurally administered ropivacaine hydrochloride solution in mares. Vet Anaesth Analg 2001;28:61–74.
76. Valverde A, Little CB, Dyson DH. Use of epidural morphine to relieve pain in a horse. Can Vet J 1990;31:211–2.
77. Natalini CC, Robinson EP. Evaluation of the analgesic effects of epidurally administered morphine, alfentanil, butorphanol, tramadol, and U50488H in horses. Am J Vet Res 2000;61:1579–86.
78. Natalini CC, Linardi RL. Analgesic effects of epidural administration of hydromorphone in horses. Am J Vet Res 2006;67(1):11–5.
79. Morgan M. The rational use of intrathecal and extradural opioids. Br J Anaesth 1989;63:165–88.
80. Yaksh TL, Rudy TA. Narcotic analgesics: CNS sites and mechanisms of action as revealed by intracerebral injection techniques. Pain 1978;4:299–359.
81. Weddel SJ, Ritter RR. Serum levels following epidural administration of morphine and correlation with relief of postsurgical pain. Anesthesiology 1981;54:210–4.
82. Hendrickson DA, Southwood LL, Lopez MJ, et al. Cranial migration of different volumes of new methylene blue after caudal epidural injection in the horse. Equine Pract 1998;20:12–4.
83. Natalini CC. Spinal anesthetics and analgesics in the horse. Vet Clin North Am Equine Pract 2010;26:551–64.
84. Sysel AM, Pleasant RS, Jacobson JD, et al. Systemic and local effects associated with long-term epidural catheterization and morphine-detomidine administration in horses. Vet Surg 1997;26(2):141–9.
85. Skarda RT, Muir WW. Continuous caudal epidural and subarachnoid anesthesia in mares: a comparative study. Am J Vet Res 1983;44:2290–8.

Advances in Laparoscopic Techniques and Instrumentation in Standing Equine Surgery

Jeremiah T. Easley, DVM[a],*, Dean A. Hendrickson, DVM, MS[b]

KEYWORDS

- Laparoscopy • Standing surgery • Equine • Advances • Minimally invasive surgery

KEY POINTS

- Advances in minimally invasive techniques have potential to improve and expand equine standing surgery.
- Advancements in equine laparoscopy rely heavily on advancements in human laparoscopic techniques and equipment.
- It is important that equine veterinarians are familiar with current techniques and equipment in both veterinary and human fields to successfully accomplish the goals of the laparoscopic surgery.

INTRODUCTION

Laparoscopy is a constantly evolving field within equine surgery. It was originally considered a surgical technique only practiced in academic hospitals by surgeons with advanced training. Laparoscopic surgery is now considered, however, an important aspect of general equine surgery and is a required part of surgical residency training. Although veterinary laparoscopy has become increasingly popular throughout the past 20 years, minimally invasive surgery (MIS) lags behind the human medical field. In the authors' opinion, the reason for this discrepancy between human and veterinary laparoscopy is decreased access to appropriate training and instrumentation. This edition of *Veterinary Clinics of North America: Equine Practice* focuses on all aspects of equine standing surgery. It is nearly impossible to cover such an important topic in equine surgery without discussing advances in laparoscopy, because without such advances the authors' think that equine standing surgery lacks potential for forward progress. Although novel standing techniques continue to be published, the addition of minimally invasive laparoscopic techniques adds an entirely

[a] Surgical Research Laboratory, Department of Clinical Sciences, Colorado State University, 300 W Drake Road, Fort Collins, CO 80523, USA; [b] Professional Veterinary Medicine, Colorado State University, 300 W Drake Road, Fort Collins, CO 80523, USA
* Corresponding author.
E-mail address: Jeremiah.easley@colostate.edu

Vet Clin Equine 30 (2014) 19–44
http://dx.doi.org/10.1016/j.cveq.2013.11.003
0749-0739/14/$ – see front matter Published by Elsevier Inc.

new dimension and provides an abundance of opportunities to surgeons practicing equine standing surgery. This article focuses on advances in both human and veterinary laparoscopy that have the potential, along with the standing procedures described in the articles elsewhere in this issue, to improve and progress equine standing surgical options.

ADVANCES IN HUMAN AND VETERINARY LAPAROSCOPY

The advancement of minimally invasive laparoscopic surgery in both human and veterinary medicine is generally due to improvement of existing and introduction of novel instrumentation combined with more developed training programs. In many cases there are specialized laparoscopic instruments developed for specific surgical procedures. Based on the authors' prior experiences, the ability to perform a laparoscopic procedure is as dependent on acquiring the appropriate instrument to perform a specific task as it is on surgical technique or talent. Although many procedures can be performed with basic laparoscopic instruments, the use of specialized instruments often improves the outcome of the surgical procedure. Unfortunately, there are only a few manufacturers that have focused on the development of instrumentation specific to the horse. Depending on the requirements of the surgery, it may be important to obtain human instrumentation to achieve a specific task.

Surgical training has also improved the outcome of minimally invasive surgical procedures. It is generally accepted that the best way to reduce complications of minimally invasive surgical procedures is to provide better training.[1] As surgical procedures become more complicated, the training methods have become more sophisticated. Newer trainers have been developed to assist surgeons in attaining the necessary skills to perform the surgeries. The availability of trainers in both number and type in the human field is impressive. Trainers range from basic systems to computerized models. One such model developed for equine MIS allows surgeons to practice equine ovariectomy (**Fig. 1**).

Endoscopic Imaging System

The imaging system consists of an endoscope, a camera, a monitor, a light transmitting cable, and a light source. An insufflator can be used to create a working space within the abdomen. Most commonly, endoscopes or telescopes for equine MIS are 10 mm in diameter and have a working length of between 33 cm and 57 cm. Manufacturers make longer telescopes to facilitate specific needs, such as thorough

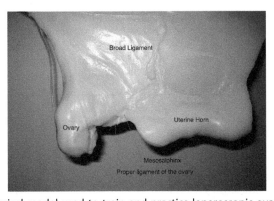

Fig. 1. Equine surgical model used to train and practice laparoscopic ovariectomies.

examination of the entire abdomen from a single-flank approach or bilateral cryptorch-idectomy. Telescopes are most commonly either 0° forward-viewing or 30° forward-oblique viewing. The 0° telescope is often easier to use, requiring less hand-eye coordination, but the 30° telescope is often more versatile due to an increased field of view. There are also single-port operating telescopes that contain an operating channel requiring only one incision site. This type of telescope has limited versatility and is most commonly used for biopsies only. Telescopes have essentially not changed throughout recent years, but advancements in the camera, light source, and monitor have improved the overall image quality obtained by the telescope. The EndoCAMeleon (Karl Storz, Tuttlingen, Germany) is the most recent and innovative advancement to telescopes and is available to veterinarians. This rigid endoscope allows surgeons to change the selected direction of view at anytime during the surgery within a range of 0° to 120° by simply rotating a wheel at endoscope head (**Fig. 2**). This endoscope currently comes in lengths of 32 cm and 42 cm and has a standard eyepiece that connects with any camera head.

One of the most recent advances to the camera is high-definition (HD) technology. HD cameras provide surgeons with higher-quality, larger, and sharper images with improved contrast and color compared with standard-definition cameras. HD technology offers 32% wider lateral views by capturing images in a wide screen 16:9 format versus the standard-definition 4:3 format.[2] HD cameras are more light sensitive, improving the ability to penetrate event the farthest reaches of the equine abdomen. As in traditional surgery, improved visualization of the surgical field aids tremendously in the overall surgical outcome.

The equine abdomen is larger than the human abdomen and requires more light to illuminate all portions of the peritoneal cavity. The most intense and white light sources available should be used for equine laparoscopy. Xenon light sources of 150 W or 175 W are available and less expensive. The authors recommend, however, a 300-W xenon light source to ensure the brightest and best-quality image. Xenon light sources produce a whiter light more closely resembling sunlight and providing a more natural color of tissues compared with halogen light sources.[2] Recently, LED light sources have become available, thus decreasing the size and energy required. LED light sources have an average lamp life of 30,000 hours, which also eliminates the need for bulb replacement.[2] Newer HD cameras that are more light sensitive allow the use of a lower-wattage light source.

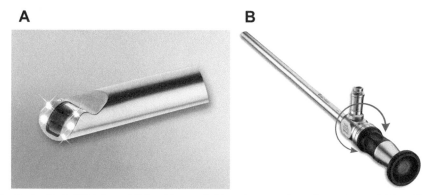

Fig. 2. An EndoCAMeleon (A) is a 10-mm rigid endoscope that allows for variable adjustment of viewing direction ranging from 0° to 120° degrees by rotating a wheel (B). (© 2013 Photo Courtesy of KARL STORZ Endoscopy-America, Inc.)

Documentation devices are becoming increasingly important in veterinary medicine. They allow surgeons to capture and archive digital images, videos, and patient data securely. Detailed and accurate digital records can provide educational opportunities to clients and colleagues and documentation for any legal needs. Digital Imaging and Communicationsin Medicine (DICOM)-compatible systems are becoming increasingly popular. DICOM is a file format that groups patient information into data sets in order to keep all patient information together in one file.[2] With regards to handling, storing, printing, and transmitting information in medical imaging, DICOM is the standard.[2] Many of the newer documentation systems provide internal storage along with the ability to store via USB, DVD, or a network. The AIDA VET (Karl Storz) is a compact data archiving system that allows digital pictures and videos to be archived onto a DVD, USB storage device, or hard disk or be sent directly to a picture archiving and communication system. In the authors' opinions, the advent of HD technology and improvements in light sources and documentation devices play a vital role in advancing equine laparoscopy by making teaching and learning easier and more accessible to veterinarians.

Access and Trocar Instruments

There have been many advancements made in access and portal instrumentation in recent years. Portals need to provide safe and easy placement and removal, stay in position, maintain pneumoperitoneum while inserting and removing instruments, and be easily cleaned and sterilized.[2] Traditionally, reusable cannulas and obturator combinations are used in veterinary medicine due to financial constraints. Although not recommended by manufacturers, most disposable cannula and trocar systems can be sterilized and reused a finite number of times. The most commonly used cannulas in equine medicine are smooth sided, 11 mm in diameter, and contain a stopcock for gas insufflation and a 1-way valve for instrument placement while maintaining insufflation (**Fig. 3**). Newer cannulas contain multifunctional valves to allow surgeons to rapidly release intra-abdominal pressure or prevent dulling of instruments or needles during insertion.[2] The EndoTIP cannula (Karl Storz) has a corkscrew system without an obturator that requires only a skin incision with a small stab incision through the fascia (**Fig. 4**). The advantage of this cannula system is that is does not use an obturator, which minimizes risk to intra-abdominal organs and remains in place much better than the traditional smooth-sided cannulas. The authors have found the EndoTIP cannula helpful when surgery requires frequent instrument or endoscope insertion and removal. It may also be a safer option in a nonfasted horse with gas-distended gastrointestinal contents. The cannula is best inserted using a 0° endoscope.

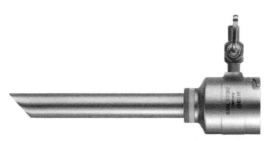

Fig. 3. An 11-mm smooth-sided titanium cannula with insufflation port. (© 2013 Photo Courtesy of KARL STORZ Endoscopy-America, Inc.)

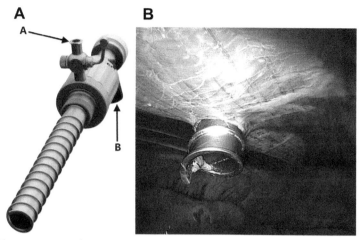

Fig. 4. (*A*) An 11-mm EndoTIP cannula with insufflation port (A) and rapid release valve (B). (*B*) Close-up image of the EndoTIP cannula spiraling through the abdominal wall, replacing the need for an obturator. (© 2013 Photo Courtesy of KARL STORZ Endoscopy-America, Inc.)

The Versaport™ V² trocars (Covidien, Mansfield, Massachusetts) and Versaport RPF trocars (Covidien) contain spring-loaded shields that advance on entry into the cavity to cover the blade or trocar tip to reduce potential injury to internal structures (**Figs. 5** and **6**). The Visiport™ optical trocars (Covidien) contain an atraumatic blunt tip with a clear window for direct visualization and controlled dissection through tissue layers (**Fig. 7**). The authors have successfully used this cannula system and found it easy, safe, and beneficial. The Visiport system may be especially useful when entering the left flank to avoid damage to the spleen or in nonfasted horses with gastrointestinal distension.

When using a 11-mm cannula and 5-mm instruments, a port reducer must be used. These are readily available for reuseable cannulas. Disposable cannula systems can

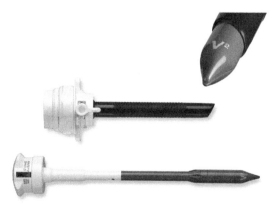

Fig. 5. The Versaport V² conventional trocar (*bottom*) and cannula (*middle*). The trocar has a spring-loaded parabolic entry shield that aids in dilation of tissue. Once the abdominal or chest cavity is entered, the shield advances to cover the trocar tip, reducing the risk of damage to internal structures. (Copyright © 2013 Covidien. All rights reserved. Used with the permission of Covidien.)

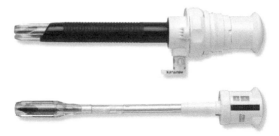

Fig. 6. Visiport Plus Optical Trocar (*top*) and cannula (*bottom*). The trocar has a spring-loaded parabolic entry shied (*top*) that aids in dilation of tissue. Similar to the Versaport V² trocars, a shield advances on entry to a cavity to cover the trocar tip. The cannula contains a self-adjusting seal to accommodate instruments ranging from 5 mm to 15 mm while maintaining insufflation. (Copyright © 2013 Covidien. All rights reserved. Used with the permission of Covidien.)

often accommodate instrumentation ranging from 5 mm to 12 mm in diameter due to a specialized flexible self-adjusting seal.

Stapling Devices

Laparoscopic stapling devices have been commercially available to equine surgeons for many years. Most of these stapling devices have been specially designed, however, for people and then adapted for equine patients. Conventional gastrointestinal anastomosis (GIA) staplers are used most commonly for mass/organ removal, jejuno-cecostomy, ileocecostomy, or side-to-side jejunojejunostomy procedures. The most commonly published equine reports using laparoscopic GIA staplers, however, are in ovariectomy/granulosa cell tumor (GCT) removal procedures. The major limitation of the GIA stapler is its high cost and inability to properly staple and divide equine tissue, which is generally thicker than human tissue. Staple sizes for the Endo GIA™ (Covidien) range in size from 2.0 mm to 4.8 mm. Even the largest cartridges, however, have difficulty stapling thick tissues providing appropriate ligation and anastomosis. The endoscopic staplers also require a larger cannula than the traditional 11-mm

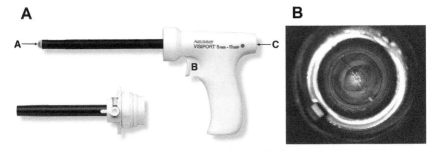

Fig. 7. (*A*) Visiport Plus Optical Trocar (*top*) and cannula (*bottom*). This optical trocar contains a blunt clear dome at the distal end (A), which encloses a crescent-shaped knife blade. As the trigger (B) is squeezed, the blade extends followed by immediate retraction, permitting a controlled sharp dissection of tissue layers. The proximal end (C) has an opening to accommodate up to a 10-mm laparoscope for visualization of tissue layers as the obturator passes through the body wall. (*B*) View through a 10-mm 0° laparoscope showing the muscle layers of the body wall as the trocar penetrates the abdomen. (Copyright © 2013 Covidien. All rights reserved. Used with the permission of Covidien.)

diameter cannula. It is imperative that equine surgeons understand which cannula diameter is required with each stapling device prior to use.

The new Tri-Staple Technology (Covidien) is likely to improve equine surgeons' ability to properly apply an Endo GIA stapler to thick tissue and feel confident in the closure. The Tri-Staple Technology contains 2 triple-staggered rows like conventional GIA staplers (**Fig. 8**). The triple-staggered rows, however, are height-progressive, which provides improved burst strength and reduced tissue compression on the outer staple row. Staples in the inner row (closest to the knife blade) form first when firing, followed by the staples in middle row, and finally the outer row. This sequential firing of staples facilitates lateral diffusion of tissue fluids during staple formation, which helps compress the tissue evenly throughout and requiring less force. The cartridges also contain a stepped face to allow its use across a broader range of tissue thicknesses. The Tri-Staple black cartridges are meant for extrathick tissues that can be compressed from 2.25 mm to 3 mm in width and are likely the most useful cartridges in the horse. The original green cartridges for the Endo GIA staplers are contraindicated for tissues any thicker than 2 mm in width. Gastrointestinal anastomoses in the horse have not been performed entirely using MIS to the authors' knowledge. This is most likely because most surgeons performing anastomoses through an open approach using stapling devices often oversew the stapled layer for additional security. The black Endo GIA cartridge with Tri-Staple Technology may, however, allow surgeons to abandon oversewing the anastomosis site, similar to human anastomoses. If oversewing is not required, more surgeons may be willing to attempt more advanced laparoscopic gastrointestinal surgery in the standing horse by minimizing intracorporeal suturing.

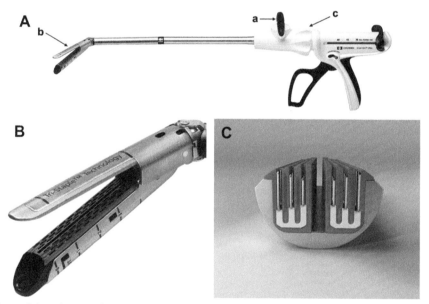

Fig. 8. (*A*) Endo GIA Ultra Universal stapler with Tri-Staple Technology. The Endo GIA Ultra Universal stapler is capable of roticulating the stapler cartridge (b) with the turn of the knob (a) and rotating by twisting the shaft (c). (*B*) A close-up image of the Tri-Staple technology black staple cartridge reload for stapling of extrathick tissues of up to 3.0 mm. (*C*) Transverse cross-sectional illustration of the Tri-Staple Technology showing the varied-height staples (2 triple-staggered, height-progressive rows of titanium staples). (Copyright © 2013 Covidien. All rights reserved. Used with the permission of Covidien.)

Energy Sources for Coagulation and Dissection

Energy sources are commonly used in equine laparoscopy for coagulation and dissection. There are many devices available to veterinarians, including monopolar and bipolar electrosurgery, electrosurgical devices, ultrasonic devices, and lasers. Each device uses the transfer of energy to tissues to achieve similar surgical effects. During electrosurgery, high-frequency current heats a metal probe placed directly on the tissue causing cutting, coagulation, and tissue ablation. Many laparoscopic instruments have an electrosurgery connection, and monopolar electrosurgery requires a passive electrode from the patient to the generator in order to work. Electrosurgery is the most easily accessible and commonly used form of energy in veterinary surgery but is limited to small vessel coagulation and soft tissue dissection. Electrosurgical devices have the ability to cut and coagulate at the same time by the production of high-frequency alternating electric current. Both single-blade and forceps-style devices exist. The basis of all electrosurgery is the production of heat at the cellular level. Electrosurgery is the only technology that provides both cutting and coagulation at the same time, making it ideal for laparoscopic surgery.[3] These modalities are recommended, however, for vessels less than 3 mm in diameter.

There are many monoboplar and bipolar electrosurgical devices that have been developed since their introduction in the 1940s. More recently, a modification of electrosurgery technology, called electrothermal bipolar vessel sealing (EBVS), has emerged as the most popular form of laparoscopic coagulation device used in veterinary medicine.[3] The LigaSure vessel-sealing device (Covidien) is capable of sealing blood vessels of up to 7 mm in diameter and withstand blood pressures up to 3 times normal (**Fig. 9**).[4] The device has a blade incorporated into the jaw to allow cutting of the tissue after tissue sealing, which in turn reduces the number of required instrument portals. Human studies have reported less postoperative pain, shorter operative times, less blood loss, and shorter hospital stays in patients where EBVS devices were used versus traditional clamps or ligatures.[5–10] A comparison study between the Olympus EBVS and a conventional bipolar electrosurgery device in a human laparoscopic hysterectomy study revealed decreased blood loss and shorter operative times in the EBVS.[11] Lakeman and colleagues[10] compared the LigaSure vessel-sealing device to traditional clamping and suturing for vaginal hysterectomy and proved that patients in the LigaSure group had significantly less pain and shorter operative times without major differences in cost. In standing horses, laparoscopic cryptorchidectomy and ovariectomy procedures have been performed successfully

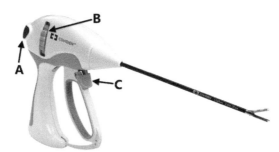

Fig. 9. LigaSure 5-mm blunt tip instrument. The power button (A) is built into that handle and no longer uses a foot pedal. The tip can rotate in either direction using the wheel (B) for improved access and control to tissues and vessels. The handle locks into place to seal the tissue and a blade activated by pulling the second trigger (C) to divide the tissues. (Copyright © 2013 Covidien. All rights reserved. Used with the permission of Covidien.)

using only electrosurgical instrumentation.[12–14] Electrosurgical instrumentation in horses replaces placement of suture loops, intracorporeal suturing, or emasculation, all of which can require tension placement on the mesorchium or mesovarium. Not only is electrosurgical instrumentation a successful replacement to traditional ligation, emasculation, or clamping but also it is less technically demanding.[13–16]

From the authors' experience, an EBVS is a valuable asset to standing laparoscopic surgery. The ability of the EBVS to seal and transect vessels and tissue replaces the need for suturing techniques or ligation devices, which leaves foreign material at the surgical site and makes the surgical procedure more invasive and challenging. Newer electrosurgical devices like the ForceTriad™ energy platform (Covidien) combine monopolar, bipolar, and the LigaSure™ tissue fusion technology into a single, all-in-one unit, potentially decreasing surgical costs and demands on staff during procedures and providing surgeons with a variety of options to use during laparoscopic surgery (**Fig. 10**).

Ultrasonic technology is increasingly popular in human laparoscopy. It works by causing cavitation in tissues with high water content, resulting in turbulence, heat, and pressure, thus denaturing the protein in the vessel wall and creating hemostasis.[4] It is capable of cutting and coagulating vessels from 3 mm to 5 mm in diameter.[2,4] One study using the harmonic scalpel to transect the ovarian pedicle and obtain hemostasis simultaneously was successful in 100% of mares.[17] All ovaries were of normal size, however, and may not successfully coagulate enlarged vessels in cases of pathologic ovaries, such as granulosa thecal cell tumors.

Most recently, the Sonicision™ cordless ultrasonic dissection device (Covidien) has become commercially available (**Fig. 11**). This handheld battery-powered device

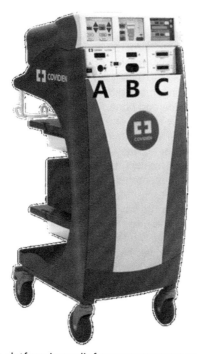

Fig. 10. ForceTriad energy platform is a radiofrequency energy system that incorporates both monopolar (A) and bipolar energy (B) along with the newer-generation LigaSure technology (C). (Copyright © 2013 Covidien. All rights reserved. Used with the permission of Covidien.)

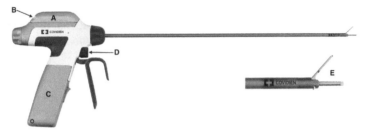

Fig. 11. Sonicision cordless ultrasonic dissection device. The cordless dissector contains a generator (A) with indicator LED (B) and removable/reusable battery with up to 100 sterilization cycles (C). The dual-mode energy button (D) and dissection tip (E) provides improved hemostasis at lower settings and rapid dissection and tissue transection at maximum settings. (Copyright © 2013 Covidien. All rights reserved. Used with the permission of Covidien.)

operates at a standard 55,500 Hz and has a dual-mode energy button, which allows for improved hemostasis at lower settings and rapid dissection and transection of tissues at maximum settings. Currently, this system can be resterilized using low-temperature hydrogen peroxide gas plasma (STERRAD, Advanced Sterilization Products, Irvine, CA). The battery and generator life are limited, however, to 100 uses only. At this time, the Sonicision may not be cost effective in the veterinary market.

Intracorporeal Knot-tying and Tacking Devices

Although laparoscopic surgery provides many advantages to both practitioners and patients, there are inherent difficulties associated with it, such as the loss of depth perception caused by the use of 2-D monitors, the altered tactile experience, and the fulcrum effect of the instruments.[18] Laparoscopic suturing is considered one of the more challenging tasks in laparoscopic surgery, often requiring specialized training. Although the steps may remain practically identical, laparoscopic suturing is a completely different overall experience from traditional suturing. Due to the challenges of laparoscopic suturing, many different training systems have been developed to enable surgeons to practice and hone their skills. Training systems are separated into physical stimulation (box trainer or animal model) and systems that use virtual software.[18] Unfortunately, the virtual training systems are currently not readily available to veterinary surgeons nor are they a large aspect of veterinary surgeon training programs. Low-fidelity suture trainers are easy to make and valuable in the training process. Even with major improvements in this area of training, however, laparoscopic suturing still has its limits.

Most recently, many instruments have been developed to either replace suturing or minimize the steps required. The Endo Stitch™ (Covidien) is a suturing device that replaces the need for needle driver and a second grasping device (**Fig. 12**). Although limited in its use, it can be especially helpful in regions that have limited space and access. The Endo Stitch consists of 2 jaws at the end of a single-handled instrument. A double-sided needle is locked in place to 1 of the jaws and then can be passed to the other jaw by squeezing the handle, releasing the needle from one of the jaws and locking in place to the opposing jaw by flipping the toggle levers. This technology prevents surgeons from having to use 2 needle drivers and continually keeps the needle in a straight position for the next pass. Initially, intracoporeal suturing with the Endo Stitch can be challenging, but there is a rapid learning curve. The Endo Stitch needle is short, limiting the thickness of tissue that can be incorporated in the closure. Recently, single-use loading units have become available containing the V-Loc™ (Covidien)

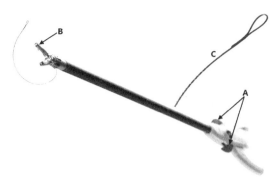

Fig. 12. Endo Stitch 10-mm suturing device contains 2 jaws (B) that grasp the single-use loading unit with the double-sided needle and suture. The needle can be passed from one jaw to the other jaw by controlled closing the handles and flipping the toggle levers (A). Single-use loading units are not available in knotless barbed suture (C). (Copyright © 2013 Covidien. All rights reserved. Used with the permission of Covidien.)

wound closure device, a barbed suture (see **Fig. 12**). It contains a welded loop on the opposite end of the needle and unidirectional barbs throughout the strand, thus eliminating the need for intracoporeal knot tying. This significantly reduces surgical time without compromising strength or security. The authors have experience with the Endo Stitch in combination with V-Loc suture to close thin tissues, such as peritoneum, and found it efficient and easy to use.

The Endo-Surgery Suture Assistant (Ethicon, Cincinnati, Ohio) is a knot-tying device with 2 levers: 1 lever to load the instrument and open the grasper and a second for controlled deployment of knots (**Fig. 13**). The Suture Assistant uses a patented pretied knot delivery system, called DURAKNOT (Ethicon). This single-patient–use instrument allows surgeons to basically tie an intracorporeal knot with the push of a button. This tool is especially useful when several interrupted sutures are required.

Pattaras and colleagues[19] compared the Suture Assistant and the Endo Stitch with conventional laparoscopic suturing by assessing suture placement accuracy, knot speed, and strength. The Suture Assistant and Endo Stitch had a significantly faster knot speed, taking only half the time compared with conventional knot tying. There was no significant difference in accuracy, and knot strength was comparable and sufficient among all techniques. This study demonstrated the advantage of the 2 suturing devices that can potentially lead to improved laparoscopic suturing/tying performance.

The LAPRA-TY Suture Clip Applier (Ethicon) is a knotless suturing device and is most beneficial when continuous patterns are used (**Fig. 14**). The LAPRA-TY Suture Clip Applier has a shaft that can rotate 360° and has a jaw angle of 22° for easy maneuverability and visibility of the clip placement. Each suture clip is made of the absorbable polymer poly (p-dioxanone) and clips onto the ends of a single strand of suture to basically act as an anchoring device. The suture clips replace the use of knots for soft tissue approximation of up to 14 days.

Surgical mesh placement procedures are commonly performed in equine laparoscopy for hernia repair.[20–22] Techniques have been described for both incisional hernioplasty and inguinal herniorrhaphy using a prosthetic mesh.[20–22] Some techniques attach the mesh in place using intracorporeal suturing, whereas others use staples to tack the mesh in place. Recently, absorbable fixation devices have become available. The AbsorbaTack and Tacker (Covidien) are 5-mm fixation devices (**Fig. 15**). The

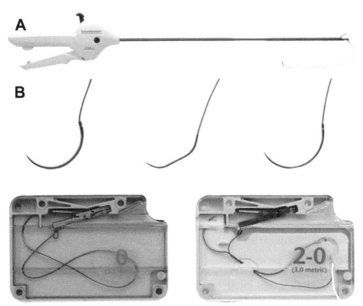

Fig. 13. (*A*) Endo-Surgery Suture Assistant simplifies intracorporeal suturing using a pretied knot delivery system, called DURAKNOT. An intracorporeal knot is deployed by the push of a button on the suture assistant handle. (*B*) The DURAKNOT system comes in various suture and needle types and sizes. (*Courtesy of* Ethicon Endo-Surgery, Inc & Ethicon, Inc, Cincinnati, OH; with permission.)

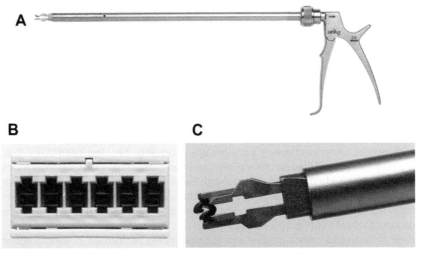

Fig. 14. (*A–C*) LAPRA-TY Suture Clip Applier is a reusable device that uses an absorbable clip to anchor and secure each end of a single strand of suture, which replaces the need for intracorporeal knot tying. The shaft rotates 360° and has a 22° jaw angle to improve maneuverability. (*Courtesy of* Ethicon Endo-Surgery, Inc & Ethicon, Inc, Cincinnati, OH; with permission.)

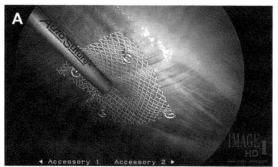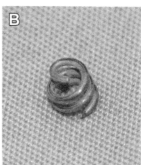

Fig. 15. (A) An intra-abdominal laparoscopic image showing the Tacker 5-mm fixation device used for surgical mesh fixation. (B) Close-up image showing the helical titanium tack.

Tacker fires a nonabsorbable titanium coil (see **Fig. 15**B) whereas the AbsorbaTack uses a tack that is constructed of an absorbable synthetic polyester copolymer derived from lactic and glycolic acid and a majority of absorption occurs within 3 to 5 months. It is available in a long version with 15 or 30 tacks that are ideal for use in the horse. Mesh placement can be challenging laparoscopically because the mesh tends to wrinkle and fold onto itself. With the use of the Tacker or AbsorbTack, the mesh can either be tacked at the corners and then sutured in place or secured entirely with tacks alone. The authors have used the Tacker fixation device and found it easy to use and efficient for mesh stabilization on soft tissue. Currently, the main limiting factor for this device's use is its high cost. Although considered disposable in humans, it may be able to be resterilized for multiple uses in veterinary surgery.

Wristed Instrumentation for Intracorporeal Suturing

The da Vinci Surgical System (Intuitive Surgical, Sunnyvale, California) consists of a surgeon's console, a patient-side cart with 3 to 4 interactive robot arms, and a vision system. With this system, the surgeon manipulates the master controllers located at the surgeon's console. The da Vinci instruments have 7° of freedom and 90° of articulation, which allow each instrument to function equivalently to the human wrist.[23] The da Vinci Surgical system has revolutionized human laparoscopic surgery and allowed surgeons to perform advanced procedures in a minimally invasive manner. The da Vinci Surgical System is unlikely be a part of veterinary laparoscopy in the near future due to its high cost and overhead. There are, however, other less sophisticated and less costly surgical systems or mechanical manipulators that provide similar wristed instrumentation that could become common to veterinary laparoscopy.

The Radius T Surgical System (Tuebingen Scientific Medical GmbH, Tubingen, Germany) was originally developed to allow improved ligation and intracorporeal suturing (**Fig. 16**).[23] The system consists of 2 hand-guided surgical manipulators, each with a deflectable and rotatable tip that provides 6° of freedom similar to the da Vinci System. The Radius T Surgical System is considered a wristed instrument but has limited articulation at the tip. It has 4 different interchangeable tips and is specially designed for suturing and tying knots. In comparison with traditional endoscopic instrumentation that has only 4° of freedom, the Radius T Surgical System provides far greater dexterity, making surgical manipulations easier and safer even in regions of limited space.[24] The authors are unaware of anyone in veterinary surgery using the Radius T Surgical System or anything similar to it currently. One of the authors, however, has evaluated a similar system in a preclinical setting and found it invaluable

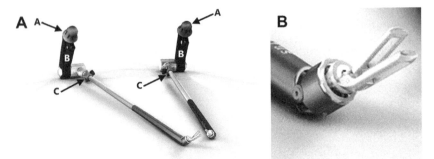

Fig. 16. (*A*) Radius T Surgical System consists of 2 (right- and left-handed) hand-guided surgical manipulators. The tip rotates when the knob (A) is rotated, and the tip is deflected when the handle (B) is deflected. The shaft (C) can also rotate around its own axis. Several interchangeable tips are available, including graspers, scissors, and needle holders. (*B*) Close-up image of the rotating and deflecting tip. (*Courtesy of* Tubingen Scientific Medical GmbH, Tubingen, Germany; with permission.)

for improving suturing and knot-tying abilities. The biggest limitation of intracorporeal suturing with traditional endoscopic instruments is the inability to perform tasks without arms colliding with one another. With the addition of instruments with increased degrees of freedom, veterinary surgeons may be able to perform complex procedures using minimally invasive techniques that have previously been performed only via an open approach. If the procedure can be performed via a minimally invasive approach, it may be more likely to be performed in a standing position as well.

Natural Orifice Transluminal Endoscopic Surgery

Natural orifice transluminal endoscopic surgery (NOTES) combines endoscopic and laparoscopic techniques to eliminate abdominal incisions and incision-related complications by performing intraperitoneal operations by way of the mouth, anus, or vagina.[25] The technique offers potential benefits, such as reduced invasiveness and increased efficacy, compared with traditional laparotomy or laparoscopy for certain indications. NOTES is a new technique in both human and veterinary medicine. Currently, there is a lack of methods for the application of NOTES, including safe methods for the closure of intraluminal incisions, avoidance of infections, and new instrumentation.[25] Alford and Hanson[26] were the first to evaluate NOTES in the equine patient in 2010. The study described a transvaginal approach to the abdomen of mares, which allowed consistent visualization of the left kidney, spleen, nephrosplenic space, stomach, cecum, duodenum, left and right ovaries, diaphragm, and caudal peritoneal reflection and inconsistent visualization of the liver on the left and right sides.[26] This study showed the potential for a NOTES technique via a transvaginal approach to be used in the diagnosis of intra-abdominal disorders in the mare.

NOTES may be most useful in surgical planning or prognosticating in chronic, nonemergency abdominal disorders. The authors see NOTES, however, potentially increasing surgeons' ability to perform a surgery in the standing position based on the information obtained. For example, uterine torsion may be more accurately diagnosed via transvaginal NOTES leading to standing flank correction instead of a ventral midline approach under general anesthesia. Two studies have been performed to evaluate transvaginal NOTES for elective bilateral ovariectomy in standing mares.[27,28] Pader and colleagues[27,28] showed that transvaginal NOTES could be successfully performed in the mare, resulting in minimal inflammation and surgical trauma. There are no published reports of transoral or transanal NOTES performed in horses to date. As NOTES evolves and becomes more established in human surgery, however, the authors see advancements made in instrumentation and safety, potentially resulting in development of new approaches to the abdomen of the horse.

Laparoendoscopic Single-Site Surgery

Laparoendoscopic single-site surgery (LESS) is also referred to as single-port access, single-incision laparoscopic surgery (SILS™), single-port laparoscopic surgery, or reduced port surgery. It is a technique where laparoscopic surgery is performed exclusively through a single entry point. In humans, the most common location of LESS is through the navel. LESS imposes obvious restrictions: maintenance of sufficient exposure, appropriate retraction, instrument and optics collision, limited instrument manipulation, and sustained pneumoperitoneum.[29,30] Recently, specially designed ports have been developed that now allow insertion of all instruments and optics along with specially designed instruments with curved or articulating arms that help to overcome many of the restrictions discussed previously. There are 2 access methods in LESS: (1) use of a single port for entry of the endoscope and all instruments or (2) several individual ports through a single incision.[29] Preference is often based on availability of specialized ports and instruments as well as cost and financial considerations. A broad spectrum of LESS procedures have been published in the human literature, including cholecystectomy, colorectal resection, inguinal hernia repair, gastric bypass, splenectomy, nephrectomy, and hysterectomy, to name a few.[31–36] In the veterinary literature, LESS procedures are less frequent and limited to exploratory laparoscopy/thoracoscopy, ovariectomy/ovariohysterectomy, and cryptorchidectomy in the dog.[37,38] No published reports are available of using LESS in the horse. This is likely due to limited access to appropriate instrumentation and ports that can accommodate 10-mm instrumentation and the thickness of the horse body wall.

The most commonly used portal system in veterinary medicine is the SILS port (Covidien). It allows the use of multiple instruments through adjustable cannulas within a malleable port. The malleable port can accommodate three 5-mm cannulas or two 5-mm and one 12-mm or 15-mm cannula along with a dedicated channel for insufflation (**Fig. 17**). The authors have experience with the SILS port in a preclinical setting performing ovariectomy and colposcopy procedures on ewes. The authors have not used this port, however, in horses to date. One limitation of the SILS port is likely

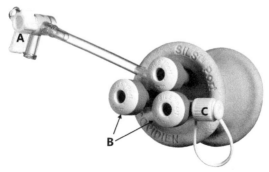

Fig. 17. SILS port for single-incision laparoscopic procedures. The low-profile malleable blue port can accommodate a channel for insufflation (A), three 5-mm cannulas (B) (or two 5-mm cannulas and a single 10-mm cannula), and channel for saline (C). (Copyright © 2013 Covidien. All rights reserved. Used with the permission of Covidien.)

the thickness of the malleable port in comparison to the thickness of the horse's body wall, especially through a flank approach. Potential uses of the SILS port may be for more simple procedures, such as standing cryptorchidectomy, ovariectomy, or inguinal herniorrhaphy, or it could be used in the vagina or anus providing a sealed cavity for insufflation (**Fig. 18**).

Despite the improvements made with curved and articulated laparoscopic instruments, severe ergonomic restrictions on surgeons exist. In order to dissociate optics from instruments and provide increased intracorporeal degrees of freedom, flexible endoscopic multitasking platforms have been developed. Few reports are available in the human literature.[30,39–41] Flexible endoscopic multitasking platforms can be classified as mechanical and robotic. Through a single port, a dual-channel flexible endoscope incorporates visual function and instrument manipulation through a multichannel access device. The Anubiscope (Karl Storz) is a purely mechanical system. It is controlled by a traction cable system actuated by hand, resulting in a lag phase to a surgeon's actions (**Fig. 19**). The Single-Port lapaRoscopy bImaNual roboT (SPRINT) is a multiarm robotic multitasking platform designed for LESS and consists of 2 robotic arms with 6° of freedom. Each robotic arm is equipped with a surgical tool, a stereoscopic camera, and a console for the execution of a surgeon's actions (**Fig. 20**). Petroni and colleagues[30] proved that the SPRINT system had a fast-learning curve for both pick-and-place and suturing exercises. In comparison to the da Vinci system, the study found the SPRINT less technically advanced with regards to precision and ease of surgical manipulation. SPRINT allows surgeons, however, to operate close to a patient, making intervention in the case of intraoperative complications easier.[30] Although this technology is highly advanced and likely some years from introduction into veterinary surgery, the authors see great potential in equine standing surgery because a LESS approach with a flexible multitasking platform can access difficult-to-reach regions and is considered less invasive, resulting in decreased pain and sedation/analgesia requirements.

Retrieval Devices

LESS, NOTES, and robotic systems eventually will become more popular in veterinary surgery, resulting in novel treatment options and improved surgical outcomes. A major limitation of these advanced minimally invasive techniques, however, is the inability to remove tissues from the surgical field. There is little point to performing a surgery

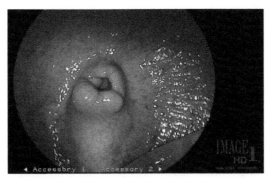

Fig. 18. An HD image of an ovine vagina and cervix. A SILS port was used to insufflate the vagina to 6 mm Hg to visualize the vaginal vault and cervix as well as localize a specific region of interest for vaginal biopsy.

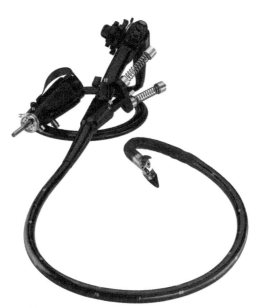

Fig. 19. Anubiscope, used for single-incision laparoscopic surgery, consists of a flexible, 110-cm long, 4-way articulating endoscope with a 16-mm articulating vertebra section and an 18-mm tip. There are 2 opposing, movable arms with 2 × 4.2 mm working channels and a central 3.4-mm channel incorporated into the distal head. (© 2013 Photo Courtesy of KARL STORZ Endoscopy-America, Inc.)

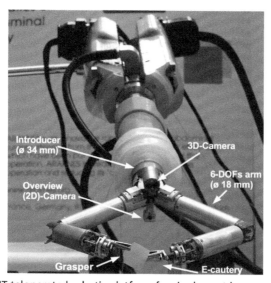

Fig. 20. The SPRINT teloperated robotic platform for single-port laparoscopic surgery. Both robotic arms are introduced through a single 34-mm introducer. There is a dedicated master console that translates hand movements of the surgeon to the robotic arms. Each robotic arm has 6° of freedom. (*Courtesy of* Paolo Dario, Scuola Superiore Sant'Anna, Italy, ARA-KNES project funded by European Commission [FP7 grant agreement n. 224565], Patent Pending PCT/IB2011/051772 and granted Italian patent IT1399603.)

through a single incision a few centimeters in size if the incision must be extended in order to remove transected tissue. This is a common scenario in laparoscopic approaches for ovariectomy, cryptorchidectomy, mass removal, and likely other surgeries as the field of laparoscopy evolves.

Morcellation provides an efficient way to remove tissue from the abdomen without requiring additional dissection beyond the original laparoscopic approach. There are many types of morcellators, but the premise is similar across all types. Morcellators typically have 2 metal hollow rigid tubes, 1 inside the other (**Fig. 21**). The mechanically driven system is usually powered by electricity that activates the rotation of the inner tube. Each tube has cutting edges on the end of the opening, and, while the tissues are cut, the tissue sucked into the tube by a vacuum source.[42] Morcellators, such as prostate and ovariohysterctomy morcellators, come in various sizes and tube lengths, depending on their intended use. The use of morcellators has been described in the veterinary literature for removal of ovarian or testicular tissue.[43]

Kummer and colleagues[43] found the morcellator a safe and effective way to remove ovarian tissue from the abdomen after GCT transection. Morcellation allowed for decreased surgical dissection and incision size but found the technique time consuming with surgeries ranging from 2 to 4.5 hours. No surgical complications were noted. The average GCT size in this study was 17 cm. Ritter and colleagues[44] evaluated 4 different morcellators to find their optimal configurations for maximum tissue morcellation speed. It was concluded that the Richard Wolf morcellators (Richard Wolf, Knittlingen, Germany) achieved the highest morcellation rates with greatest oscillation speeds. At high oscillation speeds greater than 1500 rpm, the morcellation rate of the Richard Wolf morcellator was more than twice that of the Karl Storz or VersaCut (Lumenis, Santa Clara, California). Morcellators are not commonly used in equine laparoscopy mainly due to the increased surgical time and limited availability in most equine referral hospitals. As LESS and NOTES become more common practice, the demand for morcellation devices for tissue retrieval likely will increase in popularity.

Laparoscopic retrieval bags are the most commonly used form of laparoscopic tissue retrieval in equine surgery aside from extending the surgical site for hand-assisted removal. There are many retrieval bags available to surgeons. Their use, however, can be cost prohibitive, and often the tissue retrieved in horses is larger than the

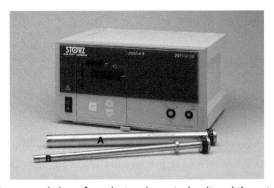

Fig. 21. A morcellator, consisting of an electronic control unit and the rotating coning knife (B) and protective stainless steel sleeve (A). The inner coning knife rotates within the protective sleeve, cutting and suctioning the tissue through the center tube and out of the abdomen. (© 2013 Photo Courtesy of KARL STORZ Endoscopy-America, Inc.)

retrieval bags commercially available. The Endo Catch™ and Endobag™ (Covidien) can be used to easily retrieve small tissue samples from the abdomen, such as biopsy specimens. In standing horses, dropped tissue, such as ovaries and testicles in the abdomen, can be especially difficult to locate. All specimen retrieval bags have a flexible device that can be compacted and passed through a 12-mm cannula, but expands only once in the abdomen to hold the bag open during specimen retrieval (**Fig. 22**). Depending on the type, size, and malleability of the tissue retrieved, the tissue can either be pulled through a 12-mm to 15-mm cannula or teased out through the small incision after the cannula has been removed from the body wall. The main advantage of the specimen retrieval bag is that it increases the likelihood of maintaining a minimally invasive approach while ensuring that the tissue is not lost or left in the abdomen. If the tissue retrieved is too large or nonmalleable, surgeons can often cut the tissue within the retrieval bag to allow the tissue to change shape to be removed through the initial incision.

If commercially available retrieval bags are not cost effective or accessible at the time of retrieval, they can be handcrafted by a surgeon. There are a few publications in human journals describing the technique to make these retrieval bags.[45,46] The

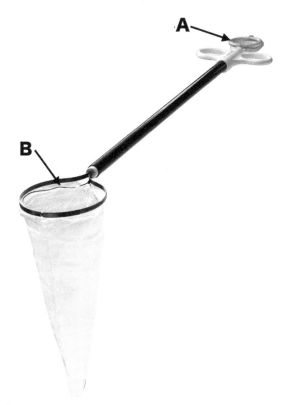

Fig. 22. Endocatch 15 mm specimen pouch. The metal ring and pouch are initially enclosed in an outer wrap for passage through a 12-mm cannula and into the abdomen. The pouch is opened within the abdominal cavity and filled with the specimen. After placement of the specimen into the pouch, the gold ring (*A*) is pulled, which pulls a string over the pouch (*B*) and closes the pouch opening. This allows the specimen to be removed through the cannula or incision. (Copyright © 2013 Covidien. All rights reserved. Used with the permission of Covidien.)

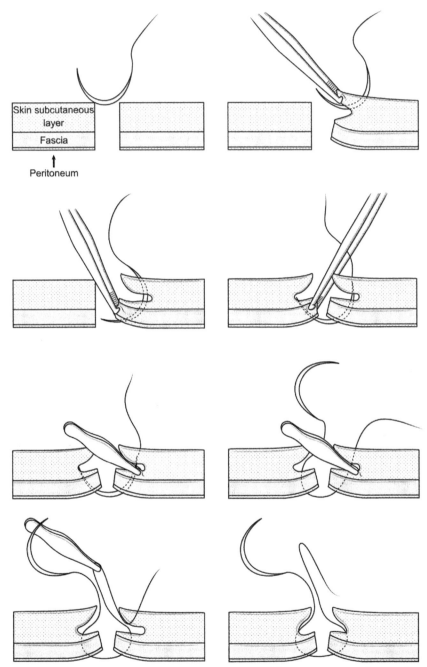

Fig. 23. One-step technique for fascial closure. (*Modified from* Botea F, Torzilli G, Sarbu V. A simple, effective technique for port-site closure after laparoscopy. JSLS 2011;15:78; with permission.)

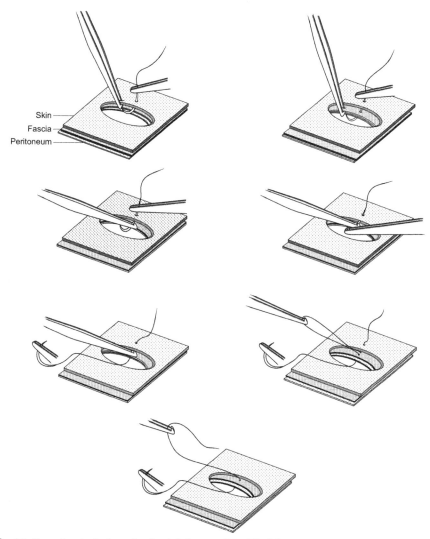

Skin
Fascia
Peritoneum

Fig. 24. Two-step technique for fascial closure. (*Modified from* Botea F, Torzilli G, Sarbu V. A simple, effective technique for port-site closure after laparoscopy. JSLS 2011;15:78; with permission.)

Nadiad bag requires a polyurethrane roll, nylon thread, and a 5F ureteral catheter and entails sewing a single folded edge of the polyurethane bag, creating a tunnel to accommodate the 5F catheter and nylon thread.[45] The study by Ganpule and colleagues successfully removed tissue in 40 cases, including prostectomy, nephrectomy, and adrenalectomy.[45] These specimens are smaller than the specimens removed in equine laparoscopy. The Nadiad bag, however, can easily be made larger by simply increasing the size of the components. Kao and colleagues[46] describe the use of homemade retrieval bag from a large sterile surgical glove. Tissue retrieval was successfully and safely performed in 110 patients without any complications.[46] Unlike commercially available specimen bags that often require only a single laparoscopic

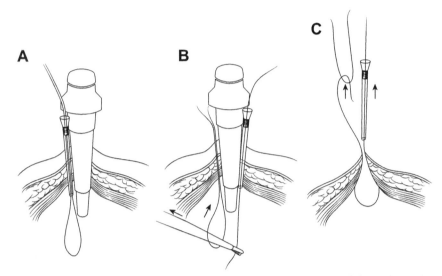

Fig. 25. (*A*) A monofilament suture is folded back onto itself and passed through a catheter into the abdominal cavity. (*B*) A suture for fascial closure is passed through the catheter into the abdominal catheter on the opposite side of the portal. A grasper from another portal is used to pull the fascial suture through the monofilament loop. (*C*) The fascial suture is drawn through the abdominal wall, by pulling up on the monofilament loop. The catheter is removed and the fascial suture is tied. (*Modified from* Nadler RB, McDougall EM, Bullock A, et al. Fascial closure of laparoscopic port sites: a new technique. Urology 1995;45:1047; with permission.)

instrument, handmade retrieval bags often require 2 laparoscopic instruments to expand the opening and place the tissue into the bag.

Portal Closure

Fascial closure at small port sites after laparoscopy can be surprisingly challenging and can lead to port site complications. A small skin incision makes standard closure of the fascia difficult, often requiring blind suturing that can lead to incomplete suturing or damage to intra-abdominal organs. There are no published reports in horses on portal site closure. The authors have experienced, however, difficulty with port site closure with complications, such as unnecessary bleeding, wound dehiscence, or hernia formation. Several reports have been published in the human literature.[47–50] Generally, port site complications occur in 1% to 6% of human cases.[48–50] Elashry and colleagues[51] reported a 17% occurrence in incisional hernia after laparoscopic nephrectomy with intact removal of the resected specimen. The lack of reported port site complications in horses may be due to the larger gastrointestinal contents compared with humans, thus preventing herniation, but more likely due to the huge discrepancy in laparoscopic caseload between the 2 species. In order to reduce port site complications and overcome the inherent challenges of blind suturing of fascia, port closure techniques have been developed.[50,52,53] Botea and colleagues[50] describes both 1-step (**Fig. 23**) and 2-step (**Fig. 24**) novel techniques for fascial closure using a transcutaneous approach and standard surgical instruments. No intraoperative or postoperative complications were noted in 34 patients and both techniques proved safe, easy to perform, and inexpensive.[50] Another technique is described by

Nadler and colleagues[52] and entails leaving the cannula in place and maintaining pneumoperitoneum while using 14-gauge venous catheters for suture placement (**Fig. 25**). A surgical sheet rolled into a plug and placed into the trocar site under direct visualization prior to skin closure was used in 500 laparoscopic robotic surgeries and proved safe and effective.[53]

Although the described port closure techniques may be more time consuming or even more technically challenging compared with traditional fascial closure, the authors think that it is important to realize the inherent risks of traditional closure and encourage surgeons to use these novel techniques in scenarios where proper fascial closure is unsatisfactory or incomplete or risk of damage to intra-abdominal organs is high.

SUMMARY

Advances in standing surgery and laparoscopy go hand in hand. As a clinician, it is important to completely use resources in both the veterinary and the human field to successfully perform the desired laparoscopic procedure. The information presented in this article is only a small percentage of the techniques and instrumentation used in human laparoscopy. Not all things are translatable to equine surgery, and it is important to realize limitations in the horse. It is also important, however, to keep an open mind and to appreciate the abundance of opportunities to advance the field of standing surgery and laparoscopy. A recent survey concluded that 99% of diplomates and 98% of residents of the American College of Veterinary Surgeons have performed MIS at some point in their career or training.[54] More than 95% of all respondents thought that postoperative morbidity was decreased as a result of MIS.[54] With a combination of improved residency training in MIS and continued development of techniques and instrumentation, the authors expect laparoscopy and standing surgery to continue to expand and flourish in equine veterinary medicine.

REFERENCES

1. Hendrickson D. Laparoscopic cryptorchidectomy and ovariectomy in horses. Vet Clin North Am Equine Pract 2006;22:777–98.
2. Chamness CJ. Reusable equipment. In: Ragle CA, editor. Advances in equine laparoscopy. 1st edition. Ames (IA): Wiley-Blackwell; 2012. p. 41–56.
3. Morris ML, Tucker RD, Baron MD, et al. Electrosurgery in gastrointestinal endoscopy: principles to practice. Am J Gastroenterol 2009;104:1563–74.
4. Hendrickson D. Minimally invasive surgery: evidence based ligation and hemostatic techniques. Proceedings of the American College of Veterinary Surgeons Symposium. Washington, 2012.
5. Hefni MA, Bhaumik J, El-Toukhy T, et al. Safety and efficacy of using the Ligasure vessel sealing system for securing the pedicles in vaginal hysterectomy: randomized controlled trial. BJOG 2005;112:329–33.
6. Elhao M, Abdallah K, Serag I, et al. Efficacy of using electrosurgical bipolar vessel sealing during vaginal hysterectomy in patents with different degrees of operative difficulty: a randomized controlled trial. Eur J Obstet Gynecol Reprod Biol 2009;147:86–90.
7. Cronje HS, de Coning EC. Electrosurgical bipolar vessel sealing during vagnal hysterectomy. Int J Gynaecol Obstet 2005;91:243–5.
8. Levy B, Emery L. Randomized trial of suture versus electrosurgical bipolar vessel sealing in vaginal hysterectomy. Obstet Gynecol 2003;102:147–51.

9. Silva-Filho AL, Rodrigues AM, Vale de Castro MM, et al. Randomized study of bipolar vessel sealing system versus conventional suture ligature for vaginal hysterectomy. Eur J Obstet Gynecol Reprod Biol 2009;146:200–3.
10. Lakeman MM, The S, Schellart RP, et al. Electrosurgical bipolar vessel sealing versus conventional clamping and suturing for vaginal hysterectomy: a randomized controlled trial. BJOG 2012;119:1473–82.
11. Cho HY, Choi KJ, Lee YL, et al. Comparison of two bipolar systems in laparoscopic hysterectomy. JSLS 2012;16:456–60.
12. Rodgerson DH, Johnson CR, Belknap JK. Laparoscopic ovariectomy in mares by using electrocautery. Proc Am Assoc Equine Practnr 44:302–3.
13. Rodgerson DH, Belknap JK, Wilson DA. Laparoscopic ovariectomy using sequential electrocoagulation and sharp transection of the equine mesovarium. Vet Surg 2001;30:572–9.
14. Hand R, Rakestraw P, Taylor T. Evaluation of a vessel-sealing device for use in laparoscopic ovariectomy in mares. Vet Surg 2002;31:240–4.
15. Hanrath M, Rodgerson DH. Laparosocpic cryptorchidectomy using electrosurgical instrumentation in standing horses. Vet Surg 2002;31:117–24.
16. Dunay MP, Nemeth T, Makra Z, et al. Laparoscopic cryptorchidectomy and ovariectomy in standing horses using the EnSeal® tissue-sealing device. Acta Vet Hung 2012;60:41–53.
17. Dusterdieck KF, Pleasant RS, Lanz OI, et al. Evaluationn of the harmonic scalpel for laparoscopic bilateral ovariectomy in standing horses. Vet Surg 2003;32:242–50.
18. Mereu L, Carri G, Florez ED, et al. Three-step model course to teach intracorporeal laparoscopic suturing. J Laparoendosc Adv Surg Tech A 2013;23:26–32.
19. Pattaras JG, Smith GS, Landman J, et al. Comparison and analysis of laparoscopic intracorporeal suturing devices: preliminary results. J Endourol 2001;15:187–92.
20. Caron JP, Brakenhoff J. Intracorporeal suture closure of the inguinal and vaginal ring in foals and horses. Vet Surg 2008;37:126–31.
21. Marien T. Standing laparoscopic herniorrhaphy in stallions using cylindrical polypropylene mesh prosthesis. Equine Vet J 2001;33:91–6.
22. Fischer AT, Vachon AM, Klein SR. Laparoscopic inguinal herniorrhaphy in two stallions. J Am Vet Med Assoc 1995;207:1599–601.
23. Ishikawa N, Watanabe G, Inaki N, et al. The da Vinci surgical system versus the radius surgical system. Surg Sci 2012;3:358–61.
24. Frede T, Hammady A, Klein J, et al. The Radius Surgical System – A new device for complex minimally invasive procedures in urology? Eur Urol 2007;51:1015–22.
25. Wang J, Zhang L, Wu W. Current progress on natural orifice transluminal endoscopic surgery (NOTES®). Front Med 2012;6:187–94.
26. Alford C, Hanson R. Evaluation of a transvaginal laparoscopic natural orifice transluminal endoscopic surgery approach to the abdomen of mares. Vet Surg 2010;39:873–8.
27. Pader K, Freeman LJ, Constable PD, et al. Comparison of transvaginal natural orifice transluminal endoscopic surgery (NOTES®) and laparoscopy for elective bilateral ovariectomy in standing mares. Vet Surg 2011;40:998–1008.
28. Pader K, Lescun TB, Freeman LJ. Standing ovariectomy in mares using a transvaginal natural orifice transluminal endoscopic surgery (NOTES®) approach. Vet Surg 2011;40:987–97.
29. Tang B, Hou S, Cuschieri A. Ergonomics of and technologies for single-port laparoscopic surgery. Minim Invasive Ther Allied Technol 2012;21:46–54.

30. Petroni G, Niccolini M, Menciassi A, et al. A novel intracorporeal assembling robotic system for single-port laparoscopic surgery. Surg Endosc 2013;27: 665–70.
31. Cuschieri A. Single-incision laparoscopic surgery. J Minim Access Surg 2011;7: 3–5.
32. Navarra G, Pozza E, Occhionorelli S, et al. One-wound laparoscopic cholecystectomy. Br J Surg 1997;84:695.
33. Cuesta MA, Berends F, Venhof AA. The "invisible cholecystectomy": a transumbilical laparoscopic operation without a scar. Surg Endosc 2008;22:1211–3.
34. Kaouk JH, Autorino R, Kim FJ, et al. Laparoscopic single-incision in Urology: worldwide multi-institutional analysis of 1076 cases. Eur Urol 2011;60:998–1005.
35. Boni L, Dionigi G, Cassinotti E, et al. Single incision laparoscopic right colectomy. Surg Endosc 2010;24:3233–6.
36. Keshave A, Young CJ, Mackenzie S. Single-incision laparoscopic right hemicolectomy. Br J Surg 2010;97:1881–3.
37. Dupre G, Fiorbianco V, Skalicky M, et al. Laparoscopic ovariectomy in dogs; comparison between single portal and two-portal access. Vet Surg 2009;38:818–33.
38. Mayhew PD, Brown DC. Comparison of three techniques for ovarian pedicle hemostasis during laparoscopic-assisted ovariohysterectomy. Vet Surg 2007;36: 541–7.
39. Ding J, Xu K, Golman R, et al. Design, simulation and evaluation of kinematic alternatives for insertable robotic effectors platforms in a single port accss surgery. In: Proceedings of the IEEE international conference on robotics and automation (ICRA). 2010. p. 1053–8.
40. Shang J, Noonan D, Payne C, et al. An articulated universal joint based flexible access robot for minimally invasive surgery. In: Proceedings of IEEE international conference on robotics and automation (ICRA). 2011. p. 1147–52.
41. Pearl J, Ponsky J. Natural orifice transluminal surgery: a critical review. J Gastrointest Surg 2008;12:1293–300.
42. Emanuel MH. New developments in hysteroscopy. Best Pract Res Clin Obstet Gynaecol 2013;27:421–9.
43. Kummer M, Theiss F, Jackson M, et al. Evaluation of a motorized morcellator for laparoscopic removal of granulosa-theca cell tumors in standing mares. Vet Surg 2010;39:649–53.
44. Ritter M, Krombach P, Bolenz C, et al. Standardized comparison of prostate morcellators using a new ex-vivo model. J Endourol 2012;26:697–700.
45. Ganpule AP, Gotov E, Mishra S, et al. Novel cost-effective specimen retrieval bag in laparoscopy: nadiad Bag. Urology 2010;75:1213–6.
46. Kao CC, Cha TL, Sun GH, et al. Cost-effective homemade specimen retrieval bag for use in laparoscopic surgery: experience at a single center. Asian J Surg 2012;35:140–3.
47. Fear R. Laparoscopy, a valuable aid in gynecologic diagnosis. Obstet Gynecol 1968;31:297.
48. Holzinger F, Klaiber C. Trocar-site hernias: a rare but potentially dangerous complication of laparoscopic surgery. Chirurg 2002;73:899–904.
49. Nezhat C, Nezhat F, Seidman DS, et al. Incisional hernias after operative laparoscopy. J Laparoendosc Adv Surg Tech A 1997;7:111–5.
50. Botea F, Torzilli G, Sarbu V. A simple, effective technique for port-site closure after laparoscopy. JSLS 2011;15:77–80.
51. Elashry OM, Guisto G, Nadler RB, et al. Incisional hernia after laparoscopic nephrectomy with intact specimen removal: caveat emptor. J Urol 1997;158:363–9.

52. Nadler RB, McDougall EM, Bullock A, et al. Fascial closure of laparoscopic port sites: a new technique. Urology 1995;45:1046–8.
53. Gaitonde K. Novel technique for port site closure during laparoscopic/robotic surgery. J Urol 2013;189:342.
54. Bleedorn JA, Dykema JL, Hardie RJ. Minimally invasive surgery in veterinary practice: a 2010 survey of diplomats and residents of the American College of Veterinary Surgeons. Vet Surg 2013;42:635–42.

Standing Equine Sinus Surgery

Safia Z. Barakzai, BVSc, MSc, DESTS, MRCVS[a],*,
Padraic M. Dixon, MVB, PhD, MRCVS[b]

KEYWORDS

- Horse • Sinusitis • Surgery • Osteotomy • Trephination

KEY POINTS

- Trephination of the equine sinuses is a common surgical procedure in sedated standing horses.
- Standing sinus flap surgery has become increasingly popular and offers several advantages over sinusotomy performed under general anesthesia, including reduced patient-associated risks and costs and less intraoperative hemorrhage.
- Other minimally invasive surgical procedures for managing equine sinusitis include sinoscopic surgery, balloon sinuplasty, and transnasal laser sinonasal fenestration.
- Regardless of the procedure used, appropriate indications for surgery, good patient selection, and familiarity with regional anatomy and surgical techniques are imperative to obtaining good results.

INDICATIONS FOR STANDING SINUS SURGERY

Standing sinus surgery is indicated in the horse to treat primary or secondary sinusitis (**Tables 1** and **2**). Sinus surgery is also performed for diagnostic reasons, such as to facilitate sinoscopy (direct sinus endoscopy), allow endoscopic-guided biopsy, or to collect samples of the sinus contents for bacterial or fungal culture or histology. Standing sinus surgeries can be divided into sinus trephination procedures and sinus flap surgery (osteoplastic flaps). Before performing either procedure, one must complete a detailed case investigation to confirm the presence of sinusitis, collect as much information as possible regarding the likely cause of the condition, determine which sinus compartments are involved, and establish the positioning of the most appropriate surgical site. Indications for sinus surgery are therefore based on the results of clinical examination, nasal endoscopy, skull radiography, and a detailed intraoral examination. If available, adjunctive advanced imaging techniques such as

Disclosures: The authors have no conflict of interests.
[a] Chine House Veterinary Hospital, Sileby, Leicestershire LE12 7RS, UK; [b] Dick Vet Equine Hospital, Easter Bush Vet Centre, University of Edinburgh, Roslin, Midlothian EH25 9RG, UK
* Corresponding author.
E-mail address: szbarakzai@gmail.com

Table 1
Indications and contraindications for sinus trephination and standing sinus flap surgery

	Indications	Contraindications
Sinus trephination	1. Sinoscopy 2. Placement of a lavage tube 3. Endoscopic fenestration of the ventral conchal bulla[10,16] 4. Sinoscopically guided sinus surgery (eg, for mass biopsy, removal of inspissated pus, conchal bone sequestrae, small sinus cysts, fungal plaques, formalin injection, or removal of small intrasinus progressive ethmoidal hematoma)	1. Bone opacity mass immediately beneath the proposed trephine site
Standing sinus flap surgery	1. Primary sinusitis unresponsive to or recurrent after conservative management (antibiotics, sinus trephination, and lavage) 2. Intrasinus mass diagnosed preoperatively (eg, sinus cyst, ethmoidal hematoma, neoplasm) 3. Inspissated pus present within the sinus (diagnosed with radiography and/or sinoscopy); cases can sometimes be treated sinoscopically using transendoscopic biopsy forceps or wire retrieval baskets 4. Sinonasal fistulation, occasionally indicated in cases of chronic sinusitis with obstruction of the nasomaxillary ostium; however, effective removal of the primary lesion from all compartments will usually reduce mucosal inflammation in these cases and allow normal drainage within a few days postoperatively (see section on minimally invasive techniques) 5. Depressed maxillary or frontal bone fractures, which require elevation and fixation or small fragments that need to be removed	1. Unsuitable patient temperament, particularly if sinonasal fenestration is likely to be required 2. Bone opacity intrasinus masses detected radiographically (eg, odontogenic tumors, osteoma); these are likely to require aggressive sectioning using chisels or bone saws to enable their removal, and this is often not well tolerated in sedated horses 3. Extraction of cheek teeth through repulsion, unless oral extraction has already been attempted with significant breakdown of the periodontal ligament; repulsion of firmly attached teeth is not tolerated in the standing horse and should not be attempted

scintigraphy, computed tomography (CT), or magnetic resonance imaging (MRI) may be indicated before surgical procedures are performed.

Endoscopy Per Nasum

The tortuous, slit-like nature of the nasomaxillary aperture in normal horses prevents direct examination of the paranasal sinuses using endoscopy per nasum. However, nasal endoscopy is required to confirm that the sinuses are the source of nasal discharge, and thereby rule out other causes of unilateral nasal discharge, such as

Table 2
Comparisons between sinus flap surgery performed standing or under general anesthesia

Form of Restraint for Sinus Surgery	Advantages	Disadvantages
Sedation in standing horse	• No risk or cost associated with general anesthesia • Surgical theater/induction box facilities not required • Less hemorrhage than when surgery is performed under general anesthesia, resulting in improved visualization and allows surgeons to take their time	• Unsuitable for some fractious patients • Unsuitable if invasive or aggressive interventions are likely to be required • Reduction in sterility of procedure (but usually a contaminated/dirty procedure anyway)
General anesthesia	• Patient is immobilized and nonresponsive during surgical interventions • Suitable for fractious patients • Concurrent dental repulsion can be performed	• Small risk of mortality or morbidity associated with general anesthetic • Cost of general anesthesia • Requires facilities such as surgical theater suite, operating table, and recovery box • Volume of hemorrhage is usually greater

disorders of the nasal cavity and guttural pouches, or lower respiratory tract infection/ inflammation, which can occasionally present as a unilateral nasal discharge.

A diagnosis of sinusitis is confirmed by recognition of mucopurulent or purulent material or blood emanating from the sinonasal ostium (sinus drainage angle), which is situated at the caudal aspect of the middle meatus. Because of the narrow, complicated drainage pathway of the ventral conchal sinus (VCS), swelling of the ventral nasal concha caused by accumulation of exudate within the VCS is common, and often causes narrowing of the common and middle meati (**Fig. 1**). If severe, distension of the VCS may also narrow the ventral meatus, and occasionally can completely occlude the ipsilateral nasal cavity and displace the nasal septum toward the contralateral side. These horses will often have respiratory stridor at rest or exercise, and careful assessment of nasal airflow may detect a reduction or absence of expired air from the affected nostril. Remodeling of the nasal conchae is also common in horses with sinusitis (**Fig. 2**), and should not be confused with primary nasal lesions.

All horses with suspected sinusitis should undergo careful endoscopic examination of the middle meatus on the affected side, because some horses with sinus disease, including more than 20% with chronic primary sinusitis, will have a fistula from the middle meatus into their VCS (see **Fig. 2**; **Fig. 3**) and less commonly into their dorsal conchal sinus (DCS).[1] If present, a small-diameter endoscope can often be passed through this fistula into the VCS, and occasionally inspissated material or conchal sequestrae can be removed from this compartment, thus allowing the sinusitis to be treated endoscopically. Additionally, some horses have pieces of necrotic ventral conchal bone (**Fig. 4**) lodged in the caudal aspect of the middle meatus, often surrounded by inspissated pus (which can be the cause of the persistent unilateral nasal discharge), and this material can usually be removed transendoscopically. Horses that have previously undergone sinus surgery with sinonasal fenestration to improve sinus drainage will have a surgically created fistula.

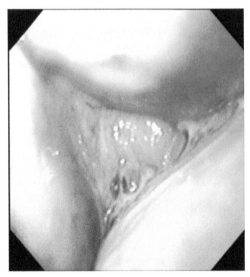

Fig. 1. Complete obstruction of the middle nasal meatus in a horse with sinusitis.

Radiography

Radiography is a well-established method of investigating sinus and dental disorders in the horse. However, the complex 3-dimensional structure of the head means that interpretation of radiographs in this region can be difficult in some cases. A minimum of 3 radiographic views should be taken of horses with sinusitis: lateral, lateral oblique (to examine individual cheek apices), and a dorsoventral view, the latter is taken specifically to establish if there is VCS involvement.[2]

Radiographs should be examined for the presence of abnormalities, such as fluid lines, intrasinus soft tissue opacity, periapical dental infection, intrasinus neoplasia, skull trauma, and distention of the VCS. Radiographs should also be

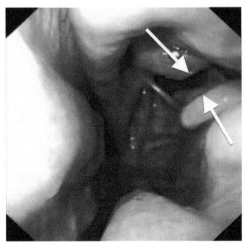

Fig. 2. Chronic destruction and remodeling of the dorsal concha in a horse with chronic sinusitis. Note the large naturally occuring sinonasal fistula (*arrows*).

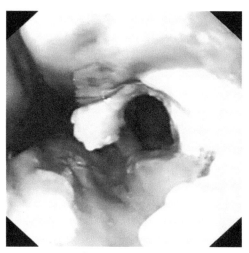

Fig. 3. Naturally occurring sinonasal fistula into the VCS in a horse with chronic sinusitis.

used to determine which sinus compartments are affected. The use of digital and computed radiography has increased in equine practice over the past few years and has helped provide higher-quality images, increasing the sensitivity and specificity of sinus radiography.

Computed Tomography

Cross-sectional imaging methods such as CT (**Figs. 5** and **6**) and MRI are extremely useful for evaluating the complex 3-dimensional structures of the equine head. The availability of CT facilities that can image the head of standing horses is increasing fast, making CT accessible to a larger number of horses. The advantages of CT over conventional radiography in horses with sinusitis include accurate identification of the sinus compartments involved, more precise identification of dental infection,[3]

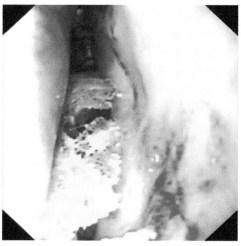

Fig. 4. Bone sequestrum in the caudal aspect of middle meatus, causing chronic clinical signs.

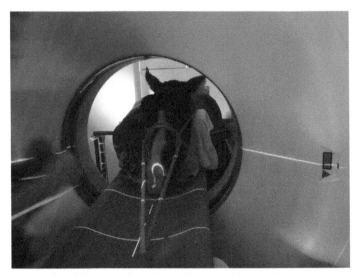

Fig. 5. Standing sedated horse undergoing a CT scan of its head.

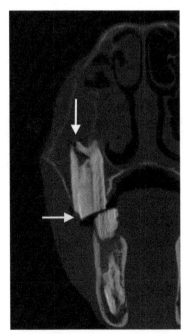

Fig. 6. Transverse CT image of a horse with dental sinusitis. Image shows a lateral "slab" fracture of 209 (*yellow arrow*), gas attenuation within the common pulp chamber, and gas around a lateral root of this tooth (*white arrow*), which confirms the diagnosis of apical infection. Disruption of the dental alveolus is also present, and soft tissue attenuating material fills the rostral maxillary and ventral conchal sinuses. The dorsal nasal concha is also filled with soft tissue–attenuating material and there is soft tissue swelling overlying the maxillary bone.

more information about the nature of sinus contents, and accurate identification of other sinonasal abnormalities that are not visible on radiographs (eg, mucosal thickening, conchal necrosis, remodeling).[3–5] In almost all cases, CT scans provide additional information that is not provided by radiography and, in the authors' experience, this extra information influences the subsequent treatment in most cases.

Oral Examination

The importance of a thorough oral examination in cases of sinusitis cannot be emphasized strongly enough. At least 41% of cheek teeth with periapical infections are now known to have occlusal pulpar exposure[6]; therefore, finding pulpar exposure in a suspect tooth on oral examination may help greatly in definitively diagnosing dental sinusitis. The teeth should be examined (preferably in the sedated horse) with a full mouth speculum in place, a strong headlamp, dental mirror or oral endoscope, and a dental pick, which is used to probe the pulp cavities. The most obvious clinical sign to note is packing of the pulp cavity with food material (**Fig. 7**). The dental pick should not normally be able to enter the occlusal aspect of the pulp cavity, which should be filled with secondary dentine. However, negative findings on oral examination do not preclude the presence of apical infection, and occasionally pulpar exposure is found in horses (particularly in older horses) without clinical signs of periapical infection.

In older horses with sinusitis, the junction of the hard palate and the maxillary cheek teeth should be carefully inspected for the presence of red, proliferative soft tissue that resembles granulation tissue. If present, this will usually be a squamous cell carcinoma that may invade the nasal cavity or sinuses after neoplastic squames migrate from their origin in the oral cavity up the periodontal spaces into the sinuses (**Fig. 8**). Biopsy results of this abnormal oral tissue in combination with radiography will allow a definitive diagnosis, and help avoid more-invasive sinus surgery.

PREOPERATIVE PREPARATION

Performing endoscopy and radiography should provide the clinician with a good idea of the horse's temperament and suitability for standing sinus surgery. Horses should be restrained in stocks for standing sinus surgery, and heavily sedated with

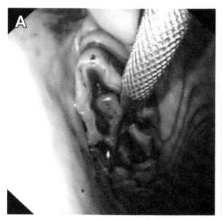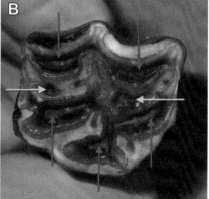

Fig. 7. (*A*) A dental probe is used to check for pulpar exposure. This 106 has multiple exposed pulps into which the probe tip can be passed. (*B*) Extracted maxillary cheek tooth with pulpar exposure of all 5 pulp horns (*red arrows*). Both infundibulae (*yellow arrows*) also have occlusal cemental defects, as is present in 90% of all cheek teeth.

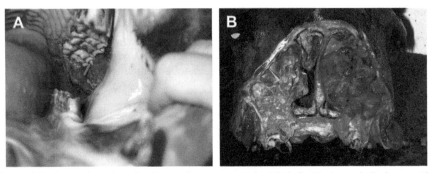

Fig. 8. (A) The oral cavity of a horse that presented with left-sided nasal discharge. The large, pink soft tissue mass lying palatally and buccally to the caudal cheek teeth is a squamous cell carcinoma that has invaded the overlying paranasal sinuses. (B) A transverse section of the affected horse after euthanasia. This image shows very extensive invasion of the sinonasal region by this aggressive oral tumor.

a combination of an α_2-agonist (romifidine or detomidine) plus butorphanol. Premedication with broad-spectrum antibiotics (the authors routinely use a combination of neomycin and procaine penicillin intramuscularly) and a nonsteroidal anti-inflammatory drug (eg, flunixin or phenylbutazone) is routine. A dental headstand is useful for resting the horse's head and keeping it steady during surgery (**Fig. 9**). The surgeon should have a good head torch.

For sinus trephination, injecting 2 mL of local anesthetic at the proposed trephination site provides adequate analgesia. For standing sinusotomy, local infiltration of skin along the incision sites on the maxilla or frontal bone is required, but a maxillary

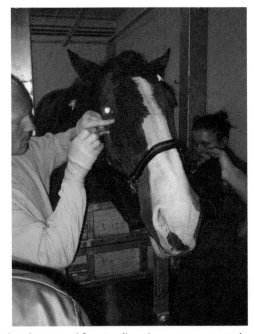

Fig. 9. Horse sedated and prepared for standing sinus surgery, restrained in stocks and head resting on a dental headstand.

nerve block[7,8] can also be useful for anesthetizing the sinus and nasal mucosa. Additionally, if fenestration into the nasal cavity is anticipated, endoscopically guided topical anesthesia of the nasal mucosa preoperatively greatly increases patient compliance when fenestrating and packing the nasal cavity. Once any degree of hemorrhage into the nasal cavity occurs, topically anesthetizing the nasal mucosa becomes very difficult.

If both nasal cavities are significantly obstructed (usually because of a unilateral lesion that is pushing the nasal septum across to the contralateral side), placing a nasopharyngeal tube via the contralateral nasal cavity is useful to maintain a patent airway during surgery and in the immediate postoperative period. In cases with severe bilateral nasal obstruction, a temporary tracheostomy tube may be required.

SURGICAL TECHNIQUES

Sinus trephination is a technique that can be easily performed by most equine practitioners in the standing sedated patient. In contrast, sinus flap surgery is a procedure that requires detailed anatomic knowledge and may be accompanied by complications such as significant intraoperative hemorrhage, damage to normal cheek teeth alveoli or the infraorbital canal, postoperative wound infection, and recurrence of clinical signs. The presence of sinus distension and mucosal inflammation frequently distorts the normal sinus anatomy, making intraoperative decision making challenging. For these reasons, sinus flap surgery should only be performed by veterinary surgeons with training in and experience with the technique.

SINUS TREPHINATION
Trephination Sites

The frontal sinus portal is often the most useful, and can be used for examining lesions in the frontal, dorsal conchal, caudal maxillary, and entrance to the ethmoidal and sphenopalatine sinuses. The site for this portal is positioned 0.5 cm caudal to a line drawn between the left and right medial canthi, and halfway between the midline and the ipsilateral medial canthus (see **Fig. 8**). This portal is particularly useful in young horses whose cheek teeth occupy much of the maxillary sinuses. It also provides access to the rostral maxillary sinus (RMS) and VCS if the ventral conchal bulla is fenestrated under endoscopic guidance.

The rostral and caudal maxillary sinuses of young horses (≤6 years of age) should not be trephined routinely, because trephination risks damaging the reserve crowns of the cheek teeth.[9] Additionally, the long reserve crowns are located close to the maxillary bone (the average distance from the maxilla to the lateral aspect of the cheek teeth is 13 mm), which limits maneuverability of the endoscope within the sinus and thus restricts visualization of the intrasinus structures. If trephination of the rostral maxillary sinus must be performed in young horses, radiographic guidance for portal positioning (lateral and dorsoventral views with markers in place) is strongly advised.

The caudal maxillary sinus (CMS) portal (for sinoscopy of the CMS, sphenopalatine, and conchofrontal sinuses) is positioned 2 cm rostral and 2 cm ventral to the medial canthus of the eye (**Fig. 10**).[10] The most reliable RMS trephine site in mature horses is positioned 40% of the distance between the rostral end of the facial crest and the medial canthus of the eye, and 1 cm ventral to a line joining the infraorbital foramen and the medial canthus (see **Fig. 10**).[10] The trephination technique involves the following (**Fig. 11**):

1. The horse is sedated routinely using an α_2-agonist plus butorphanol.
2. The skin at the trephination site is clipped and aseptically prepared.

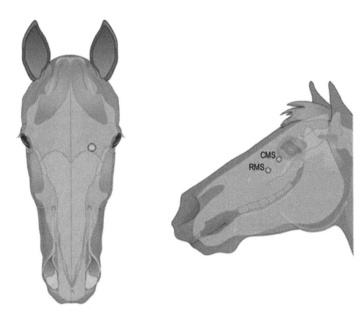

Fig. 10. (*Left*) Site for frontal sinus trephine portal. (*Right*) Sites for rostral (RMS) and caudal (CMS) trephine portals. (*From* Barakzai S. Handbook of equine respiratory endoscopy. Edinburgh, UK: Elsevier; 2006; with permission.)

3. A total of 1 to 2 mL of local anesthetic solution (eg, 2% lidocaine or mepivacaine) is infiltrated subcutaneously.
4. A 1.5- to 2.5-cm linear incision is made in the skin and the underlying periosteum; the size of the incision depends on size of the trephine being used.
5. Through this incision, the bone is trephined using a 1.0- to 1.5-cm diameter steel drill bit or a Galt trephine. Using self-retaining retractors may prevent damage to the skin and periosteum during trephination. Care should be taken that only a short length of the trephine is introduced into the sinus to avoid damaging intrasinus

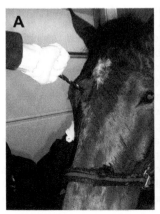
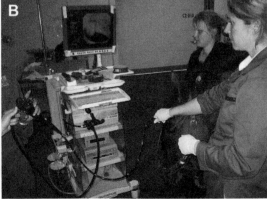

Fig. 11. (*A*) Frontal sinus trephination being performed with a modified drill bit (with T-bar welded on). (*B*) Frontal sinoscopy being performed.

structures (the ethmoid bones in particular) and inducing intraoperative hemorrhage.

6. If ventral conchal bulla fenestration will be performed, a second 8- to 10-mm diameter trephine opening can be made immediately below the original site to allow enough room for forceps/rongeurs manipulation and extraction of the bulla under endoscopic guidance.

7. The endoscope is introduced into the sinus and sinoscopy performed. A lavage tube or Foley catheter can then be placed in the sinus and secured as appropriate. If an in-dwelling tube is not left in situ, the incision may be closed primarily.

Standing Sinus Flap Surgery

Techniques for standing sinus flap surgery can be broadly split into 2 categories: those that use chisels or a bone saw to produce a 3-sided rectangular bone flap, which may be discarded or retained (**Fig. 12**), and those that use a large trephine to remove a disc of frontal bone, which is discarded (**Fig. 13**).[11] Horses require preoperative antibiosis, heavy sedation, and systemic analgesia and direct infiltration of the surgical site with local anesthetic before performing sinus flap surgery. Instillation of local anesthetic solution into the sinus lumen either before osteotomy (via a trephine hole) or after the bone flap is elevated also improves patient compliance when exploring the sinus interior and removing material from the sinuses.

Once the abnormal sinus contents have been evacuated (**Figs. 14** and **15**), the bone flap is replaced if possible (i.e., if it still has good periosteal and soft tissue attachments) and may be secured with cerclage wires before routine closure of the subcutaneous tissues and skin. Alternatively, cutting the osteoplastic flap at a 45° angle prevents depression of the flap into the sinus interior once it is replaced, and in these cases, use of cerclage wire may not be necessary. The bone flap is not retained if it is made using the large circular trephine technique.[11] Retention of the bone flap enhances the cosmetic result, particularly if a large nasofrontal osteotomy is made, which includes the curved part of the nasal bone. Inclusion of periosteum in the wound closure is believed to be important for sealing the sinus if the bone flap is not retained. Postoperative sinus lavage is nearly always indicated after sinus surgery, although overzealous lavage in the early stages (eg, within the first 24–48 hours) may be associated with increased incisional dehiscence because lavage fluid leaks into the periincisional tissues.

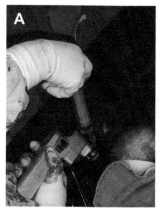
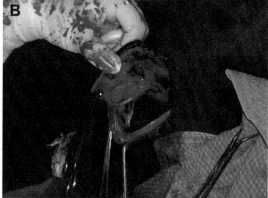

Fig. 12. (*A, B*) Oscillating bone saw being used to create hinged bone flap in the maxillary bone.

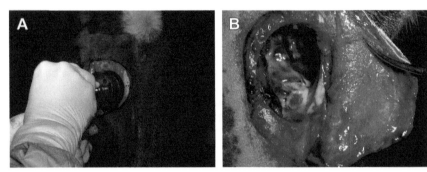

Fig. 13. (*A, B*) Frontal sinus osteotomy technique using a large Galt trephine. The disc of bone is discarded. (*Courtesy of* G. Quinn, BVSc Cert ES, Dipl. ECVS, Hamilton, New Zealand.)

MINIMALLY INVASIVE TECHNIQUES FOR ENLARGING THE SINONASAL OSTIUM
Balloon Sinuplasty

An endoscope-guided technique for enlarging the sinonasal ostium has been described as a potential treatment for horses with reduced drainage from the sinuses secondary to chronic sinusitis.[12] The technique was adapted from use in human beings and uses a dilating balloon catheter with a 12-mm diameter, 80-mm-long balloon, which is passed into the nasomaxillary ostium via the nasal cavity under endoscopic guidance. A specially modeled balloon introducer was used to facilitate correct positioning and the balloon was then dilated to a pressure of 6 atmospheres for 30 seconds. This dilatation was repeated 2 times. Inflation of the balloon effectively crushes the thin ventral conchal bulla, thus enlarging the sinonasal ostium. The results of the procedure in clinical cases of equine sinusitis have yet to be published.

Laser Vaporization of Dorsal Turbinate

Laser vaporization of dorsal turbinate effectively creates a new sinonasal ostium in the dorsal nasal concha, and thus allows for endoscopic evaluation of the sinuses with the scope passed per nasum and may also act as a portal for sinonasal drainage.[13] Under endoscopic guidance, a diode laser fiber with a contact probe was passed into the

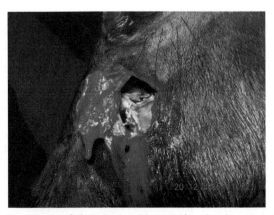

Fig. 14. Maxillary sinusotomy of chronic sinusitis case showing inspissated pus and sequestrae of nasal bones in the CMS.

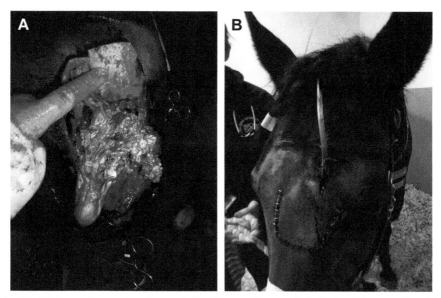

Fig. 15. (*A*) Large sinus cyst and granulation tissue with mycotic infection (diagnosed on histopathology) being removed through a bilateral frontal flap. (*B*) Postoperative appearance.

nasal passage through a custom-built laser introducer rod and used to create a stoma in the caudal, medial aspect of the turbinate overlying the dorsal conchal sinus.[13] This location in the nasal turbinates was chosen because it has the thinnest nasal mucosa, and therefore presumably the least vascularity. Sinoscopy was then performed via the new stoma to identify structures within the conchofrontal sinus and caudal maxillary sinus. The procedure was performed first in cadavers and then in standing sedated horses. In 4 of the 5 live horses, hemorrhage was reportedly minimal, and a stoma large enough to pass an endoscope through (approximately 1 cm^2) was successfully created.[13] Repeat endoscopy revealed that the stoma persisted for at least 5 weeks. Four horses had adhesion formation between the stoma and the nasal septum. The authors of this article[13] recognized that a stoma in the dorsal conchal sinus may not be optimal for sinus drainage because mucociliary clearance occurs toward the anatomic nasomaxillary ostium and not toward the surgically created stoma. Application of the technique in clinical cases and longer-term follow-up is necessary before final conclusions of this technique's efficacy can be made.

POSTOPERATIVE CARE

The sinus mucosa is extremely sensitive and only very dilute solutions of antiseptic, if any, should be used to lavage the sinuses. Solutions containing soap (ie, surgical scrubs) must not be used for sinus lavage. The primary purpose of sinus lavage is to physically dislodge and dilute material in the sinus, rather than provide antibacterial action. Lavage should therefore be performed 2 to 3 times daily with large volumes of fluid (3–5 L) (**Fig. 16**). Options for sinus lavage solutions are shown in **Table 3**.

COMPLICATIONS OF STANDING SINUS SURGERY
Hemorrhage

Hemorrhage is rarely associated with sinus trephination unless the surgeon inadvertently hits the ethmoturbinates or other intrasinus structure with the trephine. Even if

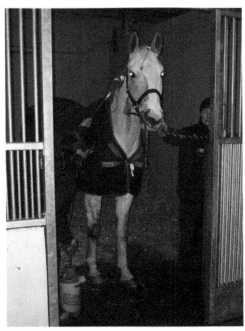

Fig. 16. Postoperative sinus lavage being performed using a large volume of nonsterile saline.

this occurs, in most cases hemorrhage will be self-limiting. Elevating the head of the sedated horse often helps reduce bleeding.

A degree of hemorrhage always occurs when sinus flap surgery is performed, because the sinus mucosa is a vascular tissue. Hemorrhage will be particularly copious if a surgical fenestration is made between the sinuses and the nasal cavity (**Fig. 17**), because the nasal mucosa is highly vascular. Sinonasal fenestration is not

Table 3 Sinus lavage solutions		
Solution	**Advantages**	**Disadvantages**
Povidone iodine 0.05%	Inexpensive, antibacterial, and antifungal activity	Irritant, particularly if inadequately diluted Solution is radio-opaque and can result in artifacts in postlavage radiographs
Sterile saline (0.9% sodium chloride)	Isotonic and least irritating to tissues	Expensive because large volumes ($\approx$3–5 L) are required bid/tid
Isotonic saline (9 g salt dissolved in 1 L water)	Inexpensive and isotonic, and therefore preferable to plain water	Not sterile and no antibacterial action
Tap water	Inexpensive	Hypotonic, and therefore increases edema of sinus mucosa Not sterile and no antibacterial action

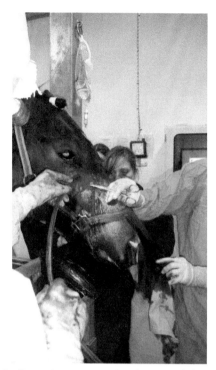

Fig. 17. Sinonasal fenestration using a stomach tube passed through the rostral aspect of the VCS. Note the end of the tube coming out of the nostril. This sinonasal fenestration technique causes minimal nasal hemorrhage, but the fistula tends to close within a month or so after surgery.

indicated often in sinusitis cases, and the free flow of blood and lavage fluid down the nasal cavity of horses undergoing sinusotomy will confirm this. We have experience of using a bipolar vessel sealing device (Ligasure TM, Covidien, Dublin, Ireland) for creating a bloodless sino-nasal fenestration in some standing surgery cases with the instrument introduced via a naso-frontal flap, however the nasal and sinus mucosa must be very well anaesthetised prior to instrument application. Hemorrhage associated with sinus surgery tends to be reduced in sedated standing horses compared with anesthetized horses, because of the elevated head position of the standing horse.

Nonetheless, hemorrhage always occurs to some degree, and measures to control it must be within easy reach during standing sinus flap surgery. These measures include local application of pressure and packing the sinuses and nasal cavity with a long sterile piece of cotton gauze (**Fig. 18**) or a sock-and-bandage pack. Use of topical adrenaline is often not effective because of the amount of hemorrhage that quickly dilutes it and carries it away from the area to which it was applied. Appropriate intravenous fluid therapy, and facilities to collect and administer whole blood, should be available in case they are required. The authors have had some success using chitosan-impregnated bandages in cases in which controlling intraoperative hemorrhage was challenging.

Patient Noncompliance

Patient noncompliance is extremely rare for sinus trephination techniques, but is observed more often during standing flap procedures, particularly during creation of

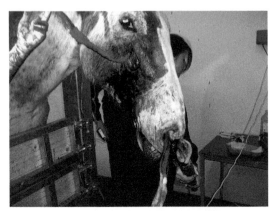

Fig. 18. Long bandage packing passed via the maxillary flap, through a surgically created sinonasal fistula, and out through the nostril. Note the horse had to be twitched for this procedure.

the osteoplastic flap if chisels or a bone saw are used. Fenestration of the nasal conchae and packing of the nasal cavity will cause resentment in most standing patients because the nasal aspect of the conchae is not only very vascular, but is well innervated. Although sinonasal fenestration and packing are possible in the standing sedated animal (see **Fig. 18**), horses with unreliable or fractious temperaments that are anticipated to require sinonasal fenestration may be better subjected to general anesthesia in the first instance. When performing standing sinus flap surgery, resources should be on-hand in case patient noncompliance results in a general anesthetic being required to complete the procedure.

Postoperative Incisional Infections

Sinus surgery in patients with active sinusitis is classified as "dirty" surgery using the National Research Council wound classification criteria (ie, transection of clean tissues performed for the purpose of surgical access to a collection of pus). In addition, suture material used to close the subcutaneous tissues may act as a foreign body and potentiate wound infections that occur. In an owner survey ($n = 178$), the authors found that the overall prevalence of surgical site infection was 10% (Dixon and Barakzai, unpublished data, 2011). Fortunately, although the prevalence of wound infection after sinus surgery is high, establishment of drainage and removal of remaining suture material (if appropriate) usually results in quick resolution of local infection with no adverse long-term consequences.

Poor Cosmetic Result

Trephination

When a small trephine hole is made, an excellent cosmetic result should be seen, with the defect being palpable but not visible. Occasionally, horses may develop suturitis at the frontonasal or frontolacrimal skull sutures, and if a large trephine hole is made, a small concavity may be visible at the surgical site.

Sinus flap surgery

Published cosmetic results of a 3-sided osteotomy technique with retention and wire fixation of the bone flap resulted in an excellent cosmetic result (no visible evidence of surgery) in 74% of cases, a good result (some discolored hair or a line in the hair) in

18% of cases, and a fair/poor result (mild or marked facial distortion) in 7% of cases.[14] In comparison, use of a large Galt trephine to remove a disc of frontal bone has been reported to result in excellent/very good surgical results in only 47% of cases (no visible evidence, irregular hair growth associated with the incision site, or a very slight concavity), a good result (mild to moderate asymmetry as a result of a slight proliferative frontonasal suture reaction or mild concavity at the surgical site) in 36%, and a poor result (because of marked periostitis or concavity of the frontal bone) in 13%.[11] Some surgeons also advocate application of a compression bandage placed around the head in a figure-of-8 pattern postoperatively to improve the cosmetic result; however, this has not been effective in the authors' experience.

Recurrence of Sinusitis

Recurrence of sinusitis after trephination and lavage is usually attributable to an ongoing underlying problem, such as failure to remove inspissated pus from some compartment, the residual presence of an intrasinus mass, or an undetected infected cheek tooth. The recurrence of clinical signs is an indication to refer the horse for further diagnostics and sinus flap surgery, if appropriate.

Recurrence of clinical signs after sinus flap surgery is reported to occur in 13% to 28% of cases.[11,14,15] These patients usually require some form of further investigation and/or surgical intervention and are often good candidates for computed tomographic examination if the cause of recurrence is not obvious.

REFERENCES

1. Dixon PM, Parkin TD, Collins N, et al. Equine paranasal sinus disease: a long-term study of 200 cases (1997-2009): ancillary diagnostic findings and involvement of the various sinus compartments. Equine Vet J 2012;44:267–71.
2. Barakzai SZ, McAllistair H. Radiography of the upper respiratory tract. In: McGorum BJ, Robinson NE, Schumacher J, et al, editors. Equine respiratory medicine and surgery. Edinburgh (United Kingdom): WB Saunders; 2006. p. 151–74.
3. Henninger W, Frame EM, Willmann M, et al. CT features of alveolitis and sinusitis in horses. Vet Radiol Ultrasound 2003;44:269–76.
4. Cissell DD, Wisner ER, Textor J, et al. Computed tomographic appearance of equine sinonasal neoplasia. Vet Radiol Ultrasound 2012;53:245–51.
5. Textor JA, Puchalski SM, Affolter VK, et al. Results of computed tomography in horses with ethmoid hematoma: 16 cases (1993–2005). J Am Vet Med Assoc 2012;240:1338–44.
6. Dacre I, Kempson S, Dixon PM. Pathological studies of cheek teeth apical infections in the horse: 5. Aetiopathological findings in 57 apically infected maxillary cheek teeth and histological and ultrastructural findings. Vet J 2008;178:352–63.
7. Staszyk C, Bienert A, Bäumer W, et al. Simulation of local anaesthetic nerve block of the infraorbital nerve within the pterygopalatine fossa: anatomical landmarks defined by computed tomography. Res Vet Sci 2008;85:399–406.
8. Bardell D, Iff I, Mosing M. A cadaver study comparing two approaches to perform a maxillary nerve block in the horse. Equine Vet J 2010;42:721–5.
9. Barakzai SZ, Knowles J, Kane-Smyth J, et al. Trephination of the equine rostral maxillary sinus: efficacy and safety of two trephine sites. Vet Surg 2008;37:278–82.

10. Barakzai SZ. Sinoscopy. In: Handbook of equine respiratory endoscopy. Edinburgh (United Kingdom): Elsevier; 2006. p. 118–32.
11. Quinn GC, Kidd JA, Lane JG. Modified frontonasal sinus flap surgery in standing horses: surgical findings and outcomes of 60 cases. Equine Vet J 2005;37: 138–42.
12. Bell C, Tatarniuk D, Carmalt J. Endoscope-guided balloon sinuplasty of the equine nasomaxillary opening. Vet Surg 2009;38:791–7.
13. Morello SL, Parente EJ. Laser vaporization of the dorsal turbinate as an alternative method of accessing and evaluating the paranasal sinuses. Vet Surg 2010; 39:891–9.
14. Dixon PM, Parkin TD, Collins N, et al. Equine paranasal sinus disease: a long term study of 200 cases (1997–2009): treatments and long-term result of treatments. Equine Vet J 2012;44:272–6.
15. Tremaine WH, Dixon PM. A long-term study of 277 cases of equine sinonasal disease. Part 2: treatments and results of treatments. Equine Vet J 2001;33:283–9.
16. Perkins JD, Windley Z, Dixon PM, et al. Sinoscopic treatment of rostral maxillary and ventral conchal sinusitis in 60 horses. Vet. Surg 2009;38:613–9.

Standing Equine Dental Surgery

Robert A. Menzies, BVSc[a],*, Jack Easley, DVM[b]

KEYWORDS

- Equine dentistry • Endodontic therapy • Tooth extraction • Buccotomy
- Mandibular fracture • External fixator • Minimally invasive surgery

KEY POINTS

- Equine endodontic therapy is a particularly challenging area of equine dentistry. An orthograde technique that has good long-term success is overviewed.
- Instrumentation and tool adaptation for tooth extraction where conventional techniques by mouth have failed are problematic. An overview of a minimally invasive buccotomy technique that allows straight-line access to a molariform tooth or fragment is presented along with a transbuccal screw extraction technique.
- Stabilization of fractures of the mandibular body are complicated by the presence of important dental structures and often contamination of the fracture site. The application of an Arbeitsgemeinschaft für Osteosynthesefragen (Association for the Study of Internal Fixation [AO]) pinless external fixator has considerable merit, particularly if combined with interdental wiring. An overview of fracture stabilization using the AO pinless external fixator is given.

INTRODUCTION

Dental surgeries in equids are procedures performed that affect the dental tissues and their supporting structures. They have been performed through the ages, and, depending on the degree of invasiveness and technologies available, with patients in a variety of positions and states of mental awareness. For many years, more-invasive diagnostic procedures and surgeries have been performed with equids under general anesthesia. Only 20 years ago, standing oral and dental procedures were limited to oral examination (with or without an oral speculum), dental floating, minor lip and gum laceration repair, wire fixation of fractures to the incisive area, and oral extraction of loose deciduous teeth, wolf teeth or loose periodontally infected incisor, premolar and molar teeth in older horses.[1] However, with a better understanding of the risks associated with general anesthesia, the availability of improved sedatives, the

[a] Dentistry & Oral Surgery Service, Faculty of Veterinary Medicine, Veterinary Teaching Hospital, University of Helsinki, PO Box 57 (Viikintie 49), FI-00014 Helsinki, Finland; [b] Equine Veterinary Practice, Easley Equine Dentistry, PO Box 1075, Shelbyville, KY 40066, USA
* Corresponding author.
E-mail address: robert.menzies@helsinki.fi

Vet Clin Equine 30 (2014) 63–90
http://dx.doi.org/10.1016/j.cveq.2013.11.002
0749-0739/14/$ – see front matter © 2014 Elsevier Inc. All rights reserved.

use of multimodal analgesia, and the continued development of equipment and surgical techniques, there are considerable advantages to performing many advanced dental diagnostic techniques and surgeries in standing sedated equids compared with recumbency under general anesthesia (see the article by Vigani and Garcia elsewhere in this issue for techniques on sedation and analgesia).

Surgery in the standing sedated patient reduces the inherent risks of general anesthesia. Anatomic orientation is made easier with the head presented in a more familiar position. Procedures typically associated with considerable hemorrhage (surgeries involving the oral mucosa, nasal passages or sinuses) are likely to bleed less with the horse in the standing position due to the head positioned above the height of the heart. The head position in a standing equid may be positioned more ergonomically for both clinician and animal and allows equal access to both sides of the head without having to move the patient. Access to the oral cavity is also optimized by not sharing the space with an endotracheal tube. However, with the presence of fluids in the oral cavity, clinicians need to be mindful of a reduced gag reflex and possible aspiration. General anesthesia may be indicated where the temperament of an equid, the invasiveness of the procedure, or inability to provide good analgesia is not conducive to a procedure performed under standing sedation.

Standing sedation in equids facilitates essential diagnostic procedures, such as a thorough oral examination and radiographic studies.[2] Equipment needed for physical restraint and examination of the head and oral cavity usually involves a set of stocks, head support, a full-mouth speculum, good intraoral lighting, soft tissue retractors, various dental picks, probes and explorers, a long-shafted dental mirror, and/or an oroscope.[3] Radiographic studies may comprise intraoral and extraoral views and be performed with and without contrast media. More-advanced diagnostics may also be undertaken in a sedated standing equid and include computed tomography (CT), scintigraphy, ultrasonography, and sinoscopy. The collection of samples for histopathologic, microbiological, viral, and parasitic analysis is also possible.

The majority of dental surgeries can be performed in a sedated standing equid. They include various odontoplastic procedures, periodontal procedures, endodontic procedures, orthodontic procedures, exodontia, orthopedic procedures, and soft tissue surgeries. The procedures have been extensively reviewed in the current veterinary literature.[4–6] This article focuses on several new and innovative techniques that have not been well disseminated in popular veterinary publications. These include (1) orthograde endodontic treatment of molariform teeth, (2) exodontia facilitated by a minimally invasive buccotomy technique and combined with a possible transbuccal screw extraction technique, and (3) minimally invasive stabilization of fractures of the mandibular body, which may involve dental or periodontal structures.

ORTHOGRADE ENDODONTIC THERAPY OF MOLARIFORM TEETH
Introduction: Nature of the Problem

Endodontic disease of the premolar and molar teeth of equids is not common in primary practice or the general equid population; however, it can make up a significant portion of cases for a dental referral practice and, when it occurs, treatment can be problematic.[7–15] Traditionally, the course of treatment has involved extraction of the affected tooth. However, exodontia is less than ideal. The treatment itself is grossly traumatic to the periodontal tissues, can be technically challenging, and has many potential complications, some of which may result in extended periods of hospitalization and further surgeries.[16–18] Long-term consequences of exodontia are inevitable and include mesial drift, malocclusion, and areas of reduced attrition.[19] Such changes are likely to increase the risk of periodontal disease and soft tissue injury and restrict rostrocaudal movement of the mandible. Removal of a loose dental fragment from an idiopathic molariform crown fracture that is not associated with apical periodontitis has a favorable prognosis.[20] Endodontic therapy avoids the problems precipitated by exodontia, is less invasive, may be repeated if unsuccessful, and does not result in tooth loss, particularly if the wrong tooth was identified and treated. It is, however, a technically challenging therapy that requires advanced dental knowledge and skills, and specialized equipment.

Clinical signs of endodontic disease are variable, ranging from none to apparently none (appreciated only in hindsight once the condition had been successfully treated) to findings, such as facial swelling, epiphoria, nasal discharge, discharging sinus tract, fetid nasal breath, weight loss, dysmastication, quidding, anorexia, pyrexia, head shyness, aversion to palpation, and lymphadenomegally. Findings on oral examination are likewise varied, from no abnormalities to subtle intraoral draining sinus tracts, changes in the occlusal secondary dentine, pulp cavity exposure, occlusal fissures, tooth fracture, caries-like lesions of infundibula, patent infundibula, and dysplastic teeth.[3,20–25]

Various techniques other than exodontia have been reported for the treatment of endodontic disease. Medical management, retrograde endodontic therapy, and apical curettage have either had unsatisfactory results, few case numbers, or inadequate long-term follow-up.[10,26–28] An orthograde approach to endodontic therapy of equine molariform teeth has recently been presented with long-term follow-up.[29] The technique is overviewed.

Preoperative Planning

Case selection is important for successful endodontic therapy. Pulp cavities that require treatment must be able to be reached properly. The affected tooth needs to have sufficient structural integrity remaining that it is unlikely to fracture or fracture further. Ideally, there should be no periodontal disease present; however, mild periodontal disease, which may be effectively treated or managed, is acceptable in equid patients. Teeth affected with periodontal-endodontic lesions have a poor prognosis. The patient must be amenable to the procedure, responding well to available sedative regimes. Concurrent disease, which decreases healing ability, such as uncontrolled Cushing's disease, reduces the prognosis for a successful outcome. Owner compliance and financial commitment are also keys for success.

A diagnosis of endodontic disease may be straightforward or challenging. Most diagnoses of endodontic disease can be made in consideration of the history, extraoral and (detailed) intraoral examination findings, and diagnostic-quality radiographs.[30] More-advanced diagnostic imaging modalities, such as CT and scintigraphy, are sometimes helpful.[11,31,32] When a diagnosis of endodontic disease is inconclusive, ongoing monitoring with repeated detailed oral examinations and ancillary diagnostics may be useful.[11,22] In contrast to endodontic disease in brachydont teeth, treatment of only the affected pulp cavities may be sufficient for a successful outcome. Pulp cavity anatomy is variable and age-dependent, often with communication between adjacent pulp horns.[33–36] Determining which pulp horns to access for treatment in an endodontically affected tooth is initially made by identification of abnormal findings in the occlusal dentin and radiographic findings but may also depend on the results of an exploratory pulpotomy if occlusal findings are within normal limits. The age-dependent changes and spatial configuration patterns of cheek teeth pulp compartments were recently described by Kopke and colleagues.[37] Knowledge of such information is helpful in planning treatment. The discovery of a vital and uninflamed pulp may necessitate only vital pulp therapy for that pulp horn. If a marked pulpitis or lack of vital tissue is discovered, the pulp should be totally removed (pulpectomy) and appropriate endodontic procedures performed.

Intramuscular procaine penicillin G (15,000–22,000 IU/kg) is administered every 12 hours starting the night before the endodontic procedure.[38]

Preparation and Patient Positioning

Endodontic therapy via an orthograde access is usually performed in equids under standing sedation. Good-quality sedation for endodontic therapy is characterized by an equid standing with minimal ataxia, not moving the head or tongue, and is relaxed and not resisting the procedure. The sedation should have only minimal cardiovascular, renal, and gastrointestinal effects and should not cause a prolonged recovery. Having appropriate equipment and necessary skills to use the equipment proficiently is important for both surgeons and anesthesiologists. Sedation should be provided in a controlled and dedicated environment. Flooring, drainage, lighting, noise, isolation from other activities, and an adjustable and sturdy head support are some of the environmental factors that require attention (**Fig. 1**). Eye covers and ear covers help reduce stimuli in sedated patients providing for more effective sedation with lower drug doses and side-effects. The working conditions should be ergonomic for both surgeons and patients. Multimodal forms of analgesia should be considered when significant discomfort is apparent or anticipated. Locoregional anesthesia may be indicated in cases of vital pulps, acute apical periodontitis, or osteomyelitis. Lavage of the oral cavity with 0.05% to 0.12% chlorhexidine gluconate solution 20 minutes

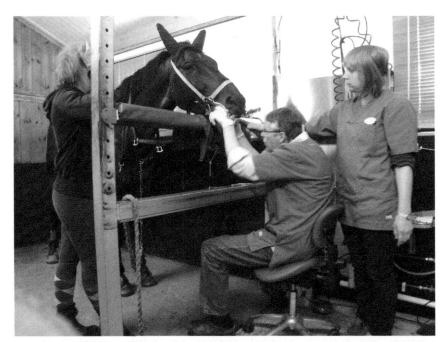

Fig. 1. Photograph illustrating a good working environment with a well-sedated horse, ergonomic positioning for the dental surgeon and patient, and a skilled dental assistant. A sturdy and adjustable headrest provides valuable support for the patient and ear covers enhance the quality of sedation achieved. (*With permission from* the Djurtandvårdskliniken [Animal Dental Clinic], Ängstugan, Västra Husby, 605 96 Norrköping, Sweden.)

prior to commencement of the endodontic procedure aids in reducing the amount of oral bacteria.

Surgical Approach

The orthograde endodontic procedure is approached via the oral cavity. Excellent intraoral lighting is necessary; however, when using composite material, appropriate steps must be taken to avoid premature polymerization. The working area is best visualized indirectly using a #4 or #5 dental mirror or an oroscope. The approach to the pulp cavity is via the occlusal surface of the affected pulp horns. The minimally invasive buccotomy approach (discussed later) can provide direct-line access to the occlusal surface of the tooth for instruments or an oroscope if needed.

Surgical Procedure

- The tooth is taken out of occlusion 1–2 mm by occlusal odontoplasty of the affected tooth and possibly the opposing tooth.
- Access to the pulp cavity is gained using a round carbide bur in a low-speed hand piece, changing to a Lindemann bur to widen it and ultimately a surgical-length fissure bur if there is a large distance between the pulp horn and occlusal surface (**Fig. 2**). Not all pulp horns may need endodontic therapy. Only the pulp horns that have evidence of pulp exposure or near-pulp exposure on oral examination or those suspected from radiographs are initially accessed. The stained occlusal secondary dentin (or unstained irregular secondary dentine or tertiary dentine) initially indicates the location of the pulp horn. Once drilled away, the direction of the pulp horn is determined by tactile sensation between the different dentine present—something easier to appreciate with a slow-speed drill

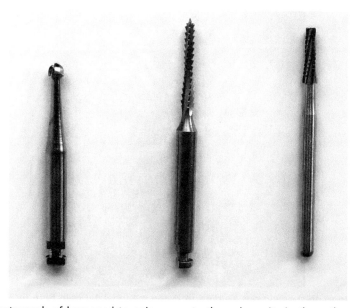

Fig. 2. Photograph of burs used to gain access to the pulp cavity in the orthograde endodontic technique. (*Left to right*) A round carbide bur, a Lindemann bur, and a crosscut tapered fissure bur on a surgical length shank. Note: the former 2 burs are latch-type, right-angle, slow-speed burs for a slow-speed handpiece whereas the latter is a high-speed friction grip bur for a high-speed handpiece—included for comparison.

compared with a high-speed drill. An endodontic file is used to access the coronal aspect of the pulp horn. A pair of large curved artery forceps is used to grasp the endodontic file (**Fig. 3**). Due to the tapering nature of pulp horns as they become more occlusal, establishing access can be considerably more challenging than for a brachydont tooth in species in which endodontic therapy is regularly performed.

- If pulp is present, it is extirpated using barbed broaches.
- Débridement and shaping of the pulp cavity are accomplished using veterinary-length endodontic files (see **Fig. 3**). The presence of denticles, intrapulpar calcifications, and calcified constrictions of the endodontic anatomy may make instrumentation challenging or impossible.[36]
- The endodontic file working length is checked using extraoral or intraoral radiography.
- The pulp cavity is irrigated alternately with a sterile isotonic solution and Dakin's solution (0.50% sodium hypochlorite) while débriding and shaping the pulp cavity. A total of 2–3 L of sterile isotonic saline solution is delivered under pressure within the pulp cavity, using a fluid pump designed for arthroscopic surgery. Irrigation is more effective if there is communication between the pulp horns accessed, such that one is for ingress and the other egress. The pulp cavity is ultimately filled with Dakin's solution, allowed to sit for 3–5 minutes, and then suctioned and flushed out. Suction and sterile paper points are used to remove excess fluid from the pulp cavity.
- Obturation is performed using an intravenous catheter to deliver calcium hydroxide paste to the apical portion of the pulp cavities. A veterinary-length spiral filler is used to obturate the pulp cavity further with calcium hydroxide. The paste is

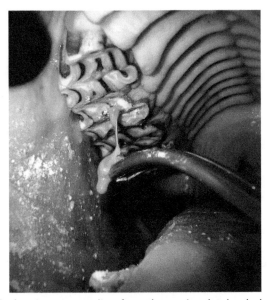

Fig. 3. Photograph showing pus exuding from the mesiopalatal pulp horn (pulp horn #3) of the right maxillary third premolar tooth during shaping and débridement with a veterinary-length Hedström endodontic file. (*Photograph courtesy of* Torbjörn Lundström, DDS, Section of Large Animal Medicine and Surgery, Department of Clinical Sciences, Faculty of Veterinary Medicine and Animal Science, Swedish University of Agricultural Sciences, 75007 Uppsala, Sweden.)

condensed with cotton pledgets and as much of the water content drawn out as possible. The coronal 8–10 mm of the pulp cavity and access are left devoid of calcium hydroxide paste.
- Restoration is accomplished by cleaning the walls of the cavity preparation and filling with a temporary cement (**Fig. 4**). The occlusal 2 mm are removed and a periodontal dressing applied to cushion the restoration.

Subsequent visit (3–4 weeks later)
- Access the previously treated pulp cavities by removing the temporary restorative cement in the same manner as described previously.
- Remove the majority of the pulp cavity filling. Observe the nature of the apical-most calcium hydroxide. If it is a pristine white powder and without odor, the pulp cavity may be obturated with calcium hydroxide paste again and a more permanent restoration may be performed. An intermediate layer of temporary cement is placed. A final restoration with wear characteristics similar to dentin is bonded in place. Space is left for a thin occlusal layer of periodontal dressing material. An important consideration is that the intermediate and final restorative layers should not bond strongly together. The intermediate layer needs to remain if the final restoration is lost.
- If the calcium hydroxide is discolored, not of a dry powder consistency, or is malodourous or any remnant pulp material is detected, the initial treatment is performed again with the flushing, débridement, sterilization, obturation, and temporary restoration. Adjacent pulp horns may also be investigated by pulpotomy for irreversible pulpitis or pulp necrosis, and, if diagnosed, then they also

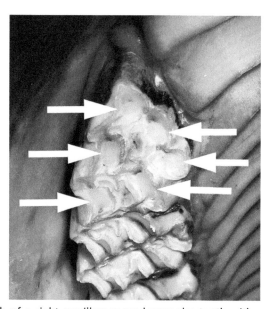

Fig. 4. Photograph of a right maxillary second premolar tooth with restorations of each pulp horn (*arrows*) after orthograde endodontic treatment. A periodontal dressing is still to be applied, used to help cushion the restorations. (*Photograph courtesy of* Torbjörn Lundström, DDS, Section of Large Animal Medicine and Surgery, Department of Clinical Sciences, Faculty of Veterinary Medicine and Animal Science, Swedish University of Agricultural Sciences, 75007 Uppsala, Sweden.)

undergo endodontic therapy in the described manner. The success of the proce-dure is again re-evaluated in 3–4 weeks.

Immediate Postoperative Care

If a purulent pulp is discovered at the first visit, intramuscular penicillin is continued for 5 days. A nonsteroidal antiinflammatory drug (NSAID) for 1 to 5 days may also be pre-scribed at the first visit depending on the degree of discomfort displayed by the equid. Food should be withheld for 2 to 3 hours after the procedure. Fresh pasture is recom-mended as a diet.

Rehabilitation and Recovery

Revisit every 3 to 4 weeks until no evidence of endodontic infection, then revisit every 6 months for 1 year, and then every 12 to 18 months for the life of the tooth. Typically, only 1 revisit of the 3 to 4-week period is necessary. If the equid is clinically improved, follow-up radiographs are usually not obtained until a year after the pro-cedure. For the first 2 years, removal of the restoration and assessment of the cal-cium hydroxide obturating material are performed. Radiographs are performed periodically. If anamnesis or clinical findings indicate possible treatment failure at any revisit, examination of the calcium hydroxide in the pulp cavity should be per-formed and radiographs obtained. Where there are no indications for further investi-gation a thorough oral examination should be performed every 12–18 months for the remainder of the equid's life.

Return to normal riding or work depends on the severity of the disease when treated and the response to treatment. If an equid was asymptomatic and no medications were prescribed after the procedure, return to work may be considered within 24 hours. At the other end of the spectrum, if an equid has a painful osteomyelitis or dental sinusitis, these conditions must be addressed and treated appropriately. A gradual return to work should occur after treatments are completed and clinical signs have resolved.

Clinical Results

Results of 501 orthograde endodontic therapies performed by the same operator at the Animal Dental Clinic and the University of Uppsala in Sweden over 3 consecutive years have been presented. The horses ranged in age from 3 to 22 years with a median age of 11 years. An overall long-term success rate of 82% was reported on 472 cases with follow-up of 3 to 6 years.[29] **Fig. 5** provides an example of radiographic findings in which endodontic treatment would be considered successful based on radiographic criteria.

Summary

Endodontic disease makes up a significant portion of the caseload in referral equine dental practices, with exodontia the most accepted form of treatment. Earlier studies have not been encouraging for the adoption of endodontic therapy as an option for molariform teeth. If endodontic therapy could be performed with good long-term re-sults, it would provide a more-conservative treatment with less morbidity for patients compared to dental extraction. The development of an orthograde endodontic therapy based on the antibacterial properties of calcium hydroxide, the ability to easily remove the calcium hydroxide to assess endodontic status and repeat the endodontic therapy at any point in time, and restorations with a similar wear rate to dentin has provided good results in a study with large numbers and long-term follow-up.[29] The endodontic treatment described is dynamic and is further condensed over time due to the occlusal

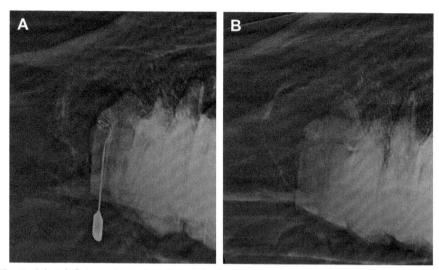

Fig. 5. (*A*) A left lateral 30° dorsal-to-right lateroventral oblique radiograph of the right maxillary second premolar tooth in an 11-year-old New Forest mare. A veterinary-length endodontic file is placed in the most mesial pulp horn (pulp horn #6) and extends into the mesiobuccal root (root canal I).[36,37,63] A large periapical radiolucency devoid of a trabecular pattern surrounds the mesiobuccal root and is bordered by an ill-defined slightly sclerotic border with a prominent trabecular pattern. The periodontal ligament space is poorly defined in the mesioapical region of the tooth with no lamina dura evident. The changes are typical of chronic apical periodontitis and are extensive enough to be classified as acute osteomyelitis. The periapical lesion is due to endodontic disease of at least the mesial portion of the second premolar tooth. (*B*) A 31-month follow-up radiograph of the same case obtained with a similar radiographic technique after orthograde endodontic treatment of all of the pulp horns and roots of the right maxillary second premolar tooth. One discrete and 3 less discrete small areas of radiopacity present along the palatocclusal aspect of the tooth are the restorations in the mesial and palatal pulp horns (pulp horns #6, #3, #4, and #5).[36,37] It is not possible to assess the quality of obturation radiographically due to: the low radiodensity of calcium hydroxide (compared with many other obturating materials); the small volumes of the pulp cavities, which are filled by the calcium hydroxide (compared with overall volume of the tooth); and the large amount of dental hard tissue comprising the tooth. An approximately circular heterogeneous radiopacity overlying the distoapical aspect of the buccal portion of the mesial root and surrounded by a thin discrete radiolucency is most likely hypercementosis. A generalized increase in radiopacity of the previously radiolucent periapical lesion with the re-establishment of a fine trabecular pattern is seen. A thin intermittent radiopaque rim outlines the extent of the earlier lesion. The mesioapical periodontal ligament space is better defined although a well-defined lamina dura is not evident. The radiographic changes indicate resolution of the osteomyelitis and periapical healing. (*Courtesy of* Torbjörn Lundström, DDS, Section of Large Animal Medicine and Surgery, Department of Clinical Sciences, Faculty of Veterinary Medicine and Animal Science, Swedish University of Agricultural Sciences, 75007 Uppsala, Sweden.)

forces of mastication. It is important to emphasize that the technique requires a veterinary dental surgeon who is knowledgeable and skilled in endodontic therapy beyond what is presented in this article, that owner compliance is key for long-term success, and that both endodontic and periodontal conditions may contraindicate the technique.

MINIMALLY INVASIVE BUCCOTOMY AND TRANSBUCCAL SCREW EXTRACTION TECHNIQUES
Introduction: Nature of the Problem

Although extraction of an equid molariform tooth or dental fragment by mouth using a noninvasive closed extraction technique is considered the optimal manner of removing a tooth, occasionally an equine clinician is challenged in doing so by a lack of clinical crown present or poor access and tool adaption.[16] Typically, such cases are selected for an open extraction technique (repulsion or lateral buccotomy) under general anesthesia. However, complication rates and long-term outcomes have been shown, to be superior for closed extraction techniques compared with open extraction techniques.[10,16,18,39,40] There are also inherent risks associated with equine general anesthesia. Addressing these 2 points, a minimally invasive surgical approach, which preserves the benefits of a closed extraction, has been developed in Germany and is usually performed in sedated standing patients.[41] The approach—a minimally invasive buccotomy—facilitates direct-line dental elevation and, when necessary, extraction via a novel transbuccal screw technique. The technique is gaining acceptance as the treatment of choice where dental extraction using oral forceps is not possible (**Fig. 6**). An overview of the technique is discussed.

Preoperative Planning

- Assess the patient's general health and risks associated with sedation. Include a review of the patient's response to previous sedation regimes.
- Ensure tetanus prophylaxis is appropriate.
- Perform a thorough oral examination (a procedure which necessitates sedation of the patient).
- Obtain an appropriate radiographic study specific to the tooth of interest. Typical extraoral radiographs include a laterolateral view, 1 or 2 lateral oblique views (including an open-mouth view), and a dorsoventral view with mediolateral displacement of the mandible. The study may also include intraoral radiography, such as occlusal, lateral bisecting angle, or lateral parallel views.

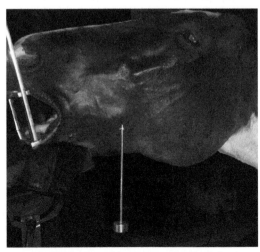

Fig. 6. Photograph of a sedated horse undergoing a transbuccal screw extraction of the left maxillary fourth premolar tooth via a minimally invasive buccotomy.

- If sufficient clinical crown is present on the tooth to be extracted or only dental fragments remain, attempt a noninvasive dental extraction or fragment removal (ie, by mouth).
- Ensure appropriate facilities: good stocks, flooring, drainage, and lighting; surgical equipment tables; and a quiet area without potential distractions outside. A solid headrest or stable suspension system is required for maintaining head position and providing support for the sedated animal.
- It is important to have appropriately trained personnel to assist and record the sedation procedure, provide surgical assistance, and monitor the patient.
- Allot an appropriate amount of time for the procedure, including time to address potential complications.
- Have an alternate plan of action if the procedure is not successful.
- The surgeon must have good anatomic knowledge of the area and a sound knowledge of surgical and dental principles.
- An appropriate surgical instrument kit is essential (**Fig. 7**).
- Appropriate surgical preparation involving cadaver training is recommended (training workshops are available).

Preoperative Preparation and Patient Positioning

- The patient is placed in well-designed stocks where sedation and surgery are performed in the standing equid.

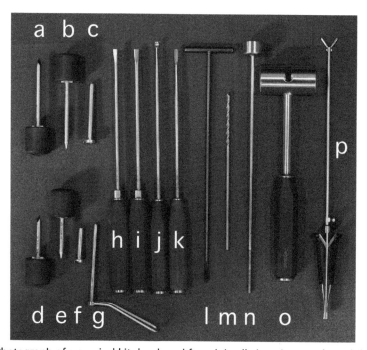

Fig. 7. Photograph of a surgical kit developed for minimally invasive transbuccal dental extractions: a, long sharp trocar; b, long blunt trocar; c, long cannula; d, short sharp trocar; e, short blunt trocar; f, short cannula; g, drill guide; h, chisel; i, osteotome; j, spoon curette; k, dental elevator; l, tap (6-mm diameter); m, drill bit (5-mm diameter); n, threaded pin with metal stopper; o, slotted mallet; and p, fragment forceps. (*Courtesy of* Frank Schellenberger, DVM, Pegasos Foundation, Sandweg 5, D-79183 Waldkirch, Germany.)

- Place an intravenous jugular catheter in an aseptic manner.
- Consider the use of broad-spectrum antibiotic therapy.[42] If selected, use appropriate spectrum of activity for common oral and skin pathogens, such as penicillin.
- A sedation protocol based on an α_2-agonist constant rate infusion with boluses as indicated is recommended. Concomitantly administer opioids, ketamine, benzodiazepines, tranquilizers, and other drugs as indicated (see article by Vigani and Garcia elsewhere in this issue).
- Administer preoperative NSAIDs.
- Ear covers or earplugs and eye covers help reduce patient stimulation and promote a more-effective sedation process.
- Perform appropriate long-acting locoregional anesthesia (ie, nerve blocks and local infiltration).
- Use an oral speculum that allows good surgical access, such as a Günther speculum.[42]
- Remove all ingesta from the oral cavity and rinse well with a weak (0.05%–0.12%) chlorhexidine solution 20 minutes prior to commencing surgery.
- Apply topical local anesthesia to oral mucous membranes to help reduce response of horse to intraoral stimuli.[42]
- Clip and surgically prepare a suitably large area of the head.
- Either visually or by palpation, identify the facial artery and vein, the dorsal and ventral buccal branches of the facial nerve (cranial nerve [CN] VII), and the parotid duct. Draw the structures onto the skin using surgical markers (**Fig. 8**).[42]
- Introduce a dog urinary catheter (2 mm in diameter and 50 cm in length) through the parotid duct papilla in a dorsoventral direction to facilitate palpation of the parotid duct if necessary.
- Maintain a patient head position that is ergonomic for both surgeon and equid.

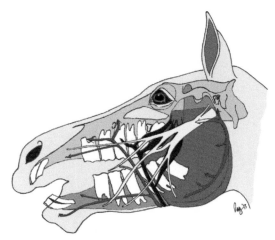

Fig. 8. A schematic drawing of a horse's head showing pertinent anatomic features for consideration when performing a buccotomy. Branches of the facial artery are on the left of the image (the masseteric branch is on the right with the transverse facial artery dorsally)—arteries are in red; the facial vein and associated sinuses are in blue (dorsal to ventral, the dilatations are part of the transverse facial vein, the deep facial vein, and the buccal vein); the parotid duct is in green; the facial nerve is in yellow; and the masseter muscle is in orange.

- Ensure that the patient does not put pressure on the ventral neck or thoracic inlet by leaning on the front of the stocks.
- Encourage the patient not to lean on the stocks.

Surgical Approach

- With the horse's mouth held open with the speculum, as for surgery, place a horizontal skin staple at both the maxillary and mandibular occlusal levels in line with the proposed buccotomy site; place 3 closely spaced (for example, 10 mm apart) vertical skin staples over the area of apex of the tooth to be extracted (**Fig. 9**).[41]
- Obtain straight lateral and oblique lateral radiographic views centered on the tooth to be extracted.
- In most cases, the transbuccal surgical approach is between the dorsal and ventral buccal branches of the facial nerve (CN VII) and, depending on the tooth of interest, either rostral or caudal to the facial artery and vein.[42]
- Rostral to the facial artery and vein and the parotid duct, the tissue layers penetrated are the skin, subcutaneous tissue, possibly the zygomaticus muscle, the buccinator muscle, submucosal tissue, and the buccal mucosa of the oral cavity.
- Caudal to the facial artery and vein and parotid duct, the tissue layers penetrated are the skin, subcutaneous tissue, possibly the zygomaticus muscle, masseter muscle, submucosal tissue, and the buccal mucosa of the oral cavity.
- An approach caudal to the facial vein requires the surgeon to be mindful of 3 large venous sinuses that branch off the facial vein. From dorsal to ventral, they are part of the transverse facial vein, the deep facial vein, and the buccal vein. The deep facial vein deserves special mention due to the lack of valves between it and the sinus cavernosus at the base of the skull, allowing blood and potentially bacteria to flow in either direction.[43] An infectious cellulitis of the buccotomy site in this area should be treated promptly and appropriately.

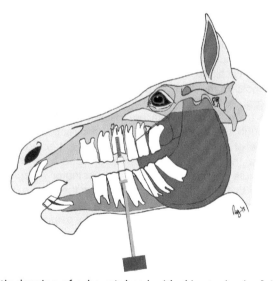

Fig. 9. A schematic drawing of a horse's head with skin staples (*red*) indicating occlusal planes and apical position of a fractured left maxillary fourth premolar tooth. A threaded metal pin is passed through the cheek tissues in a cannula (*yellow*) and screwed into the fractured tooth. The stopper at the end of the pin (*gray*) allows a slotted mallet to gently tap the loosened tooth in a ventral direction (along the path of eruption).

- The dorsal and ventral limits of the oral vestibule, and the position of the tooth to be extracted, can be appreciated externally by placing a hand in the oral cavity and pressing laterally on the buccal tissues with a digit at each of the features.[42]
- The caudal teeth are more challenging to achieve appropriate tool placement and adaptation. In particular, it may not be possible to extract the mandibular second and third molar teeth using the described technique.

Extraction of tooth or dental fragments
- All transbuccal equipment (such as the dental elevators, curettes, drill guide, drill bit, tap, threaded pin, and transbuccal fragment forceps) should be passed via the transbuccal cannula. Once the cannula is placed, it remains in place until the buccotomy is no longer needed.
- The buccotomy has the advantage of providing a straight-line approach for the implement working end, facilitating better control and instrument adaptation and increased forces in an apical direction.[42]
- An oroscope with a small diameter may also be passed via the cannula if necessary.[42]
- After mobilizing the teeth or dental fragments with the dental elevators, extraction should be attempted using conventional extraction forceps by mouth before deciding to pursue an orthograde screw extraction technique.
- An oroscope passed by mouth assists in correct instrument positioning and adaptation throughout the procedure.

Surgical Procedure

Minimally invasive buccotomy
- Despite oral surgery not able to be performed in a sterile manner, an aseptic technique should still be used and equipment cleaned to hospital surgical standards.
- To ensure desensitization of the buccotomy site, 2 mL of local anesthetic agent are injected subcutaneously and 3 mL into the deeper tissues.[41]
- A 4-mm skin incision is made with a #10 or #15 scalpel blade, taking care not to incise the subcutaneous tissues.[41] For access to the maxillary molariform teeth, the skin incision should allow entry of the trocar and cannula into the ventral aspect of the oral vestibule; conversely, for access to the mandibular molariform teeth, the skin incision should allow entry of the trocar and cannula into the dorsal aspect of the oral vestibule.
- A blunt 8-mm trocar and cannula are passed through the skin incision and continued through the deeper tissues in the direction toward the remaining occlusal surface of the tooth or fragment to be extracted.[41] To pass through the oral mucosa, the blunt 8-mm trocar is replaced by a sharp one. The short trocar and cannula are used for the transbuccinator muscle buccotomy; the longer set is used where the masseter muscle is the main muscle penetrated.
- When the sharp trocar is removed, the cannula stays in place until the end of the transbuccal procedure. All tools that subsequently pass in a transbuccal route do so via the cannula.[41]
- At the end of the procedure, the oral cavity is again lavaged with weak chlorhexidine solution, paying particular attention to the intraoral portion of the cannula. The cannula is removed and the buccotomy wound lavaged. The skin is apposed with skin sutures or staples and the oral mucosa is typically left to heal by secondary intention.[41] In approaches that involved passage through the masseter muscle, closure of the oral mucosa with dissolvable suture material is recommended.[41]

Mobilizing the tooth or dental fragment

- A long-shafted luxator or dental elevator introduced via the cannula is carefully forced into the mesial and distal interproximal spaces and into the periodontal ligament of the tooth to be extracted (see **Fig. 10**).[42] The wedge-shape displaces the tooth and creates areas of strain and compression along the periodontal ligament. Exceeding the strain limit and traumatizing the periodontal ligament help in its breakdown. Compression of the periodontal structures helps enlarge the alveolus and provides an extraction pathway for the tooth, a pathway that may also be aided by the temporary displacement of adjacent teeth away from the alveolus.
- Once the elevator is well positioned in the interproximal space or periodontal ligament, applying controlled rotational force to the handle may increase the displacement of the tooth and facilitate further periodontal destruction and alveolar enlargement.[42] Much care must be taken to not cause iatrogenic fracture of adjacent teeth.
- An oroscope is recommended to assist with correct tool placement and adaption.[42]
- Odontoplasty of the proximal surfaces of the clinical crown extending apically to include some of the reserve crown, and osteoplasty of the associated alveolar bone has been advocated to improve instrument adaption and provide a space into which the crown may be displaced further (Travis Henry, DVM, personal communication, 2012). Care must be taken not to cause iatrogenic damage to adjacent teeth and not to cause thermal necrosis of the alveolar bone. A sterile isotonic irrigating solution should be used during the osteoplastic procedure.
- Extraction of the tooth or tooth fragment should not be attempted until sufficient alveolar enlargement and periodontal ligament destruction have occurred and the tooth or tooth fragment has considerable mobility.

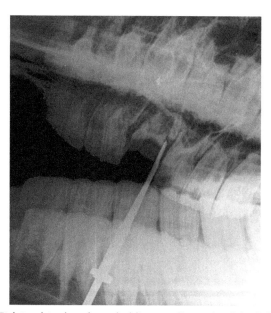

Fig. 10. Ventral 45° lateral-to-dorsolateral oblique radiograph of the left maxilla showing placement of a transbuccal dental elevator via the buccotomy cannula and into the distal periodontal ligament space of the fourth premolar tooth.

Transbuccal screw extraction technique
- Prior to initiating the transbuccal screw extraction technique, but after the tooth or tooth fragment has been mobilized, extraction should again be attempted using oral dental forceps.[42] If unsuccessful, proceed with the next step.
- Drill a superficial guide hole starting on the buccal aspect of the occlusal surface of the tooth or fragment using either a bur inserted at right angles into a dental machine hand piece (by mouth) or a 3-mm diameter drill bit via the transbuccal approach.[41] Visualize the process using an oroscope. With the transbuccal approach, a drill sleeve is passed through the cannula to the tooth. For a maxillary tooth, the drill hole is started on the buccal aspect of the occlusal surface and is directed slightly in a palatal direction.[44] For a mandibular tooth, the drill hole is started in the buccal wall of the clinical crown and directed slightly in a lingual direction. Using the previous radiographs with markers as a guide, direct the drill in a direction close to the axial direction of the tooth. Drill to a depth of approximately 5 mm, then take a lateral oblique radiographic view with the drill bit in place to check positioning.
- From the radiographs, estimate the distance from the external aspect of the cannula to the apex of tooth or a depth of 40 mm from the occlusal surface (whichever comes first), and set the drill stop at the same distance on the 3-mm diameter drill bit.[41]
- Enlarge the hole in the same manner using the 5-mm diameter drill bit with an adjustable stop to control drill depth (see **Fig. 11**).[41] Drill to the apex of the tooth or a depth of 40 mm, whichever comes first (penetration of alveolar bone should be avoided). Be cognizant that in the transverse plane, the drill is partially

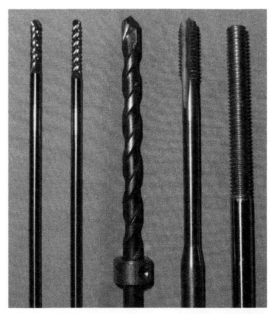

Fig. 11. Photograph (*left-to-right*) of 3-mm bur for proximal crown odontoplasty, 3-mm drill bit for making a guide hole in the tooth crown, 5-mm drill bit with adjustable stop, 6-mm tap, and 6-mm threaded pin with large stop at end of shaft. These long shaft instruments are used sequentially in the transbuccal screw extraction technique.

directed in a palatal or lingual direction. Use irrigation to cool the bit while drilling to reduce the risk of thermal damage either to the periodontal or buccal tissues and also to improve cutting efficiency. Repeat radiographic control with drill in place. Irrigate the drill hole to remove all tooth chips.

- Tap the drill hole with the 6-mm tap (**Fig. 11**). Do not use the tap to further loosen the tooth because the tap may break.
- Screw in a 6-mm threaded pin with a metal stopper attached to the free end (**Figs. 11** and **12**).[41] Further disruption of the periodontal ligament and enlargement of the alveolus may be achieved with careful manipulation of the tooth using the pin as a handle. Once the tooth is considerably mobile and surrounded by a bloody froth, extraction of the tooth may proceed.[42]
- A metal mallet with a slot created in it for the 6-mm pin is positioned around the pin. Many small stokes of the mallet are used to percuss the metal stopper at the free end of the pin until the tooth is gently removed from the alveolus.[42]
- Once the tooth has been extracted from the alveolus, the threaded pin is unscrewed from the tooth and the tooth removed via the mouth (**Fig. 13**).[44]
- Examine the tooth for indications of missing root tips that may have fractured off. Using a dental mirror or oroscope, examine the alveolus for tooth and bony fragments. Repeat examination with digital palpation, wearing a sterile glove.
- Obtain postoperative radiographs and examine closely for retained root tips, bony fragments, and iatrogenic damage to adjacent teeth and their periodontia.
- Perform standard postextraction alveolar care. In some cases, this may involve packing the alveolus or placing an obturator to prevent ingress of ingesta.

Complications

- If the tooth disintegrates during the extraction process, remove the fragments using fragment forceps and dental elevator.

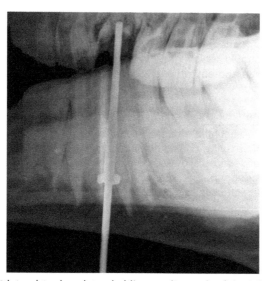

Fig. 12. Ventral 45° lateral-to-dorsolateral oblique radiograph of the left maxilla showing a 6-mm transbuccal pin screwed into the fourth maxillary premolar. Note the pin has been placed more apically than ideal due to its likely engagement of periapical bone. This was corrected by backing the screw out several millimeters before attempting extraction.

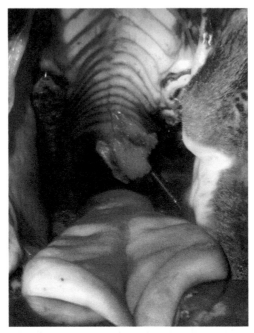

Fig. 13. An intraoral photograph showing the extraction of the left maxillary fourth premolar tooth using the transbuccal screw extraction technique.

- If the threaded pin pulls out of the tooth, there is usually room to drill an adjacent hole and repeat the extract process.
- If the tooth is too weak to sustain the screw extraction technique, the tooth may be fractured into multiple pieces by drilling more holes and using a small osteotome or chisel to fracture it.[44] The pieces may then be extracted using dental elevators and fragment forceps.
- The alveolus should be lavaged, oroscopically inspected, radiographed for retained fragments and any other abnormalities, and treated in the standard way for postextractions.

Immediate Postoperative Care

- Muzzle the horse until the effects of sedation have worn off.
- Reversal agents may be considered if recovery from sedation is protracted.
- When no longer sedated allow the horse to graze fresh pasture or eat soft moistened feed. Avoid dry pellets; grains; dry chopped fibrous matter, such as chaff; and hay with a high stalk component.

Rehabilitation and Recovery

- Feed soft feed, such as fresh pasture or bran gruel, for at least 3 days while oral wounds begin to heal.
- Continue NSAIDs for 3–7 days.[42]
- Consider gastric protectant measures if the horse is kept in stall confinement.
- Consider antibiotic therapy.[42] If good surgical preparation and technique are used, however, minor oral surgery should not routinely necessitate antibiotic therapy in an otherwise healthy horse. Consider lavage of oral wound with

0.05%–0.12% chlorhexidine gluconate solution once or twice daily using an oral dosing syringe for 3–7 days.
- Treat concurrent disease, such as dental sinusitis, if necessary.
- Recommend keeping horse in hospital 1 night postoperatively if a prolonged procedure.
- Recommend revisit at 10–14 days to assess healing of alveolus (particularly for the presence of sequestra) and to remove skin sutures or staples.
- Scheduled rechecks should be in 1 month, 3 months, and 6 months.
- Owner needs to be aware of likely increased oral care needs with regards to long-term health of mouth—hypereruption and supereruption of unopposed tooth, mesial drift, malocclusion, occlusal areas of reduced attrition, soft tissue interference, diastemata formation, and periodontal disease.

Clinical Results

The results of 26 minimally invasive transbuccal surgeries performed in 22 horses have been presented in a pilot study involving 100 horses which were referred for dental extraction by mouth by one veterinary surgeon in Germany. All teeth (or their fragments) that underwent minimally invasive transbuccal surgery were successfully extracted. The surgeries involved 2 maxillary premolar teeth, 19 maxillary molar teeth, 3 mandibular premolar teeth, and 2 mandibular molar teeth. Complications were 70% mild peribuccotomy edema, 27% transient facial nerve paresis, 4% sinus penetration with subsequent nasal discharge, and 4% purulent discharge from the buccotomy site. All complications resolved without additional treatment.[41]

Summary

For teeth and dental fragments that cannot be extracted by mouth in a noninvasive manner, the minimally invasive buccotomy and associated transbuccal surgeries provide an attractive option to traditional techniques. The documented complications are minor when the technique is performed in a skilled manner and when compared with the complication rates of more-invasive procedures, such as dental repulsion. Specialized equipment and surgical skills are required that are worthy investments for those with a significant dental referral caseload.

APPLICATION OF AN AO PINLESS EXTERNAL FIXATOR FOR MANDIBULAR FRACTURE STABILIZATION
Introduction: Nature of the Problem

Fractures of the body of the mandible occasionally occur and are usually traumatic in origin. The teeth make up a significant portion of the mandible, particularly in younger equids. Therefore, a suspected jaw fracture should be thoroughly investigated to determine whether there is involvement of dental or periodontal structures. Mandibular fractures that are stable and minimally displaced, and the equid is able to eat and drink without difficulty, may not require further stabilization. However, for those fractures requiring fixation, repair can be challenging, which is partly due to the necessity to avoid iatrogenic damage to existing teeth. There are many techniques for stabilizing mandibular jaw fractures and often a combination of techniques is most appropriate.[45–53] Each jaw fracture is unique and requires a tailored approach.[50] The application of an AO pinless external fixator for mandibular fractures has been used with success in Switzerland and Germany.[54,55] Although originally applied with patients under general anesthesia, recently it has been performed in standing sedated patients, thus providing surgeons with more treatment options.[55]

There are 2 important objectives of jaw fracture repair. The first is to re-establish an equid's normal occlusion. The second objective is to provide a stable environment in which callus formation and healing may occur. Many mandibular fractures are open, and treatment planning needs to address a contaminated environment. Overall, resolve of discomfort and a rapid return to normal function is the main goal.

The AO pinless external fixator was developed as a first-stage treatment of severe open fractures of the tibia in humans, primarily to avoid pin tract infection of conventional external fixators (**Fig. 14**).[56,57] It has been successfully adapted for the stabilization of mandibular fractures in cattle and equids.[54,58,59] The advantages in equids include the following: (1) the clips used do not penetrate the cortex and, therefore, avoid iatrogenic damage to teeth; (2) in cases of open fractures, an implant is not placed in a contaminated environment; (3) placement is minimally invasive; (4) the fixator is easily combined with other types of fixation when necessary; (5) surgery time is short; and (6) the procedure may be performed in a standing sedated equid. Disadvantages are the AO pinless external fixator is applied on the compression side of the fracture line; it is not the most stable of fixation devices available; and clip loosening, sequestration, and localized cellulitis associated with the clips are common.[47,54] A report on 6 equids using locking compression plate osteosynthesis to repair severely comminuted and open mandibular fractures showed healing without sequestrum formation.[46] It is

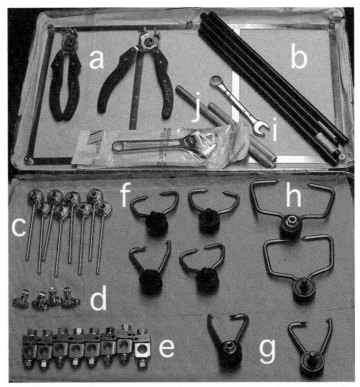

Fig. 14. Photograph of the OA pinless external fixator surgical set (Synthes): a, removable clip handles; b, carbon fiber rods; c, fixation posts; d, small clamps; e, adjustable AO clamps; f, small symmetric clips; g, asymmetric clips; h, large symmetric clips; i, wrench; and j, brass rods. (*Courtesy of* Manfred Stoll, DVM, Bleidenstadter Weg 7, 65329 Hohenstein, Germany.)

suggested that this may be due to improved fracture stabilization; thus, combining the AO pinless external fixator with interdental wiring may be advantageous.[47,54]

Surgical Technique

Preoperative planning

Anamnesis should include when the animal was last noted to be asymptomatic, changes in eating habits, and current tetanus vaccination status. Record the stimulus for seeking veterinary attention—the iatropic stimulus. The general health status of the animal should be determined through a physical examination with attention to CN abnormalities, facial asymmetry, and presence of discharges (nasal, ocular, and wound). Determination of the mandibular fracture, both clinically and radiographically, is important. An oral examination should be performed with the animal sedated. Avoid the use of a full-mouth speculum or device that could potentially further displace the fracture. Some clinicians may be able to palpate the oral cavity without a speculum but this carries considerable risk for clinicians. Oroscopy may be useful in determining involvement of oral soft tissues, presence of fractured clinical crowns, and malocclusion. A thorough extraoral examination may help determine if a fracture is displaced (although associated swelling may make the technique unreliable) and should include palpation of the temporomandibular joint. An uncommon differential for malocclusion in the horse is luxation of the temporomandibular joint.[60,61] Pain relief and antibiotics should be considered.

Characterization of the fracture is usually best determined using CT with subsequent computerized 3-dimensional modeling. CT machines designed to accommodate a standing equid are increasingly popular in Europe and the United States. Standard radiographic views of the head complemented with additional views specific to the location are recommended. A minimum of 2 radiographic views with perpendicular projections is required for fracture characterization. Determining dental involvement can be challenging.

Standard fracture assessment applies, such as determining whether the fracture is displaced or nondisplaced, simple or comminuted, closed or open, and favorable or nonfavorable along with the fracture pattern. Specific to the head, the degree of dental and alveolar involvement and the presence of malocclusion are important. Ultrasonography may be useful in determining displacements of the mandible, which are concealed by the associated swelling. The degree of morbidity associated with the fracture should also be assessed.

If fixation is necessary, appropriate equipment and skills are required. Potential patients need to be good candidates for a standing surgical procedure. If a procedure is not successful, an alternative plan needs to be prepared, which may involve general anesthesia. Adequate fracture reduction may be difficult to achieve in some cases without general anesthesia.

The repair is planned using information gained from the clinical examination and diagnostic imaging modalities. With a fracture of the body of the mandible, the dorsal aspect of the mandible is under tension while the ventral aspect experiences compression. Ideally, neutralization of the tension side of the fracture is sought, but doing this without damaging the teeth may be difficult. Interdental wiring and intraoral splinting have been used successfully to counteract such forces. Stabilization of the fracture using AO pinless external fixation is limited to the compression side of the fracture and, therefore, less than ideal. A minimum of 2 and preferably 3 clips should be positioned on either side of the fracture line. If the fractured mandible is still unstable, fixation to the other mandible may be necessary. Clips may be positioned to encompass both mandibles where the symphysis is formed.

Initially, all teeth involved in the fracture line should remain in place unless they are markedly mobile.[52] Once a mandibular fracture has healed, further assessment and treatment of the teeth are required. Occlusal forces on the affected teeth should be reduced by occlusal odontoplasty to reduce the clinical crown height of the teeth and/or their opposing number by 1 to 2 mm. A similar procedure should be considered for the incisor teeth on the affected mandible and/or the opposing maxillary incisor teeth.

Patient preparation and positioning

The standing procedure should be performed in a dedicated area free of potential distractions. There should be adequate room, good flooring, drainage, and lighting. Patients are placed in well-designed stocks and the head supported with a sling placed in the maxillary physiologic interdental space (**Fig. 15**).

The bifurcated ends and trocar tips of the clips should be examined for signs of damage. The AO pinless external fixator is intended for single use in humans. Repeated use has been documented, however, without implant failure.[62] Some clips have been used consecutively in cattle up to 7 times while still useable.[59] Due to the inability to sharpen the trocars while maintaining their working length, thus increasing the risk of clip loosening, the clips are recommended to be used no more than 3 times in equids.[54]

Intravenous access is aseptically gained and maintained. Intravenous antibiotics and antiinflammatory medication is administered. Sedation is provided and monitored as described in the article by Vigani and Garcia elsewhere in this issue.

Open fractures should be copiously lavaged with a 0.05% to 0.12% chlorhexidine solution until all gross contamination is removed. The area of the mandible (or mandibles) in which clips are to be positioned is clipped and surgically prepared. Inferior

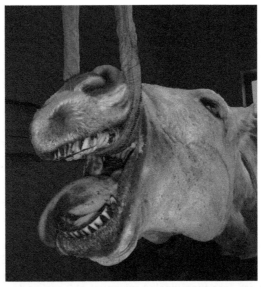

Fig. 15. Photograph of a horse with a fractured mandible illustrating suspension of the head with a sling, the ventrally displaced rostral mandible, and a surgical clip in preparation for fracture reduction and fixation performed under standing sedation. (*Courtesy of* Manfred Stoll, DVM, Bleidenstadter Weg 7, 65329 Hohenstein, Germany.)

alveolar nerve blocks are administered using local anesthetic agents. Local anesthetic agent is infiltrated subcutaneously and intramuscularly at the sites of clip penetration.

Surgical Approach

The main anatomic features that a surgeon needs to avoid when placing the clips are the facial artery and vein and parotid duct, which course along the rostral edge of the masseter muscle; branches of the facial nerve; the hypoglossal neurovascular bundle medially; and the neurovascular bundle, which exits the mental foramen rostrally.

In some cases, interdental wiring is combined with external fixation. The wiring procedure should be performed using instruments and techniques described in the previous minimally invasive buccotomy section to aid in accurate atraumatic wire placement between the clinical crowns of the cheek teeth. Wires should be placed before but not tightened until after the external fixation is complete.

The AO pinless external fixator is positioned on the ventral aspect of the fractured mandible (**Fig. 16**). Hypodermic needles (20 gauge) are placed at the proposed sites for clip placement and the position checked radiographically. The clips are positioned approximately 5 cm rostral and caudal to the fracture line, the most rostral clip involves the symphysis, the remaining clips are distributed along the length of the mandible.[54,59] A large clip is required to span the mandible at the level of the symphysis; either asymmetric or symmetric small clips are used along the remainder of the mandible.

Surgical Procedure

The technique is obtained from 3 sources.[54,55,59]

A stab incision is made in the transverse plane through the skin down to the periosteum using a #11 or #15 scalpel blade at the position of insertion of the working ends of the clips. Avoid arteries, veins, nerves, and ducts.

- The hinge nut on the clip is loosened with a wrench.
- The handle is applied to the clip and the knob tightened.
- Each clip is positioned by inserting the trocar ends through the skin incisions to contact the periosteum.
- The clips are gently squeezed while rocking the handle back and forth to drill the trocars into the cortical bone approximately 3 mm.
- The hinge nut is tightened with a wrench while maintaining the pressure of the trocars on the bone.

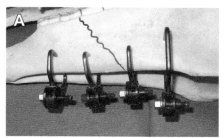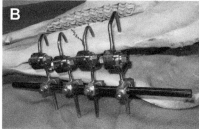

Fig. 16. (*A*) Photograph of the AO pinless external fixator clips applied to a simulated mandibular body fracture in an equid skull. (*B*) Photograph of the AO pinless external fixator applied to a simulated mandibular body fracture in an equid skull. (*Courtesy of* Manfred Stoll, DVM, Bleidenstadter Weg 7, 65329 Hohenstein, Germany.)

- The grab test is performed to check whether the working ends of the clips have penetrated the cortices sufficiently to provide stable fixation. If so, the handle is then removed.
- Once all clips are positioned in this manner, the fixation posts are loosely attached to each clip.
- The graphite rod is inserted through each fixation post to connect them all together.
- The fracture is reduced.
- All the nuts in the assemblage are tightened.
- The fracture reduction is checked by palpation, assessment of occlusion, and radiographically.
- If the alignment of the mandible is unsatisfactory, loosen all but the hinge nuts, repeat reduction, and tighten nuts again. Fracture reduction is again checked in the same manner.
- If intraoral wire fixation is used to aid support to the external fixation, the wires should be tightened after proper fracture alignment and fixator tightening.

Immediate Postoperative Care

- Skin incisions are dressed with an antibiotic ointment.
- The AO pinless external fixator apparatus is wrapped in a bandage or covered in rubber tubing to reduce the risk of damage caused to the fixation device, the animal, or personnel (**Fig. 17**).

Rehabilitation and Recovery

- Skin incisions are cleaned and dressed once or twice daily with antibiotic ointment. Open oral wounds are lavaged after each meal.
- Systemic antibiotics are continued for 5–7 days.
- The stable environment is modified to reduce the risk of the AO pinless external fixator being caught on protruding objects. Feed troughs are removed and automatic watering devices covered. The equids are fed from a large bowl and water is provided in a large bucket.

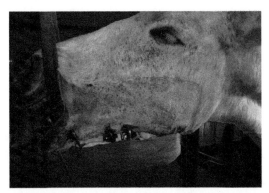

Fig. 17. A postoperative photograph of a horse that had fractured the body of both mandibles. Under standing sedation the fractures were reduced and stabilized using bilateral interdental wiring and an AO pinless external fixator that incorporated both mandibles. The horse's head was supported using a sling placed in the maxillary interdental space. The AO pinless external fixator was padded and bandaged after its placement. (*Courtesy of* Manfred Stoll, DVM, Bleidenstadter Weg 7, 65329 Hohenstein, Germany.)

- Unrestricted access to hay is provided and supplemented with bran mash and soaked pellets.
- Equids are stall confined and hand walked using a head collar. They are not permitted to exercise freely with the fixator in place.
- Fracture healing is assessed radiographically prior to removal of the AO pinless external fixator.
- The AO pinless external fixator is removed under sedation after approximately 6 weeks.
- The skin incisions are bathed daily and dressed with antibiotic ointment until healing has progressed.

Clinical Results in the Literature

Clinical results in the literature are limited to 1 study of unilateral mandibular fractures in equids in which the procedure was performed under general anesthesia.[54] Anecdotal success has been reported when the procedure was performed for unilateral and bilateral mandibular fractures in standing sedated equids, with clip loosening the major complication.[55]

Summary

The AO pinless external fixator applied in the standing sedated equid provides a good option for repair of unstable or misaligned unilateral and some bilateral mandibular fractures. Fracture stability may be improved with concurrent interdental wiring and cross-fixation between both mandibles. A closed reduction technique and lack of implant against an open-type fracture may promote improved healing. Complications are common but manageable. Importantly, the risks of inadvertently involving dental structures in the repair technique, and those risks inherent with general anesthesia are avoided.

ACKNOWLEDGMENTS

The authors would like to thank Torbjörn Lundström, DDS (Sweden), Manfred Stoll, DVM (Germany), and Frank Schellenberger, DVM (Germany) for their assistance in preparing this article.

REFERENCES

1. Ford TS. Standing surgery and procedures of the head. Vet Clin North Am Equine Pract 1991;7(3):583–602.
2. Menzies R. Oral examination and charting: setting the basis for evidence-based medicine in the oral examination of equids. Vet Clin North Am Equine Pract 2013;29(2):325–43.
3. Menzies RA, Lewis JR, Reiter AM, et al. Essential considerations for equine oral examination, diagnosis, and treatment. J Vet Dent 2011;28(3):204–9.
4. Rawlinson J, Earley E. Advances in the treatment of diseased incisor and canine teeth. Vet Clin North Am Equine Pract 2013;29(2):411–40.
5. Tremaine WH. Advances in the treatment of diseased equine cheek teeth. Vet Clin North Am Equine Pract 2013;29(2):441–65.
6. Easley J, Schumacher J. Basic equine orthodontics and maxillofacial surgery. In: Easley J, Dixon PM, Schumacher J, editors. Equine dentistry. Edinburgh (United Kingdom): Elsevier; 2011. p. 289–317.
7. Wafa N. A study of dental disease in the horse, in Faculty of Veterinary Medicine. Dublin (Ireland): National University of Ireland; 1988. p. 215.

8. Taylor L, Dixon PM. Equine idiopathic cheek teeth fractures: part 2: a practice-based survey of 147 affected horses in Britain and Ireland. Equine Vet J 2007; 39(4):322–6.

9. Baker GJ. A study of dental disease in the horse, in Department of Veterinary Surgery. Glasgow (Scotland): University of Glasgow; 1979. p. 181.

10. Dixon PM, Tremaine WH, Pickles K, et al. Equine dental disease part 4: a long-term study of 400 cases: apical infections of cheek teeth. Equine Vet J 2000; 32(3):182–94.

11. Dixon PM, Dacre I. A review of equine dental disorders. Vet J 2005;169:165–87.

12. Dixon PM, Hawkes C, Townsend N. Complications of equine oral surgery. Vet Clin North Am Equine Pract 2008;24(3):499–514.

13. du Toit N, Burden FA, Dixon PM. Clinical dental findings in 203 working donkeys in Mexico. Vet J 2008;178(3):380–6.

14. du Toit N, Burden FA, Dixon PM. Clinical dental examinations of 357 donkeys in the UK. Part 1: prevalence of dental disorders. Equine Vet J 2009;41(4):390–4.

15. du Toit N, Gallagher J, Burden FA, et al. Post mortem survey of dental disorders in 349 donkeys from an aged population (2005-2006). Part 1: prevalence of specific dental disorders. Equine Vet J 2008;40(3):204–8.

16. Dixon PM, Dacre I, Dacre K, et al. Standing oral extraction of cheek teeth in 100 horses (1998-2003). Equine Vet J 2005;37(2):105–12.

17. Dixon PM, Parkin TD, Collins N, et al. Equine paranasal sinus disease: a long-term study of 200 cases (1997-2009): treatments and long-term results of treatments. Equine Vet J 2012;44(3):272–6.

18. Tremaine WH, Dixon PM. A long-term study of 277 cases of equine sinonasal disease. Part 2: treatments and results of treatments. Equine Vet J 2001;33(3): 283–9.

19. Townsend NB, Dixon PM, Barakzai SZ. Evaluation of the long-term oral consequences of equine exodontia in 50 horses. Vet J 2008;178(3):419–24.

20. Dixon PM, Barakzai SZ, Collins NM, et al. Equine idiopathic cheek teeth fractures: part 3: a hospital-based survey of 68 referred horses (1999-2005). Equine Vet J 2007;39(4):327–32.

21. Casey MB, Tremaine WH. The prevalence of secondary dentinal lesions in cheek teeth from horses with clinical signs of pulpitis compared to controls. Equine Vet J 2010;42(1):30–6.

22. Menzies RA, Lundström TS, Lewis JR, et al. Diagnostic imaging in veterinary dental practice. J Am Vet Med Assoc 2012;240(4):379–81.

23. Menzies RA, Lundström TS, Reiter AM, et al. Diagnostic imaging in veterinary dental practice. J Am Vet Med Assoc 2012;240(8):949–51.

24. van den Enden MS, Dixon PM. Prevalence of occlusal pulpar exposure in 110 equine cheek teeth with apical infections and idiopathic fractures. Vet J 2008; 178(3):364–71.

25. Dacre I, Kempsot S, Dixon PM. Equine idiopathic cheek teeth fractures. Part 1: pathological studies on 35 fractured cheek teeth. Equine Vet J 2007;39(4): 310–8.

26. Carmalt JL, Barber SM. Periapical curettage: an alternative surgical approach to infected mandibular cheek teeth in horses. Vet Surg 2004;33(3):267–71.

27. Simhofer H, Stoian C, Zetner K. A long-term study of apicoectomy and endodontic treatment of apically infected cheek teeth in 12 horses. Vet J 2008; 178(3):411–8.

28. van Foreest AW, Wiemer P. Veterinary dentistry (15). Apex resection in the horse. Tijdschr Diergeneeskd 1997;122(23):670–9 [in Dutch].

29. Lundström, T. Orthograde endodontic treatment of equine teeth with periapical disease - a long-term follow-up. In: Proceedings of the 51st British Equine Veterinary Association Congress. Birmingham, United Kingdom: BEVA. September 12–15, 2012.

30. Townsend NB, Hawkes CS, Rex R, et al. Investigation of the sensitivity and specificity of radiological signs for diagnosis of periapical infection of equine cheek teeth. Equine Vet J 2011;43(2):170–8.

31. Weller R, Livesey L, Maierl J, et al. Comparison of radiography and scintigraphy in the diagnosis of dental disorders in the horse. Equine Vet J 2001;33(1):49–58.

32. Archer DC, Boswell JC, Voute LC, et al. Skeletal scintigraphy in the horse: current indications and validity as a diagnostic test. Vet J 2007;173(1):31–44.

33. Windley Z, Weller R, Tremaine WH, et al. Two- and three-dimensional computed tomographic anatomy of the enamel, infundibulae and pulp of 126 equine cheek teeth. Part 1: findings in teeth without macroscopic occlusal or computed tomographic lesions. Equine Vet J 2009;41(5):433–40.

34. Windley Z, Weller R, Tremaine WH, et al. Two- and three-dimensional computed tomographic anatomy of the enamel, infundibulae and pulp of 126 equine cheek teeth. Part 2: findings in teeth with macroscopic occlusal or computed tomographic lesions. Equine Vet J 2009;41(5):441–7.

35. Kirkland KD, Baker GJ, Manfra Marretta S, et al. Effects of aging on the endodontic system, reserve crown, and roots of equine mandibular cheek teeth. Am J Vet Res 1996;57(1):31–8.

36. Dacre IT, Kempson S, Dixon PM. Pathological studies of cheek teeth apical infections in the horse: 1. Normal endodontic anatomy and dentinal structure of equine cheek teeth. Vet J 2008;178(3):311–20.

37. Kopke S, Angrisani N, Staszyk C. The dental cavities of equine cheek teeth: three-dimensional reconstructions based on high resolution micro-computed tomography. BMC Vet Res 2012;8(173):1–16.

38. Love DN, Rose RJ, Martin CA, et al. Serum concentrations of penicillin in the horse after administration of a variety of penicillin preparations. Equine Vet J 1983;15(1):43–8.

39. Orsini PG, Ross MW, Hamir AN. Levator nasolabialis muscle transposition to prevent an orosinus fistula after tooth extraction in horses. Vet Surg 1992; 21(2):150–6.

40. Prichard MA, Hackett RP, Erb HN. Long-term outcome of tooth repulsion in horses. A retrospective study of 61 cases. Vet Surg 1992;21(2):145–9.

41. Stoll M. Minimally invasive transbuccal surgery and screw extraction. In: Proceedings of the 22nd European Congress of Veterinary Dentistry and the 12th World Veterinary Dental Congress. Prague, Czech Republic: EVDS. May 23–26, 2013.

42. Stoll M. How to perform a buccal approach for different dental procedures. In: Proceedings, 53rd Annual AAEP Convention. Orlando, Florida: AAEP. December 1–5, 2007.

43. Staszyk C, Bienert A, Bäumer W, et al. Simulation of local anaesthetic nerve block of the infraorbital nerve within the pterygopalatine fossa: anatomical landmarks defined by computed tomography. Res Vet Sci 2008;85(3):399–406.

44. Stoll M. Minimalinvasive Bukkotomie mit bukkaler Schraubextraktion nach Stoll. In: Vogt C, editor. Lehrbuch der Zahnheilkunde beim Pferd. Stuttgart (Germany): Schattauer; 2011. p. 208–13.

45. Belsito KA, Fischer AT. External skeletal fixation in the management of equine mandibular fractures: 16 cases (1988-1998). Equine Vet J 2001;33(2):176–83.

46. Kuemmerle JM, Kummer M, Auer JA, et al. Locking compression plate osteosynthesis of complicated mandibular fractures in six horses. Vet Comp Orthop Traumatol 2009;22(1):54–8.

47. Peavey CL, Edwards III RB, Escarcega AJ, et al. Fixation technique influences the monotonic properties of equine mandibular fracture constructs. Vet Surg 2003;32(4):350–8.

48. Murch KM. Repair of bovine and equine mandibular fractures. Can Vet J 1980; 21(3):69–73.

49. Little CB, Hilbert BJ, McGill CA. A retrospective study of head fractures in 21 horses. Aust Vet J 1985;62(3):89–91.

50. Beard W. Fracture repair techniques for the equine mandible and maxilla. Equine Vet Educ 2009;21(7):352–7.

51. Caldwell FJ, Davis HA. Surgical reconstruction of a severely comminuted mandibular fracture in a horse. Equine Vet Educ 2012;24(5):217–21.

52. Tremaine WH. Management of equine mandibular injuries. Equine Vet Educ 1998;10(3):146–54.

53. Auer JA, Watkins JP. Instrumentation and techniques in equine fracture fixation. Vet Clin North Am Equine Pract 1996;12(2):283–302.

54. Haralambus RM, Werren C, Brehm W, et al. Use of a pinless external fixator for unilateral mandibular fracture repair in nine equids. Vet Surg 2010;39(6):761–4.

55. Stoll M. How to stabilize mandibular fractures with pinless external fixation. In: Proceedings of the 22nd European Congress of Veterinary Dentistry and the 12th World Veterinary Dental Congress. Prague, Czech Republic: EVDS. May 23–26, 2013.

56. Stene GM, et al. Biomechanical evaluation of the Pinless external fixator. Injury 1992;23(Suppl 3):S9–27.

57. Remiger AR, Magerl F. The pinless external fixator–relevance of experimental results in clinical applications. Injury 1994;25(Suppl 3). p. S-C15–29.

58. Lischer CJ, Fluri E, Auer JA. Stabilisation of a mandibular fracture in a cow by means of a pinless external fixator. Vet Rec 1997;140(9):226–9.

59. Lischer CJ, Fluri E, Kaser-Hotz B, et al. Pinless external fixation of mandible fractures in cattle. Vet Surg 1997;26(1):14–9.

60. Devine DV, Moll HD, Bahr RJ. Fracture, luxation, and chronic septic arthritis of the temporomandibular joint in a juvenile horse. J Vet Dent 2005;22(2):96–9.

61. Hurtig MB, Barber SM, Farrow CS. Temporomandibular joint luxation in a horse. J Am Vet Med Assoc 1984;185(1):78–80.

62. Schutz M, Buhler M, Swiontkowski M, et al. Documentation. Injury 1994; 25(Suppl 3). p. S-C34–7.

63. Du Toit N, Kempson SA, Dixon PM. Donkey dental anatomy. Part 1: gross and computed axial tomography examinations. Vet J 2008;176(3):338–44.

Standing Ophthalmic Surgeries in Horses

Michala de Linde Henriksen, DVM, PhD[a],*,
Dennis E. Brooks, DVM, PhD, DACVO[b]

KEYWORDS

- Standing surgery • Ophthalmology • Horse • Eye

KEY POINTS

- Ophthalmic procedures are performed on very delicate, sensitive, and thin ocular tissues, such that one wrong movement by the horse or surgeon could cause catastrophic problems resulting in blindness and/or loss of the globe.
- Ophthalmic nerve blocks should be performed when ophthalmic procedures are being performed on the standing sedated horse.
- Surgical eyelid procedures that can be performed on standing sedated horses include entropion in the foal, traumatic eyelid laceration repair, and biopsy/therapy for eyelid neoplasia.
- A corneal biopsy or superficial keratectomy can be performed on the standing sedated horse and should be performed when cytology is inconclusive and a superficial corneal disease is present.
- An exenteration refers to the removal of the globe and as much of the ocular contents as possible – this surgical procedure is a little more challenging than an enucleation on a standing horse but can still be performed.

INTRODUCTION

Standing surgery in horses is gaining popularity among horse owners and veterinarians, primarily because of elimination of the risks and costs of general anesthesia. More types of standing ophthalmic procedures and surgeries in the horse have therefore been attempted and described in recent years. Disadvantages of performing standing ophthalmic surgeries in the horse include the increased risk of causing tissue damage arising from the inability to eliminate eye and head movements, which preclude one's proficiency in using an operating microscope to complete the often

[a] Comparative Ophthalmology Service, Department of Veterinary Clinical Sciences, College of Veterinary Medicine, University of Minnesota, 1352 Boyd Avenue, Saint Paul, MN 55108, USA; [b] Comparative Ophthalmology Service, Departments of Large and Small Animal Clinical Sciences, College of Veterinary Medicine, University of Florida, 2015 Southeast 16th Avenue, Gainesville, FL 32608, USA
* Corresponding author.
E-mail address: mhenriks@umn.edu

Vet Clin Equine 30 (2014) 91–110
http://dx.doi.org/10.1016/j.cveq.2013.11.012
0749-0739/14/$ – see front matter © 2014 Elsevier Inc. All rights reserved.

precise surgeries. Ophthalmic procedures are performed on very delicate, sensitive, and thin ocular tissues, such that one wrong movement by the horse or surgeon could cause catastrophic problems resulting in blindness and/or loss of the globe. Local anesthesia, heavy sedation, nose twitches, and orbital and local nerve blocks of the involved motor and sensory nerves are therefore essential in achieving a good outcome after a standing equine ophthalmic procedure or surgery. Most of these standing ocular procedures in horses should not be attempted by inexperienced surgeons. **Table 1** gives an overview of the ophthalmic procedures and surgeries that can be performed on a standing sedated horse.

ANALGESIA AND BLOCKS

Tetracaine and proparacaine are the 2 topical anesthetics that have most commonly been investigated for their ability to perform anesthesia of the equine cornea.[1–3] These agents are used to locally desensitize the conjunctiva and cornea when procedures are performed in these tissues.[4] It has been shown that 0.5% tetracaine and 0.5% proparacaine will have their maximal effect in horses after 5 to 10 minutes, and the effective duration will be 20 to 30 minutes.[1–3] It has also been shown that whereas proparacaine does not have a complete anesthetic effect on the equine cornea, tetracaine does achieve complete anesthesia.[1,3] Topical tetracaine is therefore a better topical anesthetic for standing equine ophthalmic procedures. A recent study by Pucket and colleagues[5] looked at the duration and efficacy of 4 different topical anesthetics on corneal sensitivity; 0.5% proparacaine hydrochloride, 0.5% bupivacaine hydrochloride, 2% lidocaine hydrochloride, and 2% mepivacaine hydrochloride solutions. The study concluded that 0.5% proparacaine and 2% lidocaine solutions induce an adequate level of short-duration corneal anesthesia (respectively 35 minutes and 45 minutes for the 2 topical anesthetics), whereas the use of 0.5% bupivacaine solution showed usefulness for longer-duration corneal procedures, owing to the longer efficacy of this topical anesthetic (duration 60 minutes). The topical 2% mepivacaine solution never reached maximal anesthetic impact in the study, and was therefore the least effective topical anesthetic.[5] Application of the local anesthetic to the conjunctiva and cornea can be achieved with 0.5 to 1 mL of the topical anesthetic in a syringe with a 25-gauge needle. For safety and to make it easier to apply the anesthesia, the needle tip should be removed by bending the needle tip a couple of times to each side.

The nerve blocks used in veterinary ophthalmology for standing surgeries are normally performed with either 2% lidocaine for short procedures, or a half-and-half solution of 2% lidocaine and 2% mepivacaine (carbocaine) for procedures that take longer than 30 to 45 minutes, owing to the rapid effect of lidocaine and the longer-lasting effect of mepivacaine.[6] The auriculopalpebral nerve block is the most used nerve block for equine ophthalmic procedures.[4] This block is normally performed with 1 to 2 mL of 2% lidocaine, and blocks the motor branch of the facial nerve (cranial nerve nucleus [CNN] VII), which innervates the orbicularis oculi muscle of the upper and lower eyelids of the horse. The auriculopalpebral nerve block can be performed in 3 places in the horse. The lower portion of the facial nerve can be palpated over the zygomatic arch, where it is easiest to perform the block (point A in **Fig. 1**). The higher type of this block can be performed superior to the zygomatic arch and inferior to the ear cartilage (point B in **Fig. 1**). This type of auriculopalpebral nerve block reduces the activity of most branches of the facial nerve and will therefore be more effective than blocking the lower portion. Lastly, auriculopalpebral nerve block can be performed at the base of the ear (points C and D in **Fig. 1**). This location for

Table 1
Standing surgical procedures that are possible to perform in a sedated horse in equine practice

Eyelid	Third Eyelid	Conjunctiva	Cornea	Anterior Chamber	Vitreous	General
Entropion, temporary tacking (foals)	Third eyelid laceration, repair	Conjunctival biopsy	Cytology sample	Aqueous paracentesis	Intravitreal injection	Enucleation with orbital nerve block
Eyelid laceration, repair	Third eyelid removal	Conjunctival mass removal	Corneal biopsy	Intracameral injection		Exenteration with orbital block
Eyelid mass, removal			Corneal laceration repair			
Temporary Tarsorrhaphy			Superficial keratectomy			
			AMT placement with tissue glue			

Abbreviation: AMT, amniotic membrane transplant.
Data modified from Gelatt KN. Surgical instruments. In: Gelatt KN, Gelatt JP, editors. Veterinary ophthalmic surgery. 2nd edition. Elsevier Saunders; 2011. p. 1–15; and Provost PJ. Surgical instruments. In: Auer JA, Stick JA, editors. Equine surgery. 2nd edition. WB Saunders Company; 1999. p. 71–84.

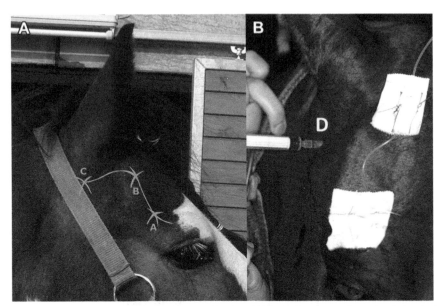

Fig. 1. (*A, B*) The auriculopalpebral nerve block will block the motor branch of the facial nerve (cranial nerve VII), and the block can be performed in 3 places. A: the lower portion, over the zygomatic arch; B: the higher portion of the block, superior to the zygomatic arch and inferior to the ear cartilage; C and D: the base of the ear.

achieving akinesia of the orbicularis oculi muscle can be used when head movement from face or eye pain is such that the horse does not allow the other blocks to be performed. Other nerve blocks useful for standing ophthalmic surgeries on horses are those that block the sensory stimulation to the upper and lower eyelids innervated by the trigeminal nerve (CNN V). These blocks include the supraorbital nerve block (frontal nerve branch of CNN V) that innervates the central aspect of the upper eyelid, the lacrimal nerve block (ophthalmic branch of CNN V) that innervates the medial aspect of the upper eyelid, the infratrochlear nerve block (ophthalmic branch of CNN V) that innervates the medial canthus, and the zygomatic nerve block (maxillary branch of CNN V) that innervates most of the lower eyelid.[4] **Fig. 2** shows the areas where the sensory nerves should be blocked to cause denervation of the nerves. The blocks can be performed by injection with 1 to 2 mL of the local anesthetic as a line block in the area of the nerve.

A retrobulbar nerve block (RBNB) should be performed when the globe has to be immobilized. The RBNB will temporarily block the extraocular muscle innervation by blocking the oculomotor nerve (CNN III), the abducens nerve (CNN VI), and the trochlear nerve (CNN IV). An RBNB will also cause temporary blindness by blocking the function of the optic nerve (CNN II), as well as temporarily blocking the sensation of the medial cornea by affecting the function of the maxillary and ophthalmic branches of the trigeminal nerve (CNN V). The skin area near the block should be clipped if possible and aseptically prepped with 5% betadine solution (one must never use alcohol solutions close to the eye). The RBNB is performed by injecting 10 to 12 mL of lidocaine into the retrobulbar space. A 22-gauge, 9-cm spinal needle is placed into the supraorbital fossa just posterior to the posterior aspect of the dorsal orbital rim.[4] A 4-point block will cause akinesia of the extraocular muscles. A curved 20-gauge, 9-cm spinal needle can be used for the 4-point block (**Fig. 3**).[7]

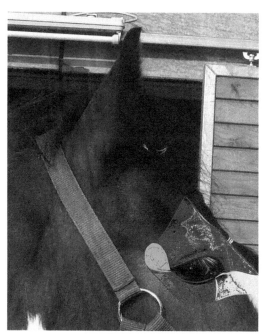

Fig. 2. The supraorbital nerve block (*pink*) will block the sensation to the central aspect of the upper eyelid. The lacrimal nerve block (*yellow*) will block the sensation to the medial aspect of the eyelids. The infratrochlear nerve block (*green*) will block the sensation to the lateral aspect of the eyelids. The zygomatic nerve block (*blue*) will block the sensation to the lower eyelid.

The conjunctiva and cornea should also be aseptically prepped and a local anesthetic administered to the conjunctiva and cornea. The 4-point block can be performed by injecting 5 mL anesthetic solution at the 12 o'clock, 2 or 4 o'clock, 6 o'clock, and 8 or 10 o'clock positions of the globe through the conjunctiva; the 3 and 9 o'clock

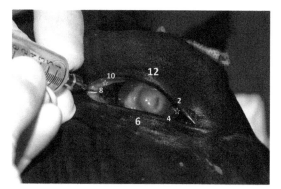

Fig. 3. The 4-point block can be performed by injecting 5 mL of anesthetic solution in the retrobulbar space with a curved spinal needle. The places for injection should be 12 o'clock, 2 or 4 o'clock, 6 o'clock, and 8 or 10 o'clock (3 and 9 o'clock [*green stars*] should be avoided because of the proximity of blood supply to the eye).

positions are not used owing to the proximity of the major blood vessels (long posterior ciliary arteries). This 4-point block is easier to perform than the retrobulbar nerve block, but will only block the extraocular muscles and will cause more tissue damage and swelling. This block is therefore only recommended for enucleation or exenteration.

SURGICAL INSTRUMENTS USED FOR OPHTHALMIC SURGERIES ON STANDING HORSES

Table 2 gives an overview of surgical instruments and sutures recommended for ophthalmic procedures performed on a standing sedated horse. The skin near the surgical area should be clipped if possible, and be aseptically prepared with a 5% betadine solution, which can be used on the periocular skin, the conjunctiva, and cornea. No alcohol or surgical scrub solutions should be used close to the eye.

EYELID

Surgical eyelid procedures that can be performed on standing sedated horses include entropion in the foal, traumatic eyelid laceration repair, and therapy for eyelid neoplasia. Entropion in foals should be treated with temporary tacking so that the eyelid margin and its eyelashes are not touching the cornea. This procedure reduces ocular discomfort and decreases the risk of developing corneal ulcers.[8] The temporary tacking procedure can be performed on a sedated foal with entropion when a sensory nerve-line block has been performed to the area of the eyelid that needs to be tacked. Nonabsorbable 4-0 to 5-0 monofilament sutures are recommended (**Fig. 4**). Vertical mattress sutures are placed along the eyelid beginning 1 to 2 cm away from the eyelid margin. The first suture is placed in the central aspect of the eyelid[8,9] with the next 2 sutures placed on each side of the central suture. In many foals, 3 to 5 sutures are enough to roll out the eyelid margin from the cornea.[10] The knots should be secured with 4 throws; the suture tag nearest the cornea should be cut short and the suture tag away from the cornea should be cut long, such that no suture touches the cornea. Leaving a long suture end will help in removing the suture later. The sutures will normally stay in place for 2 to 4 weeks.[10]

Traumatic eyelid lacerations should be sutured without removing any lid tissue if possible.[8,9] Traumatic eyelid lacerations can generally be sutured on a standing sedated horse. The area should be clipped and aseptically prepared for surgery, and a nerve block of the involved sensory nerve, an auriculopalpebral nerve block, and local topical anesthesia performed.[8,9] The edges of the lid laceration should be gently debrided with a #15 scalpel blade so that fresh vascularization can increase the healing process. The laceration should be repaired in 2 layers with the surgery divided into 3 steps. The first step is to reposition the lacerated margins back together, using a figure-of-8 suture pattern with nonabsorbable 4-0 to 5-0 monofilament suture with a P3 needle (small needle). The second step should be closure of the deeper layer of the lid laceration with an absorbable 3-0 to 4-0 suture as either a single interrupted or simple continuous suture pattern. No suture should penetrate the conjunctiva on the ocular surface because suture material rubbing against the cornea will cause corneal ulcers. The third and last step should be closing the skin with a simple interrupted suture pattern (**Fig. 5**).[8,9] A hard cup hood should be placed on the horse to avoid any rubbing of the suture site. The horse should be treated with an antibiotic ointment to the cornea and on the suture incision 3 to 4 times a day until sutures have been removed. Systemically administered nonsteroidal anti-inflammatory drugs (NSAIDs) can be used for 5 days in addition to systemically administered antibiotics. The sutures should stay in place for 14 days, and the owner should monitor the horse for any signs of blepharospasm or epiphora in case

Table 2		
Surgical instruments and sutures used for standing ophthalmology surgeries in horses		
Eyelid/Third Eyelid Surgery	**Conjunctival/Corneal Surgery**	**Enucleation/Exenteration**
Bishop-Harmon forceps	Eyelid speculum for equine	Adson tissue forceps (with
Adson tissue forceps (rat	Caliper	teeth)
tooth)	Bishop-Harmon forceps	Adson tissue forceps (tooth
Adson tissue forceps (tooth	0.12-mm and 0.3-mm tying	smooth)
smooth)	tooth microforceps	Small hemostat
Small and medium-sized	Stevens tenotomy scissors	Medium-/large-sized
curved Mayo/	(curved/straight)	curved Mayo/
Metzenbaum scissors	Small needle holder	Metzenbaum scissors
Stevens tenotomy scissors	Castroviejo needle holder	Curved vessel pattern
(curved/straight)	Beaver scalpel handle for a	clamp
Large curved hemostat	#64 beaver blade	Standard needle holder
Allis forceps	Skin biopsy trephines in	(Castroviejo/Barraquer)
Standard needle holder	different sizes (3–6 mm)	Blade scalpel handle for a
(Castroviejo/Barraquer)	Tissue-adhesive glue	#15 blade
Blade scalpel handle for a	(cyanoacrylate tissue	Spratt curettes
#15 blade	glue)	Periosteum elevator
4-0 or 5-0 nonabsorbable	Hair dryer	3-0 nonabsorbable
monofilament suture	7-0 absorbable suture	monofilament suture
material (nylon)	(Vicryl)	material (nylon)
3-0 or 4-0 absorbable suture		2-0 absorbable suture
(Vicryl)		(Vicryl)

Data modified from Gelatt KN. Surgical instruments. In: Gelatt KN, Gelatt JP, editors. Veterinary ophthalmic surgery. 2nd edition. Elsevier Saunders; 2011.p. 1–15; and Provost PJ. Surgical instruments. In: Auer JA, Stick JA, editors. Equine surgery. 2nd edition. WB Saunders Company; 1999. p. 71–84.

the sutures should cause corneal ulcers. A tetanus shot is recommended in cases of an unknown tetanus vaccination status.

Removal of small eyelid masses such as melanomas or squamous cell carcinomas (SCC) can be performed on a standing horse. Eyelid masses under one-third of the eyelid margin length can be removed with either a simple wedge or 4-sided ("house") technique.[9] The more sophisticated and challenging blepharoplastic surgical procedures that are used when more than two-thirds of the eyelid has to be removed should be done with the horse under general anesthesia, owing to the need for undermining and removal of facial skin in a larger area.[11]

A temporary tarsorrhaphy can be placed in a standing sedated horse (**Fig. 6**). This procedure is used to prevent blinking of the eyelids over an indolent corneal ulcer, or to apply lid pressure to a fragile thin cornea or cornea that has received a corneal transplant or conjunctival or amnion graft. A temporary tarsorrhaphy can also be placed in horses with facial nerve paralysis whereby the horse is not able to blink and the corneal surface dries out, leading to corneal ulcers caused by exposure keratitis.[8,9] An auriculopalpebral nerve block together with a sensory nerve block along the superior and inferior eyelid margins is used. The eyelashes can be cut off with Metzenbaum scissors, and the eyelid and conjunctiva aseptically prepped for surgery with 5% betadine solution. Topical anesthesia should also be administered. The temporary tarsorrhaphy can be performed with nonabsorbable 4-0 monofilament (nylon) sutures. The suture pattern used is a horizontal mattress pattern with the starting point for the initial needle skin entry 2 to 4 mm from the superior eyelid margin (A in **Fig. 6**A), exiting by the eyelid-margin meibomian glands (B in **Fig. 6**A), crossing over to the inferior eyelid margin

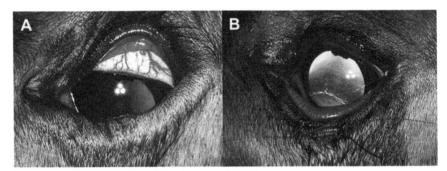

Fig. 4. (*A*) Entropion in foals should be treated with temporary tacking sutures. (*B*) The tacking sutures are placed as vertical mattress sutures with a 4-0 to 5-0 monofilament suture.

where the needle enters at the meibomian glands (C in **Fig. 6**A), then exiting the skin 2 to 4 mm from the eyelid margin (D in **Fig. 6**A). Pieces of rubber bands or catheter tubes can be used as stents to minimize suture irritation to the skin (**Fig. 6**B). One end of the superior rubber band needs to be placed on the suture before the mattress suture is started; both ends of the inferior rubber band will be placed on the suture when the suture comes through the inferior eyelid margin at the meibomian glands and exits 2 to 4 mm from the eyelid margin, and then again before it is placed back into the eyelid 2 to 4 mm from the eyelid margin and 2 to 4 mm away from the needle entry into the skin (E, F in **Fig. 6**A). The last end of the superior rubber band will go onto the suture when the suture goes back into the superior eyelid margin precisely at the meibomian glands (G in **Fig. 6**A) and exits 2 to 4 mm from the eyelid margin (H in **Fig. 6**A). A 3-throw surgeon's knot can be used, and the suture should be tight enough so that the suture material is not rubbing against the cornea thus potentially causing a corneal ulcer, but not too tight to cause necrosis of the eyelid margin.[8,9] The suture ends should be cut short so that no suture material can rub against the cornea.[10]

THIRD EYELID

Third-eyelid lacerations can be repaired on a standing sedated horse with local anesthesia and local sensory nerve blocks in the area of the third eyelid. The laceration can normally be closed in one layer, and it is important that the sutures are not penetrating

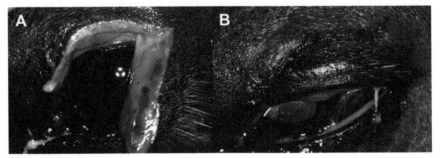

Fig. 5. (*A*) Eyelid lacerations should be sutured without removing any eyelid tissue. (*B*) The eyelid laceration should be closed in 2 layers with a figure-of-8 suture pattern at the eyelid margin.

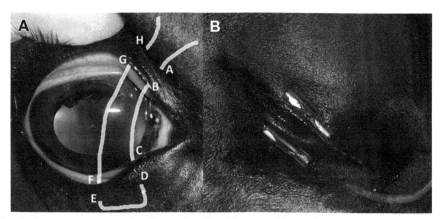

Fig. 6. A temporary tarsorrhaphy can be placed in a standing sedated horse. (*A*) A horizontal mattress suture pattern is placed with a 4-0 monofilament (nylon) suture. Letter A to H is described in the text. (*B*) Rubber bands or a 1- to 2-cm piece of a catheter tube can be used as stents.

the bulbar side of the third eyelid such that they are touching the cornea. The third eyelid margin should be closed with a figure-of-8 suture pattern.[12]

Resection of the third eyelid can be done in a standing sedated horse (**Fig. 7**). The procedure is most commonly performed in eyes with third-eyelid neoplasia such as SCC. A study by Labelle and colleagues[13] showed no significant differences in the outcome of third-eyelid resection performed in standing horses or those under general anesthesia. Aseptic preparation of the third eyelid, conjunctiva, and skin surrounding the medial aspect of the globe is first performed. Local anesthesia and local sensory nerve blocks in the area of and into the base of the third eyelid are initially performed. Allis tissue forceps are placed at each end of the third eyelid, and a large curved hemostat placed as close to the base of the third eyelid as possible (including the base of the cartilage). The hemostat stays in place for 60 to 90 seconds. The resection of the third eyelid occurs in the groove from the removed hemostat using curved Metzenbaum scissors or a #15 blade.[12] The third-eyelid cartilage has to be removed completely so that no cartilage edges can rub against the cornea and thus cause corneal ulcers. Prolapse of retrobulbar fat is a rare complication of resection of the third eyelid in horses.[8] In the authors' experience, this complication can be avoided by closing the conjunctival edge of the incision with absorbable 4-0 suture. The horse should have a hard cup hood placed after surgery; topical ophthalmic antibiotic ointment should be applied 3 times daily for 2 to 3 weeks, along with a systemically administered regimen of NSAIDs and antibiotic for 5 and 10 days, respectively. Discharge from the surgical site is a minor complication, and the owner should be advised on how to keep the periocular area clean with water or 5% betadine solution.[13]

CONJUNCTIVAL

Conjunctival biopsies or masses can be removed in a standing sedated horse. An auriculopalpebral nerve block is placed, and the conjunctiva is aseptically prepared with 5% betadine solution and topical anesthesia. The conjunctiva is grabbed with Bishop-Harmon forceps or Adson forceps, and Stevens tenotomy scissors or small Metzenbaum scissors are used to resect a piece of the conjunctiva for a biopsy sample or to remove a conjunctival mass (**Fig. 8**). A punch biopsy can also be used for the

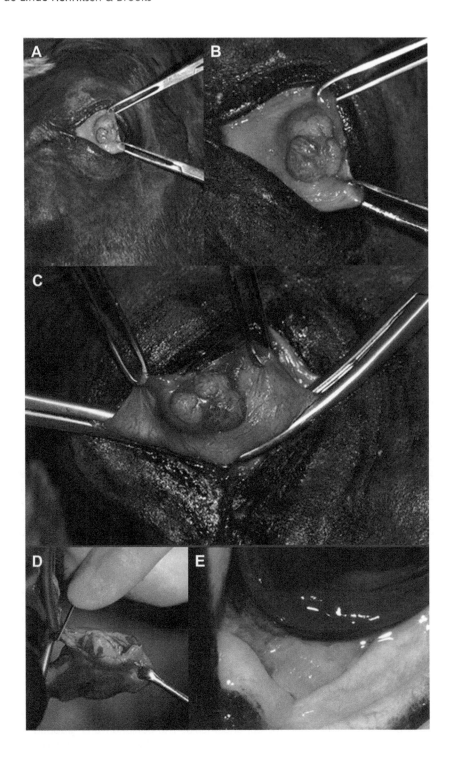

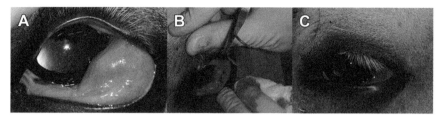

Fig. 8. Removal of a lower eyelid conjunctival mass. (*A*) The mass before surgery. (*B*) The mass has been removed and the conjunctiva left to heal by secondary-intention healing. (*C*) The conjunctiva was mildly swollen postoperatively. Medical treatment included systemic nonsteroidal anti-inflammatories (NSAIDs) and antibiotics, as well as topical antibiotics to the eye and, in the event of no contraindications, topical steroids or NSAIDs, in some cases a subpalpebral lavage system can be placed to make the medical treatment easier for the owner. The mass was sent to histopathology and was diagnosed as granulation tissue.

removal of a biopsy area.[12] The conjunctiva can be either left for primary healing or sutured with a simple continuous suture pattern using absorbable 4-0 or 5-0 suture material. It is important that sutures are not touching the cornea, and the simple continuous suture needs to be buried in the conjunctiva.

CORNEA

Surgeries performed on the equine cornea that require extensive corneal suturing are recommended to be performed under general anesthesia so that any unexpected globe or horse movements can be avoided. The authors would also recommend that the more delicate surgical procedures be performed by experienced microsurgeons. However, some surgical procedures can be attempted and accomplished in a standing sedated horse. Corneal cytology is used together with a corneal swab for microbiology to diagnose infectious corneal diseases as well as inflammatory and neoplastic changes in the cornea.[8] Corneal cytology can be obtained with an auriculopalpebral block and the cornea locally anesthetized. A cytobrush, a Kimura spatula, or the metallic back side of a #15 scalpel blade can be used to collect the corneal sample from a corneal lesion (**Fig. 9**).

A corneal biopsy or superficial keratectomy should be performed when cytology is inconclusive and a superficial corneal disease is present. A corneal biopsy and a superficial keratectomy can be performed when an auriculopalpebral block, supraorbital block, and local topical anesthesia have been used together with aseptic preparation of the cornea. A retrobulbar nerve block is also recommended to block the extraocular muscles so as to avoid movements of the globe. Corneal anesthetics reduce the stimulus for nictitans movement and prevent the third eyelid from covering the corneal surgical site when the corneal procedure is being performed. Placing a lid speculum will help prevent the upper and lower eyelid from interrupting the surgical

◀——————————————————————————————————

Fig. 7. Resection of the third eyelid can be performed in a standing horse. (*A*) A horse with a third eyelid mass (squamous cell carcinoma) (*B*) A close-up of the third eyelid. (*C*) The margins of the third eyelid are held with Allis tissue forceps, and a large curved hemostat is placed at the base of the third eyelid and kept in place for 60 to 90 seconds. (*D*) The third eyelid is resected at the groove from the removed curved hemostat. The resection can be performed with curved Metzenbaum scissors or with a #15 scalpel blade. (*E*) Same horse 4 weeks after the resection of the third eyelid. The area has healed and only mild discharge can be seen.

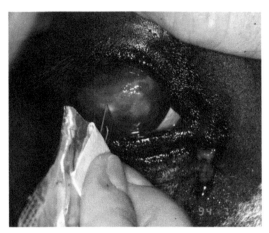

Fig. 9. The metallic back side of a #15 scalpel blade is used to take a cytology sample from an infected corneal ulcer.

procedure by covering the corneal surface. Measurement of the diseased corneal area can be carried out with a caliper. A punch biopsy (trephine) 1 mm larger than the diseased corneal area can be used for the procedure. Bishop-Harmon forceps or 0.3-mm tooth microforceps should be used to grasp the conjunctiva and thereby stabilize the globe, and 0.12-mm tooth microforceps should be used to handle and manipulate the corneal tissue. The punch biopsy is placed perpendicular to the cornea, and soft pressure to the punch biopsy cuts the margins of the biopsy/keratectomy area. When the margins of the biopsy/keratectomy area have been cut, the 0.12-mm tooth microforceps are used to grasp the corneal tissue to be removed. This maneuver causes less trauma to the healthy cornea and aids in quicker healing without complications. A corneal dissector or a #64 beaver scalpel blade can be used to gently dissect under the cornea (**Fig. 10**). The removed corneal piece should be placed in a biopsy cassette and into formaldehyde, and submitted for histopathologic evaluation. In the case of a linear superficial corneal stromal condition with normal epithelial involvement, the area can be removed by making a linear incision at the epithelial level, exposing the stroma, removing a stromal piece, and then either suturing the linear corneal epithelial incision (7-0 or 8-0 absorbable suture) such that no ulcer is present, or allowing the incision to heal by secondary wound healing. The equine cornea is 0.8 to 1.0 mm in thickness, and the surgeon should be very careful not to perforate the cornea. A biopsy or a superficial keratectomy whereby no conjunctival flap or other tissue is placed to cover the corneal defect should not extend deeper than one-third of the corneal thickness.[14] A subpalpebral lavage system and a hard cup hood are recommended after this procedure. The horse should be on topical antibiotics, antiproteinases, and atropine. Topical antifungal treatment should be considered in areas with increased risk of fungal keratitis. The horse should also be treated with systemically administered NSAIDs. A recheck of the cornea with fluorescein stain should be performed 3 to 5 days after surgery, and the corneal defect should be healed within 7 to 10 days.[8,14]

Amniotic membrane transplant (AMT) is being used in equine ophthalmology as a self-sacrificing corneal bandage supplying the cornea with growth factors, anti-inflammatory substances, and antiangiogenic cytokines, as well as having a bandaging function.[15] The AMT has been documented to cause less scarring of the cornea than a conjunctival graft, and the AMT will therefore in many cases provide

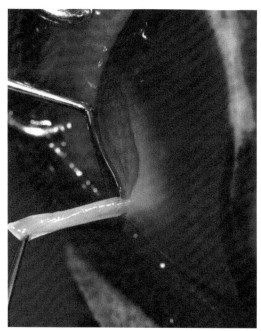

Fig. 10. A corneal biopsy or a superficial keratectomy can be performed on a standing sedated horse.

the horse with better vision after surgery.[16] The AMT can be glued on to the equine cornea, and the procedure can be performed on a standing horse as an extra procedure after superficial keratectomy or in the case of a deep corneal ulcer whereby economic factors or the horse's condition preclude the use of general anesthesia. The cornea has to be completely dry for the glued AMT to stick to the corneal tissue. A hair dryer has been used to dry out the equine cornea, although the cornea has to be locally anesthetized and the horse well sedated for it to accept this procedure. The surgeon needs to be aware of the risk of burning the cornea with the hair dryer, and it should therefore be kept 20 to 30 cm away from the cornea during the procedure. While an assistant dries the cornea, the surgeon and another assistant prepare the AMT by holding it with 2 Bishop-Harmon forceps (**Fig. 11**). When the cornea is dry (average time 1–2 min), the second assistant applies Tissuemend II or cyanoacrylate tissue glue to the epithelial side of the AMT and to the corneal defect. In the authors' experience, Tissuemend II has a better adhesive effect on the equine cornea and AMT.[17,18] The surgeon then places the AMT over the corneal defect while the first assistant continues to dry the cornea, now with the AMT applied as well, for 1 more minute. A complication of this procedure is that equine tears seem to break down tissue glue very quickly, such that it can be a problem to keep the AMT glued to the cornea. An equine contact lens can be applied over the glued AMT to keep the AMT attached to the cornea. A partial temporary tarsorrhaphy is also recommended, and should stay in place for the next 5 to 7 days to give the corneal area time to heal.[9] The same medical treatment as described for the corneal biopsy and superficial keratectomy should be used for horses with a glued AMT.

In the authors' opinion, corneal lacerations can be sutured in the standing sedated horse if the horse is calm, the surgeon has experience in corneal surgery, and the

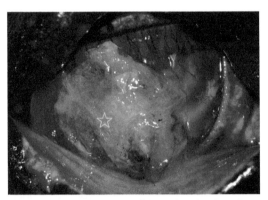

Fig. 11. An amniotic membrane transplant (AMT) can be glued to the cornea on a standing sedated horse (*green star*). This horse underwent corneal transplant surgery (*red star*). The transplant had an infected area and an AMT glued over the infected area.

laceration is small in length. Auriculopalpebral and supraorbital nerve blocks should be performed, and topical anesthetics applied to the cornea. Simple interrupted 7-0 absorbable suture can be used to close the corneal laceration. The sutures should be placed at three-fourths corneal thickness, and it is important that the sutures do not penetrate the cornea because of the risk of infection and leakage of aqueous humor through the placed sutures.[8,19] It is recommended that a Seidel test be performed after the sutures have been placed to ensure that the sutured laceration has been completely closed and no aqueous humor is leaking from the incision site.[4]

ANTERIOR CHAMBER

An aqueous paracentesis or tissue plasminogen activator (TPA) injection can be performed on a sedated standing horse. Auriculopalpebral and supraorbital nerve blocks should be performed. A high-risk complication of this procedure is infectious endophthalmitis, and aseptic preparation with 5% betadine is therefore very important before the application of the topical anesthetics to the cornea and conjunctiva, and the insertion of the needle into the anterior chamber.[20] Placement of a needle in the anterior chamber should never be attempted in a nonsedated horse. The needle can be accidentally placed into the lens and iris, causing bleeding and severe blinding phacolytic or phacoclastic uveitis. The peripheral anterior chamber is very shallow in the horse, and it is easy to tear the iris and cause hyphema during needle insertion.[4,8] An eyelid speculum is placed and the globe stabilized with Bishop-Harmon forceps. A 25- to 27-gauge, 0.75- to 1-inch (2–2.5 cm) needle is used for the injection into the anterior chamber. The needle is placed 1 to 2 mm posterior to the limbus at the 10- to 2-o'clock position (depending on whether the surgeon is right or left handed). The needle tip is aimed away from the iris but should not touch the corneal endothelium. The area where the needle will penetrate the limbus should also be locally anesthetized, which can be done by holding a sterile cotton swab or Q-tip soaked in local anesthetic solution to the specific area of needle placement, and insertion for 30 seconds directly before the needle touches the limbus. The needle and attached 2.5-mL syringe is placed in the anterior chamber by the surgeon, and an assistant then slowly aspirates up to 0.2 to 0.5 mL of the aqueous humor.[4] There will be a risk of increased intraocular pressure (IOP) if no aqueous humor is removed, depending of the amount of solution injected into the anterior chamber. When the aqueous humor has been aspirated, TPA (0.2–0.4 mL, 50–150 µg/eye solution) can be injected into the anterior chamber to break down fibrin that will otherwise cause anterior and posterior synechia, corneal edema, or cataract formation.[21] Because of the risk of increased IOP after an aqueous paracentesis, the IOP should be monitored before and after the procedure. Topical and systemic antibiotic and systemic NSAIDs should be added to the treatment plan for horses that have had an aqueous paracentesis/injection performed, as well as topical steroids or topical NSAIDs, in cases where it is not contraindicated to use topical steroids or NSAIDs.

INTRAVITREAL INJECTION

Intravitreal injection can be used for delivering medication into the posterior segment of the eye, and has been used to treat equine vitritis seen in cases of equine recurrent uveitis (ERU). Steroids (triamcinolone acetonide) or other immunosuppressive medications (rapamycin) have been injected into the vitreous to decrease the inflammatory reaction.[20,22] Small amounts of gentamicin (4 mg) have been injected into the equine vitreous for successful treatment of suspected leptospirosis inflammatory/infectious reactions in eyes with ERU, but this treatment should be performed with extreme caution because gentamicin in large volumes can cause retinal degeneration, cataracts and endophthalmitis, and a blind eye as the final result.[8] Intravitreal injection can also be used as the final option in uncontrolled glaucoma under the term chemical ciliary body ablation (CBA). Gentamicin (50 mg) and steroids (1 mg dexamethasone) are injected into the vitreous to cause nonpainful phthisis bulbi.[23] A CBA procedure should only be performed in a blind eye. Intravitreal injections can be performed on the standing sedated horse. Auriculupalpebral and supraorbital nerve blocks are used together with aseptic preparation of the globe and local anesthesia. Topical phenylephrine (2.5% ophthalmic solution) can also be used to prevent conjunctival and scleral bleeding. An eyelid speculum is placed, and the surgeon's assistant tilts the horse's head so that the dorsal-lateral aspect of the sclera is free of the eyelid margin. The surgeon stabilizes the globe with Bishop-Harmon forceps, holding the conjunctiva and episclera, while the other hand places a 27- to 23-gauge, 1-inch needle attached to a 2.5-mL syringe into the sclera 10 to 12 mm from the dorsal-lateral limbus at a 45° angle toward the optic nerve and away from the lens (**Fig. 12**). When the needle and syringe are in place in the vitreous, an assistant can aspirate vitreous (up to 2.5 mL) and then inject the medication into the vitreous.[6] While the needle is being removed from the vitreous, the Bishop-Harmon forceps can clamp the area around the needle site to avoid vitreous or medication leaking from the puncture hole. In cases where no vitreous can be aspirated, an aqueous paracentesis can be performed to lower the acute increased IOP that a CBA will cause owing to the amount of solution injected into the vitreous. Complications seen with an intravitreal injection include cataracts or even lens rupture with severe uveitis caused by the needle touching or penetrating the lens, infectious endophthalmitis and blindness, vitreal hemorrhage, and retinal detachment, as well as corneal ulcers, corneal edema, and a possibility of no reduction in IOP from the CBA.[6]

STANDING ENUCLEATION

Enucleation of the globe can be performed on a well-sedated standing horse. The sedation protocol for this 45-minute to 1-hour long standing procedure is explained in an article elsewhere in this issue by Vigani and colleagues. The horse has its head on a head stand and is prepared for surgery by clipping a square area around the globe. The area can be prepared for surgery with aseptic standard protocols using betadine scrub and alcohol on the skin area. The globe should be aseptically

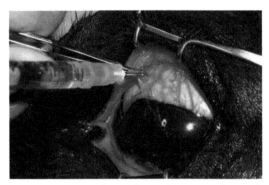

Fig. 12. A vitreal centesis/injection can be performed on a standing sedated horse. The needle (23–27 gauge, 1 inch [2.54 cm] long) is inserted into the sclera 10 to 12 mm from the limbus at 12 o'clock.

prepared for surgery with a 5% betadine solution. It is important to clean under the third eyelid. Auriculopalpebral, supraorbital, and 4-point nerve blocks are used for standing enucleation with the 50:50 2% lidocaine and 2% mepivacaine analgesic solution. A double subcutaneous ring block is placed with a 25-gauge needle around the superior and inferior eyelids with 8 mL lidocaine/mepivacaine for each ring, and topical anesthesia is applied to the cornea and conjunctiva. The halter can be covered with sterile towels, and the surgery area should be kept as sterile as possible, but a standing enucleation is not a completely sterile procedure. Tetanus status should always be discussed with the owner before any equine ophthalmic surgery, but is especially important for standing enucleation. The horse should have systemically administered antibiotics after surgery and, if possible, 1 day before surgery as well. The transpalpebral enucleation approach is recommended for standing equine enucleation. The eyelids are sutured closed with a nonabsorbable 2-0 monofilament suture (nylon) in a simple continuous suture pattern. A knot is placed in the medial and lateral aspect of the eyelids and 5-cm long suture ends are left on each side (**Fig. 13**). Each of the suture ends is grasped with a small hemostat and used to stabilize the surgery site. A full-thickness skin incision is made 5 to 7 mm from the eyelid margin with a #15 scalpel blade. The incision is made all the way around the closed eyelids. Dissection through the subcutaneous tissue toward the curvature of the bony orbit is performed in the superior, inferior, medial, and lateral aspects with curved Metzenbaum scissors. Dissection is continued deeper to the fornix, and frees the globe from its surrounding tissue envelope. The extraocular muscles and the medial and lateral canthal ligaments are resected, which loosens the globe inside. The optic nerve is clamped with a curved-vessel pattern clamp for 30 to 60 seconds and the optic nerve cut with curved Metzenbaum scissors. The globe in its tissue envelope can now be removed and placed in formaldehyde for further histopathologic diagnostics. The surgery site is closed with either 3 or 2 layers of sutures. The first closure layer (optional) is a mesh placed as a simple continuous suture pattern in the periosteum with an absorbable 2-0 suture (Vicryl). The second closure layer uses an absorbable 3-0 suture (Vicryl) opposing the subcutaneous tissue with a simple continuous suture pattern. The third layer of closure is carried out with nonabsorbable 2-0 suture (nylon) in a cruciate suture pattern. A standard-pressure head bandage is placed over the surgical site for 2 days (**Fig. 14**), and the horse treated with a systemically administered antibiotic for 7 days and systemic NSAIDs for 5 days after surgery. The sutures

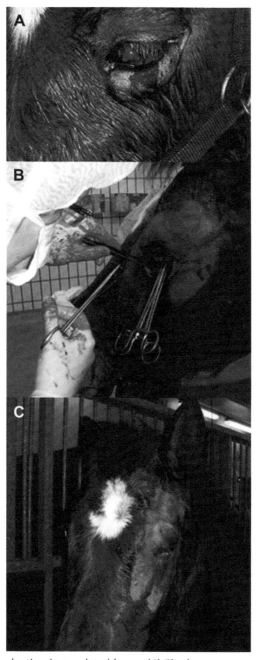

Fig. 13. Standing nucleation in a sedated horse. (*A*) The horse was presented with a trau-matic perforated blind globe. (*B*) The head is on a head stand and the surgical area has been clipped. The surgery area should be kept as sterile as possible, but a standing enucle-ation is not a completely sterile procedure. (*C*) The horse 2 days after surgery. The head bandage has been removed, and only mild swelling can be appreciated in the surgery area.

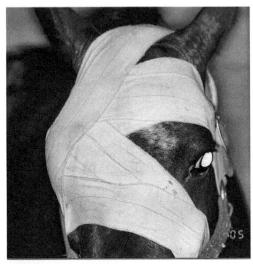

Fig. 14. A standard pressure head bandage should be placed over the surgical site for the first 2 days after an enucleation.

are removed after 10 days during which the horse should be wearing a flue mask or hard cup hood for protection of the surgery site.[7]

An exenteration refers to removal of the globe and as much of the ocular contents as possible. This procedure is performed in cases with periorbital or retrobulbar neoplasia or in cases with orbital infection.[24] Exenterations are best performed under general anesthesia, because an exenteration can be a long procedure. More tissue has to be removed and, because of the possibility of bone involvement, periosteal elevators may be needed during an exenteration.[24] Some horses will not allow the surgeon to perform these needed steps in a standing exenteration, and there will be a risk of not being able to remove all the neoplastic or infectious/necrotic tissue during surgery. The surgical approach for an exenteration is the same as that for transpalpebral enucleation, and can be carried out as a standing equine surgery in cases where the horse is not able to undergo general anesthesia. When the globe in the tissue envelope has been removed (see transpalpebral enucleation), a curette and periosteal elevator can be used to remove the remaining tissue in the orbit. In some cases intraoperative injection of local analgesia is necessary for the surgeon to continue to remove retrobulbar tissue during the exenteration procedure. In cases where the eyelids and tissue around the orbit are removed during surgery, the surgical site can be left to heal by secondary wound healing. In the case of secondary-intention healing, it is recommended to place iodoform gauze or a Penrose drain in the orbit for days to weeks and to keep a head bandage in place until the wound is healed. The head bandage should be changed according to normal bandaging techniques, every day for the first couple of days and thereafter according to the degree of healing at the surgical site.[25]

REFERENCES

1. Kalf KL, Utter ME, Wotman KL. Evaluation of duration of corneal anesthesia induced with ophthalmic 0.5% proparacaine hydrochloride by use of a Cochet-Bonnet aesthesiometer in clinically normal horses. Am J Vet Res 2008;69(12):1655.

2. Monclin SJ, Farnir F, Grauwels M. Duration of corneal anaesthesia following multiple doses and two concentrations of tetracaine hydrochloride eyedrops on the normal equine cornea. Equine Vet J 2011;43(1):69.
3. Sharrow-Reabe KL, Townsend WM. Effect of action of proparacaine and tetracaine topical ophthalmic formulation on corneal sensitivity in horses. J Am Vet Med Assoc 2012;241:1645.
4. Gilger BC, Stoppini R. Equine ocular examination routine and advanced diagnostic techniques. In: Gilger BC, editor. Equine ophthalmology. 2nd edition. Elsevier Saunders; 2011. p. 1–51.
5. Pucket JD, Allbaugh RA, Rankin AJ, et al. Comparison of efficacy and duration of effects on corneal sensitivity among anesthetic agents following ocular administration in clinical normal horses. Am J Vet Res 2013;74(3):459.
6. Hessermer V. Peribulbar anesthesia versus retrobulbar anesthesia via facial nerve block. Techniques, local anesthetics and additives, akinesia and sensory block, complications. Klin Monbl Augenheilkd 1994;204(2):75.
7. Pollack PJ, Russell T, Hughes TK, et al. Transpalpebral eye enucleation in 40 standing horses. Vet Surg 2008;37:306.
8. Brooks DE, Matthews AG. Equine ophthalmology. In: Gelatt KN, editor. Veterinary ophthalmology. 4th edition. Blackwell Publishing, Ames, Iowa; 2007. p. 1165–274.
9. Gelatt KN, Whitley RD. Surgery of the eyelids. In: Gelatt KN, Gelatt JP, editors. Veterinary ophthalmic surgery. 2nd edition. Elsevier Saunders, Maryland Heights, Missouri; 2011. p. 89–140.
10. Giuliano EA. Equine ocular adnexal and nasolacrimal disease. In: Gilger BC, editor. Equine ophthalmology. 2nd edition. Elsevier Saunders; 2011. p. 133–80.
11. Brooks DE. Complications of ophthalmic surgery in the horse. In: Goodrich LR editor. Surgical Complications and Management Strategies. Elsevier Sauders, Maryland Heights, Missouri; 2008,24(3):697.
12. Gelatt KN, Brooks BE. Surgical procedures for the conjunctival nictitating membrane. In: Gelatt KN, Gelatt JP, editors. Veterinary ophthalmic surgery. 2nd edition. Elsevier Saunders, Maryland Heights, Missouri; 2011. p. 157–90.
13. Labelle AL, Metzler AG, Wilkie DA. Nictitating membrane resection in the horse: a comparison of long-term outcomes using local vs. general anaesthesia. Equine Vet J Suppl 2011;(40):42–5.
14. Gelatt KN, Brooks BE. Surgery of the cornea and sclera. In: Gelatt KN, Gelatt JP, editors. Veterinary ophthalmic surgery. 2nd edition. Elsevier Saunders, Maryland Heights, Missouri; 2011. p. 191–236.
15. Plummer CE, Ollivier F, Karllberg M, et al. The use of amniotic membrane transplantation for ocular surface reconstruction: a review and series of 58 equine clinical cases (2002-2008). Vet Ophthalmol 2009;12(Suppl 1):17–24.
16. Ollivier FJ, Karllberg ME, Plummer CE, et al. Amniotic membrane transplantation for corneal surface reconstruction after excision of corneolimbal squamous cell carcinomas in nine horses. Vet Ophthalmol 2006;9(6):404.
17. Vote BJT, Elder MJ. Cyanoacrylate glue for corneal perforations: a description of a surgical technique and a review of the literature. Clin Experiment Ophthalmol 2000;28:437.
18. Tsujita H, Brennan AB, Plummer CE, et al. An ex vivo model for suture-less amniotic membrane transplantation with a chemical defined bioadhesive. Curr Eye Res 2012;37(5):372.
19. Clode AB. Disease and surgery of the cornea. In: Gilger BC, editor. Equine ophthalmology. 2nd edition. Elsevier Saunders, Maryland Heights, Missouri; 2011. p. 181–266.

20. Yi NY, Davis JL, Salmon JH, et al. Ocular distribution and toxicity of intravitreal injection of triamcinolone acetonide in normal equine eyes. Vet Ophthalmol 2008;11(Suppl 1):15–9.
21. Brooks DE. Equine ophthalmology. AAEP Proceedings 2002;48:300.
22. Douglas LC, Yi NY, Davis JL, et al. Ocular toxicity and distribution of subconjunctival and intravitreal rapamycin in horses. J Vet Pharmacol Ther 2008;31:511.
23. Utter ME, Brooks DE. Glaucoma. In: Gilger BC, editor. Equine ophthalmology. 2nd edition. Elsevier Saunders, Maryland Heights, Missouri; 2011. p. 350–66.
24. Brooks DE. Orbit. In: Auer JA, Stick JA, editors. Equine surgery. 2nd edition. WB Saunders Company, Philadelphia, Pennsylvania; 1999. p. 497–508.
25. Henridrickson DA. Second-intention healing. In: Hendrickson DA, editor. Wound care management for the equine practitioner. 1st edition. Teton New Media, Jackson, Wyoming; 2005. p. 99–137.

Standing Equine Surgery of the Upper Respiratory Tract

Phil A. Cramp, BSc, BVM&S, MS, MRCVS[a],*, Timo Prange, DVetMed, MS[b],
Frank A. Nickels, MS, DVM[c]

KEYWORDS

- Equine • Upper airway • Guttural pouch • Endoscopy • Laser • Epiglottis • Larynx
- Pharynx

KEY POINTS

- Upper respiratory surgery can be successfully performed in the horse.
- Appropriate case selection and equipment are imperative to successful outcome.
- Accessibility to the upper respiratory tract is improved in the standing horse due to appropriate anatomic positioning and superior visibility.

INTRODUCTION

The purpose of this article is to review the literature and personal experiences of equine surgeons so as to describe procedures that can be performed in the standing sedated horse to alleviate conditions that result in upper respiratory tract obstruction. Performing many upper respiratory tract surgeries in the standing sedated horse is advantageous because accessibility to the head is improved, the anatomy is in the appropriate position, and visibility is superior. However, these advantages must be weighed against the fact that upper respiratory tract surgery requires attention to detail, meticulous planning, and careful dissection and execution with little room for error. The ability to flex and extend the head, and move the head and neck to the left and right, can facilitate better accessibility to various parts of the upper airway, and procedures can be performed with greater ease. Although standing upper airway surgery is very appealing to the surgeon and the animal owner, as it eliminates the need for general anesthesia and thereby the associated

---

[a] Hambleton Equine Clinic, 20 Linden Close, Hutton Rudby, North Yorkshire, England, TS15 0HX, UK; [b] Equine and Farm Animal Veterinary Center, NC State College of Veterinary Medicine Veterinary Health Complex, 1052 William Moore Drive, Raleigh, NC 27607, USA; [c] A203 Veterinary Medical Center, College of Veterinary Medicine, Michigan State University, East Lansing, MI 48824, USA
* Corresponding author.
E-mail address: philcramp@yahoo.co.uk

costs and risks, it often requires special equipment, such as a videoendoscope and laser.

This article describes a selection of standing upper airway procedures, the indications for and possible complications of these surgeries, and advantages and disadvantages of a particular method.

NASAL SURGERIES
Surgical Extirpation of Nasal Atheromas (Epidermal Inclusion Cysts of the Nasal Diverticulum)

Dissection and en bloc removal
The local area is infiltrated subcutaneously with local anesthetic solution (2% mepivacaine-hydrochloride; Zoetis, Kalamazoo, MI) over the cyst (**Fig. 1**). A linear incision is made directly over the cyst extending 0.5 to 1.0 cm rostrally and caudally. Careful dissection with Metzenbaum scissors is performed around the margin of the cyst making every effort to leave the thin cystic wall intact. Although rupturing of the wall is not a significant complication (**Fig. 2**), it does make removal of the entire cyst more difficult. Following complete removal, the site is lavaged with saline and the skin closed in a routine fashion.

Removal with a laryngeal burr
Schumacher and Dixon[1] described a technique that involves making a stab incision into the rostroventral aspect of the cyst via the nasal cavity and inserting a laryngeal burr. The burr is then rotated to engage the lining of the cyst. Once the lining is firmly engaged, the burr is slowly everted, exposing the attached lining that can then be transected and removed. The incision is then left to heal by secondary intention. This procedure is performed following either local anesthesia of the ipsilateral infraorbital nerve or local infiltration of the cyst with a local anesthetic solution (2% mepivacaine-hydrochloride). The latter is preferred to desensitize the rostral aspect of the cyst within the nasal diverticulum.

Chemical ablation
Regression of epidermal inclusion cysts can be achieved by injecting 2 to 4 mL of a 10% formalin solution into the lumen of the cyst.[1,2] After initial enlargement, the cysts generally disappear within 2 weeks after the injection. Local anesthesia is not required for this procedure.

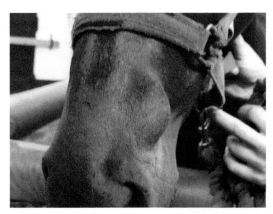

Fig. 1. Nasal atheroma. (*Courtesy of* R. Ordidge, North Yorkshire, UK.)

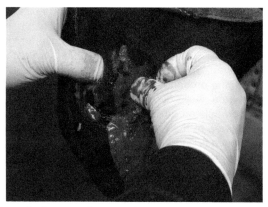

Fig. 2. A ruptured nasal atheroma showing the typical appearance of the contents, which often has a "fishy" smell. (*Courtesy of* R. Ordidge, North Yorkshire, UK.)

Advantages and disadvantages

Dissection and en bloc removal will typically ensure that the complete cyst is removed. These procedures prevent recurrence, but scar formation is a common sequel of this technique. The latter is not a concern when using the transnasal burr, but this procedure is slightly more complicated and may leave a "tag" of lining behind, possibly resulting in recurrence of the cyst. Chemical ablation is a simple and anecdotally very successful technique. It is important that the owner and veterinarian are aware that resolution may take up to 2 weeks, during which time the cyst can become significantly enlarged before ultimately disappearing.

Complications

Overall, there are few complications reported and the recurrence rate is very low with these methods.

GUTTURAL POUCH SURGERIES
Transendoscopic Laser Fenestration of the Median Septum of the Guttural Pouches

Disease treated

Unilateral Guttural pouch tympany; bilateral cases are not suitable candidates for this treatment, as it relies on one of the guttural pouch ostia functioning normally.

Procedure

This procedure allows the treatment of unilateral guttural pouch tympany in foals without the need for general anesthesia. Furthermore, the creation of a surgical approach to the guttural pouch is not necessary, decreasing the risk of inadvertent tissue trauma, especially nerve damage. The original publication[3] described the use of an Nd:YAG laser to perform the fenestration, but a diode laser is equally effective and has less potential for latent thermal damage. The power output for the laser is set at 100 W, continuous mode (Nd:YAG) or 20 W (Diode). After adequate chemical restraint, a flexible endoscope is placed up the nostril opposite the affected guttural pouch until the pharyngeal opening of the guttural pouches can be seen. A Chambers catheter is then introduced into the opposite nostril and, under endoscopic guidance, directed into the affected guttural pouch. The endoscope is passed into the unaffected guttural pouch and the median septum is brought into view. The Chambers catheter is now rotated until its curved tip tents the septum toward the endoscope. The laser fiber is advanced through the instrument channel of the endoscope and brought in contact with the membranous septum directly over the tip of the Chambers catheter. In this position, the catheter functions as a barrier to prevent inadvertent irradiation of other tissues. The laser is now fired until the end of the Chambers catheter is protruding through the median septum. The catheter is then repositioned behind the septum next to the opening and the procedure is repeated until a fistula of about 2.5 cm in diameter has been created. A Foley catheter is inserted into one of the guttural pouches and the balloon inflated so that it remains in place and the distal end of the Foley catheter is sutured to the naris. The Foley catheter provides a conduit for lavage of the guttural pouches and this should be performed every 2 to 4 days after surgery to remove any necrotic debris. Once the lavage is clear, the catheter can be removed.

Advantages and disadvantages
The main advantage of this procedure is that it reduces the risk of damage to the sympathetic trunk and cranial nerves IX to XII, which pass through the guttural pouch, and carries a relatively good success rate of 70%, with only 30% requiring a second procedure.[4] The main disadvantage is that it can be more technically challenging to perform in a foal that is not under general anesthesia.

Complications
Few complications are reported but the most significant risk is inadvertent damage to the neurovascular structures, including the internal carotid artery, sympathetic trunk, and cranial nerves IX to XII.

Salpingopharyngeal Fistulation Using a Transendoscopic Laser

Disease treated
Bilateral or unilateral guttural pouch tympany.

Procedure
An Nd:YAG or diode laser works well for this procedure. Similar to septal fenestration, an endoscope is passed up the nostril opposite the affected guttural pouch. A Chambers catheter is then inserted into the affected guttural pouch and rotated so that the medial wall of the guttural pouch is tented into the pharynx. The laser fiber is passed through the instrument channel of the endoscope and used in contact fashion over the tented mucosa to create a 1-cm diameter[3] fistula into the guttural pouch. Once created, a Foley catheter (size 16) is inserted into the guttural pouch via the fistula, the balloon is inflated, and is left in place to ensure that the fistula does not close. This Foley catheter also can be used to lavage the guttural pouch in cases in which there is a degree of mucus accumulation or infection. The Foley catheter should remain in place for 10 to 14 days or until the infection has resolved and then removed. The procedure is repeated on the opposite side if bilateral tympany is present.

Advantages and disadvantages
This procedure is more amenable to being performed in a foal under sedation and carries an equally good prognosis as fenestration of the median septum.

Complications
Few complications are reported, but the most significant risk is inadvertent damage to the neurovascular structures. Premature closure of the fistula can occur, requiring a second procedure.[3]

In cases of bilateral guttural pouch tympany, a combination of these 2 laser procedures can be used; for example, fenestration of the median septum and salpingopharyngeal fistulation of one or both guttural pouches.

Transarterial Coil Embolization of the Internal Carotid Artery

Disease treated
Guttural pouch mycosis.

Procedure
Benredouane and Lepage[5] reported a modified technique for transarterial coil embolization (TACE) of the internal carotid artery in the standing sedated horse (**Fig. 3**). The investigators used a set of mobile stocks with the head and neck in extension and the mandible resting on a head support with a technician in front of the horse to steady the head. The investigators also note that they used a customized drape extending from the base of the neck to the tail. In their study, 8 adult, healthy horses underwent TACE to assess safety and feasibility of the procedure. Subsequently, 5 horses with guttural pouch mycosis (GPM) were treated using the following surgical protocol. First, a 10-cm skin incision is made at the junction of the proximal and middle third of the neck, dorsal to the jugular vein. The common carotid artery (CCA) is located following sharp dissection through the cutaneous coli, brachiocephalicus, and omohyoideus muscles. It is then separated from the vagosympathetic trunk and elevated with umbilical tape.[5] A 6-F introducer system (Check Flo Performer introducer set; Cook, Inc, Limerick, Ireland) is placed into the CCA via an 18-G angiographic needle, and a 5-F single end-hole nylon angiographic catheter (Slip-Cath Beacon Tip Catheter; Cook, Inc) is advanced under fluoroscopic guidance rostrally into the CCA.[5] Using meglumine ioxithalamate contrast boluses, the internal (ICA) and external carotid artery (ECA), as well as the occipital artery are identified (see **Fig. 3**). Following the ICA, the catheter is advanced to the level of the basisphenoid bone at the level of the

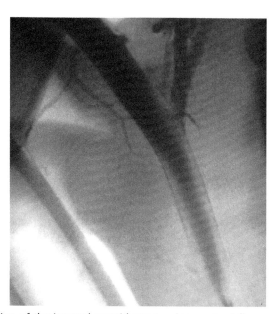

Fig. 3. Identification of the internal carotid artery using contrast fluoroscopy. (*Courtesy of* JT Easley, Shelbyville, KY.)

ICA sigmoid flexure, before another bolus of contrast is used to establish the diameter of the artery.[5] Next, a Dacron fiber-covered, stainless steel occluding spring embolization coil (Nester Embolization Coil; Cook, Inc) is introduced. The diameter of the first coil should be slightly larger than the estimated arterial diameter. Injection of contrast material is used to assess the degree of occlusion. It might be necessary to place 1 or 2 smaller additional coils to accomplish complete embolization of the artery. The CCA is closed with 4-0 polypropylene suture, the muscles and skin are closed routinely.[5] The same standing technique could be performed using transarterial nitinol vascular occlusion plugs instead of embolization coils (**Fig. 4**).

Advantages and disadvantages
The avoidance of general anesthesia, particularly in cases that have suffered significant blood loss and are in an advanced stage of shock, makes this technique very attractive for a select number of horses. However, it requires considerable expertise and equipment, including fluoroscopy, which is available only at certain specialist centers.

Complications
Benredouane and Lepage[5] did not report any surgery-related complications in the 5 horses with guttural pouch mycosis they treated using this method. However, one horse died following a cardiac infarction 9 days after surgery and another horse died within 3 days of surgery due to a diaphragmatic hernia and incarceration of the large colon. In all horses, the coils were placed accurately and in the 3 surviving horses the epistaxis resolved and the mycotic lesion regressed within 2 to 4 months.[5]

Transendoscopic Removal of Inspissated Material with Basket Forceps or a Snare

Disease treated
Guttural pouch empyema with chondroid formation (**Fig. 5**).

Procedure
With the horse sedated and the head supported, a videoendoscope is passed into the affected guttural pouch. After removal of liquid purulent material by guttural pouch

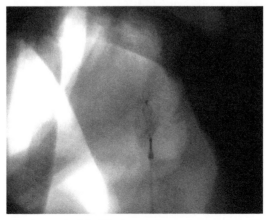

Fig. 4. Application of a transarterial nitinol vascular occlusion plug. (*Courtesy of* JT Easley, Shelbyville, KY.)

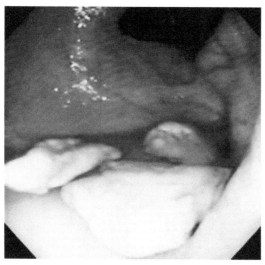

Fig. 5. Endoscopic appearance of multiple chondroids lying on the floor of the guttural pouch. (*Courtesy of* S. Barakzai, Sileby, Leicestershire, UK.)

lavage, basket forceps or a snare (**Fig. 6**) are deployed via the instrument channel. Individual or small groups of chondroids (**Fig. 7**) are retrieved before removing the endoscope and basket together from the guttural pouch. The basket/snare is cleaned and the process is repeated until all chondroids have been removed. Small chondroids or remaining debris can be readily lavaged out of the guttural pouch. It is also possible to break down larger chondroids by use of the snare, and then remove these fragments via lavage.

Advantages and disadvantages

Although this technique can be time-consuming, it is an effective, noninvasive method of removing chondroids and, when combined with a lavage, can be effective in 44% to 66% of cases.[6]

Complications

None.

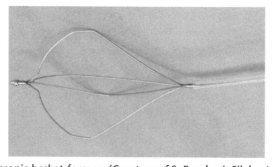

Fig. 6. Transendoscopic basket forceps. (*Courtesy of* S. Barakzai, Sileby, Leicestershire, UK.)

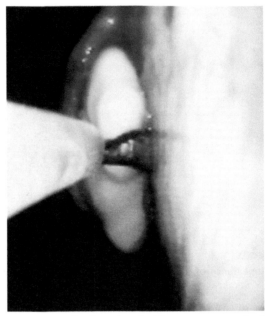

Fig. 7. Transendoscopic removal of a chondroid using a snare/basket forceps device. (*Courtesy of* S. Barakzai, Sileby, Leicestershire, UK.)

Modified Whitehouse Approach

Disease treated
Guttural pouch empyema with chondroid formation.

Procedure
Perkins and colleagues[7] described the use of a modified Whitehouse approach in 10 standing horses with guttural pouch chondroids. For this procedure, the patient should be placed in stocks with the head in an extended position. After the patient has been sedated, the subcutaneous tissues at the surgery site are infiltrated with 30 mL of 2% mepivacaine hydrochloride. A 10-cm to 12-cm incision is then made ventral and parallel to the linguofacial vein as it runs between the caudal aspect of the vertical ramus of the mandible and the ventral border of the sternocephalicus muscle. Next, the omohyoideus muscle attachment to the jugular vein is severed and dissection is continued lateral to the larynx in a rostrodorsal direction. Once the ventrocaudal aspect of the medial compartment of the guttural pouch has been reached, chondroids or a previously inserted Chambers catheter can be palpated and the pouch opened.[7] The investigators describe 2 methods of entering the guttural pouch:

1. If possible, the caudal wall of the guttural pouch should be grasped by 2 Allis tissue forceps approximately 5 mm apart and perforated with Metzenbaum scissors. The initial hole is then widened by expanding the jaws of the scissors.
2. If the guttural pouch cannot be grasped, a Chambers catheter is inserted into the medial compartment of the affected guttural pouch by a nonsterile assistant. The catheter tip is then bluntly forced through the caudomedial wall of the pouch into the surgeon's hand. A strand of 3.5-metric suture material is then attached to the catheter and is drawn back through the guttural pouch. Following the suture, the surgeon can locate the hole and enlarge it digitally to about 4 cm.

An endoscope is inserted through the pharyngeal ostium and the inspissated material is visualized. Sponge forceps are introduced via the newly created opening and is used to remove the chondroids under endoscopic guidance. On completion of this procedure, a 28-F Foley catheter is inserted through the incision into the lumen of the pouch and sutured to the skin.[7] The guttural pouch is lavaged daily for 3 to 5 days before the catheter is removed. The horses in this study were maintained on routine perioperative antibiotics and phenylbutazone for 3 to 7 days. The wounds healed well by secondary intention within 2 to 3 weeks after surgery.

Advantages and disadvantages
With 8 of 10 horses returning to their previous levels of competition,[7] the success rate for this procedure is reportedly high. Complications in the remaining 2 horses (1 horse died from unknown reasons, 1 suffered from persistent dysphagia that had already been present before surgery) did not appear to be related to the procedure. However, a surgeon planning to perform the modified Whitehouse approach in a standing patient should have sufficient experience with this surgery in recumbent horses. The complex anatomy of the guttural pouches and adjacent structures poses the risk of inadvertent damage to large blood vessels and cranial nerves. Gaining control of severe bleeding during the standing surgery is more difficult than in an anesthetized horse and can result in life-threatening blood loss.

Complications
As described previously, inadvertent damage to relevant neurovascular structures (cranial nerves, internal and external carotid artery) is a risk when performing the modified Whitehouse approach in horses. However, performing the procedure standing does not appear to increase this risk.

Modified Garm Technique

Disease treated
Persistent guttural pouch empyema of the lateral compartment, refractory to aggressive medical treatment.

Procedure
In 1946, Garm described a surgical approach to the lateral compartment (LC) of the guttural pouch.[8] He proposed that an opening in the rostroventral aspect of the LC would allow better and more complete drainage than conventional approaches. Furthermore, the nasopharyngeal guttural pouch opening is located too dorsal to allow complete drainage from the LC. Munñoz and colleagues[8] modified the original technique by making the incision more rostral. Although this increases the depth of dissection to the guttural pouch, it reduces the risk of inadvertent damage to blood vessels that lie between the salivary gland and facial artery. For the surgery, the horse is sedated and placed in stocks with the neck and head in an extended position. The incision site is infiltrated with 5 mL of local anesthetic. A 6-cm skin incision is made, beginning 2 cm caudal to the point where the linguofacial vein crosses the mandible, continuing rostrally medial to and parallel with the facial artery, vein, and parotid duct. The mylohyoid and digastric muscles are bluntly separated and dissection is carefully continued in a 45° angle toward the base of the ear until contact is made with the lateral aspect of the stylohyoid bone.[8] At this point, an endoscope is passed into the guttural pouch and the head of the horse is brought into a slightly flexed position. This change effectively increases the size of the lateral compartment. A 50-cm-long, 0.7-mm diameter metal tapered trochar within a 45-cm-long, 0.9-mm blunt rigid plastic sheath is then inserted into the incision, following the previously established

dissection plane. During the passage of this cannula, it is important to remain close to the stylohyoid bone and medial to the pterygoid muscle, so as to avoid damage to the hypoglossal nerve or mandibular gland duct.[8] Once the endoscopic image confirms contact of the cannula with the wall of the LC, the metal trochar is advanced through the wall into the guttural pouch. Using the trochar as a guide, a 16-mm mucosal dilator is introduced and then replaced with a 16-mm blunt end silicone drainage/lavage tube. The egress end of this tube is sutured to the skin.[8]

Advantages and disadvantages
This modification of the original Garm technique provides a safe and effective method for entering the LC of the guttural pouch, as it avoids the myriad of neurovascular structures that traverse the LC, which include the external carotid artery and its branches, part of the facial nerve, mandibular nerve, and auriculopalpebral nerve. However, careful dissection and detailed knowledge of the surrounding anatomy is of utmost importance to avoid inadvertent damage to cranial nerves. Once completed successfully, the surgical opening facilitates high-volume lavage and drainage of the LC of the guttural pouch. Because of its long and narrow shape, the approach is not suitable for the insertion of instruments into the guttural pouch. In cases in which purulent material is also present in the medial compartment, an additional opening into the medial compartment may be required.[8]

Complications
Reported complications include the inability to remove all chondroids from the guttural pouch, local emphysema (resolved without complication), and submandibular lymph node enlargement, which resolved by 3 days postoperative.[8]

Salpingopharyngeal Fistulation of the Guttural Pouch

Disease treated
Guttural pouch empyema refractory to aggressive medical treatment.

Procedure
The horse is sedated and placed in stocks, the mucosa surrounding the pharyngeal opening of the affected guttural pouch is topically anesthetized using 2% lidocaine (lidocaine hydrochloride injection 2%, AgriLabs, Bedford, TX) hydrochloride. Similar to the salpingopharyngeal fistulation that is described for guttural pouch tympany, an endoscope is passed up the opposite nasal passage opposite to the affected guttural pouch. A Chambers catheter is then inserted into the nasal passage of the affected side and placed under the cartilage of the guttural pouch opening. Using a laser, the cartilage directly over the catheter is incised and the fistula created. A Foley catheter is then inserted through the newly created opening and left in place to prevent premature closure and allow daily lavages of the guttural pouch. This treatment was reported in 2 cases by Hawkins and colleagues[9] in 2001. In both horses, the investigators noted that the ventral aspect of the cartilage underwent latent thermal necrosis and left the animal with a large and wide pharyngeal opening of the guttural pouch.

Advantages and disadvantages
This is a simple procedure that allows drainage and lavage of infected guttural pouches. However, the removal of chondroids might not be possible using this approach.

Complications
Although Hawkins and colleagues[9] did not report any significant complications, one horse required removal of a 2-cm mass of granulation tissue that obstructed outflow from the fistula.

Laser Fenestration of the Medial Septum

Disease treated
Guttural pouch empyema.

Procedure
Gehlen and Ohnesorge[10] described the use of a transendoscopic Nd:YAG laser to fenestrate the medial guttural pouch septum and remove multiple chondroids from the guttural pouch of a pony. The opening of the affected pouch appeared malformed and fibrotic adhesions did not allow passage of the endoscope or a catheter into the guttural pouch. Under sedation, the endoscope was passed into the normal guttural pouch and the laser fiber of the Nd:YAG laser was used to penetrate the medial septum.[10] Enlargement of the fenestration can be accomplished by use of the laser or a transendoscopic monopolar electrosurgery loop. Several standing procedures were necessary to completely remove the chondroids by use of grasping and/or basket forceps from the infected pouch.

Advantages and disadvantages
The main advantage to this procedure is avoiding surgical approaches, which run the significant risk of complications from inadvertent damage to neurovascular structures.[10] Additionally, the investigators suggest that this method leaves the pharynx undisturbed, which avoids subsequent complications such as soft palate displacement, altered airway dynamics, pharyngeal function, and guttural pouch function.[11] This is a good "backup" option should there be complications to more routine approaches. The disadvantages are the same as those already listed and also include a perceived difficulty with achieving adequate lavage of any remaining inspissated material.

Complications
None were reported in the literature, but they are potentially the same for all procedures associated with the medial, or median septum (ie, inadvertent damage to neurovascular structures).

EPIGLOTTIC SURGERIES
Endoscope-Guided, Transoral Axial Division of the Entrapping Epiglottic Membrane

Disease treated
Epiglottic entrapment (**Fig. 8**).

Procedure
Following a diagnosis of epiglottic entrapment via endoscopy, the horse is sedated and placed in the stocks. The entrapping fold is sprayed with 2% lidocaine hydrochloride along with the surrounding mucosal surface. With the head in extension and a Haussmann gag in place, a hand is inserted into the mouth and the soft palate is displaced dorsally. The entire oropharynx is the sprayed with local anesthetic[12] before a videoendoscope, protected by an endotracheal tube, is passed through the oral cavity. Once the entrapped epiglottis can be seen, a curved, hooked bistoury (**Fig. 9**) is placed behind the caudal edge of the entrapping membrane. It might be necessary to further extend the head to facilitate accurate positioning of the bistoury. The bistoury is then pulled rostrally to divide the entrapping membrane and free the epiglottis. The postoperative management includes phenylbutazone for 5 to 10 days along with broad-spectrum antibiotics. The horses are restricted to hand walking for 2 weeks before a return to work.

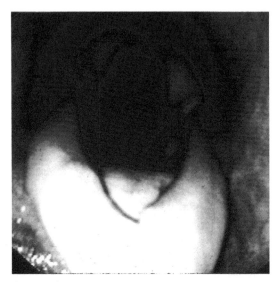

Fig. 8. Epiglottic entrapment.

Advantages and disadvantages

Compared with the transnasal use of a bistoury, this technique eliminates the risk of damaging the soft palate during transection of the entrapping tissue. The procedure is also easier to perform from an ergonomic perspective, and no reentrapment was documented in a group of 15 horses that underwent the surgery. However, some horses will not tolerate the procedure and might need to be anesthetized to complete the surgery.[12]

Complications

No complications were recorded and no evidence of reentrapment was documented in the study by Perkins and colleagues.[12] A general concern when treating epiglottic entrapments is that only a partial release of the entrapment is accomplished. This tends to occur when the transection of the entrapping membrane is not performed on the midline (**Fig. 10**). This complication can be reduced by using custom-made

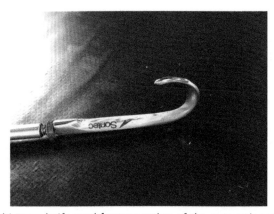

Fig. 9. A hooked bistoury knife used for transection of the entrapping membrane.

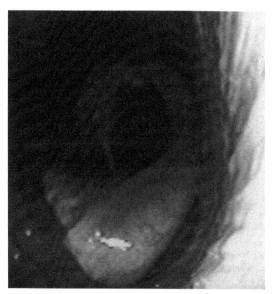

Fig. 10. Partial release of an epiglottic entrapment.

bistoury hooks that have an elongated ventral arm. This ensures that the cut that is made extends throughout the entire entrapping membrane.

Endoscope-Guided, Transnasal Axial Division of the Entrapping Epiglottic Membrane

Disease treated
Epiglottic entrapment.

Procedure
The surgical technique of transecting the entrapping membrane is similar to the one described for the transoral approach, with the exception that the endoscope and hook bistoury are introduced through the nostrils.[13]

Advantages and disadvantages
Using the standard, transnasal approach to examine the nasopharynx, it is easy to identify the entrapment and position the hook bistoury in the correct location. The disadvantages are associated with the complications that can occur.

Complications
Serious complications can occur when using this technique, including lacerations of the epiglottis, the soft palate, and/or pharynx. Although this makes the procedure somewhat unattractive, a recent modification described the use of a shielded hook bistoury, which successfully avoided inadvertent trauma to the surrounding tissues **(Fig. 11)**.[14]

Videoendoscopy-Assisted Laser Transection of the Entrapping Membrane

Disease treated
Epiglottic entrapment.

Procedure
The horse is sedated, placed in stocks, and the head is placed in an extended position. Local anesthetic solution is applied to the surface of the entrapping membrane and the

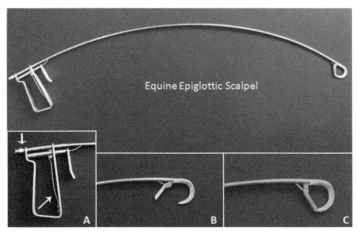

Fig. 11. A shielded hooked bistoury: the "equine epiglottic scalpel." (*A*) Overview of handle with *long arrow* indicating spring in the handle that keeps the shield closed with pressure on the trigger opening the shield. The *short arrow* indicates a luer lock flushing system to allow for cleaning of the instrument. *B* indicates the open position and *C* indicates Closed position. (*Courtesy of* M. Marcoux, Montreal, QC.)

videoendoscope is positioned on the midline, just rostral to the tip of the epiglottis. The laser fiber of a diode or Nd:YAG laser is advanced for approximately 2 to 3 cm so that it can reach the caudal aspect of the entrapping membrane. The laser fiber is fired and transects the entrapping membrane from caudal to rostral.[15,16] There is usually sufficient tension on the membrane to facilitate transection with the laser. It is important to ensure that the laser fiber, as it is being retracted, can reach the rostral aspect of the entrapping membrane to allow for completed transection. Further extension of the head might be necessary in some cases to accomplish this task. Multiple gentle passes along the membrane will allow gradual transection of the membrane until it slides rostrally and ventrally and the epiglottis is freed. Following release of the entrapped epiglottis, the endoscope should be kept in place so that normal swallowing can be observed several times. If reentrapment does not occur, then the procedure can be considered complete.

Advantages and disadvantages
This technique allows the surgeon to identify reentrapment immediately after completion of the surgery by observing swallowing.

Complications
The biggest risk associated with this procedure is inadvertent damage to the epiglottis. This risk can be reduced by using bronchoesophageal forceps (**Fig. 12**) to elevate the membrane off of the epiglottis.[13] The use of a custom-made hooked shield that is placed between the entrapping membrane and the epiglottis during the use of the laser is also a valid option to avoid epiglottic injury. The overall reentrapment rate is approximately 4%, and dorsal displacement of the soft palate (DDSP) can occur in 10% to 15% of the cases following surgery. Some surgeons will remove 2 small triangles of mucosa from either side of the transected membrane,[13] but removal of too much tissue can increase the chances of DDSP. An additional complication that this author has witnessed is granuloma formation in the subepiglottic folds, which results in DDSP and upper airway obstruction.

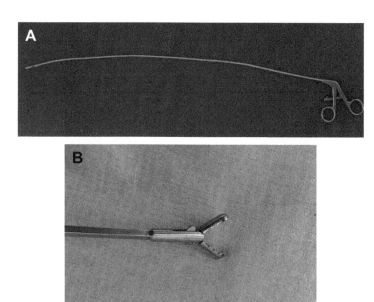

Fig. 12. (*A*) Endoscopic forceps. (*B*) A close-up of the jaws of a pair on endoscopic forceps.

Videoendoscopy-Assisted Laser Resection of Subepiglottic Cysts/Granulation Tissue/ Dorsal Epiglottic Abscess

Disease(s) treated
Subepiglottic cysts (**Fig. 13**), granulation tissue, and dorsal epiglottic abscesses.

Procedure
Diagnosis of these masses can readily be made via videoendoscopy (see **Fig. 13**), and treatment is based on removal of the structures. After sedation and application of a topical anesthetic, a videoendoscope with a diode or Nd:YAG laser fiber in the working channel is introduced through the nasal passage. The laser is then used in a contact fashion to remove or drain the mass. In cases of subepiglottic cysts, it is considered ideal to remove the complete lining to prevent recurrence of the cyst. Drainage of the purulent contents is the goal when treating dorsal epiglottic abscesses. Postoperative treatment involves broad-spectrum antibiotics and nonsteroidal anti-inflammatory drugs, along with throat spray. Following treatment, horses should be confined to box rest with hand walking for 10 days and then normal training can resume.

Advantages and disadvantages
The main advantage is that direct visualization of the structure before and during resection or drainage is possible. However, some subepiglottic masses will flip between the nasal and oral aspects and make it difficult to keep the mass within the field of vision. If it is possible to hold on to the structure by use of bronchoesophageal forceps, removal with technique is still possible. However, in some cases the procedure has to be abandoned in favor of a laryngotomy or a laser resection under general anesthesia.

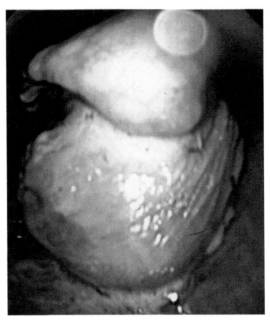

Fig. 13. Endoscopic appearance of a large epiglottic cyst.

Complications
The risk of complication is low, but care must be taken not to resect an excessive amount of tissue and thereby damage either the epiglottis or the soft palate.

LARYNGEAL AND PHARYNGEAL SURGERIES

A number of diseases can be treated with videoendoscopy-assisted laser resection or cautery. This section looks at the various techniques available and the indications of each procedure.

Videoendoscopy-Assisted Laser Resection of Granulation Tissue, Cysts, and Neoplastic Lesions in the Nasopharynx

Disease(s) treated
Nasopharyngal masses (granulation tissue, cysts, and/or neoplastic structures).

Procedure
Resection of tissues of various origins and in different locations can be performed with either an Nd:YAG or a diode laser in contact fashion. Under sedation, the videoendoscope is passed up the nostril that provides the best access to the structure of interest, and 20 to 30 mL of local anesthetic solution is used topically to desensitize the mass, nasopharynx, and both nasal passages. A pair of bronchoesophageal forceps is passed up the nostril opposite to the endoscope and the laser fiber is passed down the biopsy channel of the videoendoscope. The forceps are used to grasp the mass and apply tension. The latter is critical, as laser resection is more easily completed when the tissue is under moderate tension. These authors would recommend performing a couple of "practice" passes with the laser fiber to accustom one's self to the movements of the endoscope and laser fiber required. Good preparation will pay off during surgery, especially when the lasing begins to distort landmarks. With

upward traction applied to the mass, its base is gradually transected by consecutive side-to-side sweeps of the endoscope and laser. Once the mass has been freed, it is retrieved via the nostril with the forceps. Larger masses may need to be divided into smaller sections for removal.[13] With the videoendoscope still in place, a "throat spray" solution should be applied directly to the region. Various concoctions, exist but the authors have good success by using the following combination of drugs: 250 mL glycerin, 250 mL dimethyl sulfoxide (DMSO), and 500 mg of prednisolone. This mixture is applied twice daily for 5 days, using a catheter that is passed up the nasal passage. Antibiotics are not necessary, but phenylbutazone is given for up to 10 days postoperatively and dexamethasone should be given at the time of and 24 hours after surgery.

Advantages and disadvantages
This is a straightforward procedure that allows for accurate removal of various masses in the upper airway. Complete removal of the cyst and its lining, necessary to prevent recurrence, can be challenging, as these fluid-filled structures tend to burst during laser resection. In most cases, the procedure can still be completed successfully if the forceps have maintained traction on the remainder of the cyst, which can then be removed.

Laser Thermopalatoplasty

Disease treated
Palatal instability and intermittent dorsal displacement of the soft palate (**Fig. 14**).

Procedure
A videoendoscope is introduced into either nostril and 15 to 20 mL of local anesthetic solution is applied to the surface of the soft palate and a further 30 mL is sprayed along both nasal passages. A pair of bronchoesophageal forceps, or a custom-made alternative (**Fig. 15**), is passed up the other nostril and used to push the epiglottis dorsad and caudad. This exposes the most caudal aspect of the soft palate and prevents inadvertent damage to the epiglottis. The laser fiber (diode or Nd:YAG laser) is passed down the biopsy channel and used in contact fashion to "spot weld" the surface of the soft palate. The laser fiber should be in contact for only 1 to 2 seconds until the mucosa puckers and blanches and each point of contact should be approximately 5 mm apart (**Fig. 16**).

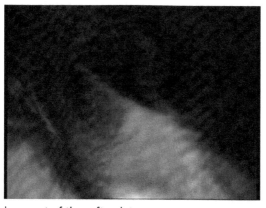

Fig. 14. Dorsal displacement of the soft palate.

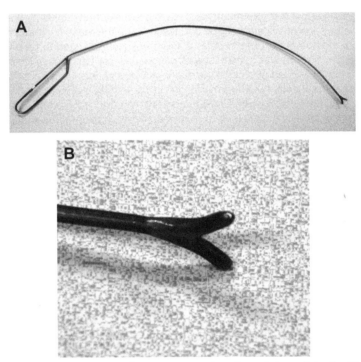

Fig. 15. (*A*) Custom-made device for atraumatic elevation of the epiglottic. (*B*) Close-up view of the atraumatic "Y"-shaped end piece of the custom-made device for elevating the epiglottis.

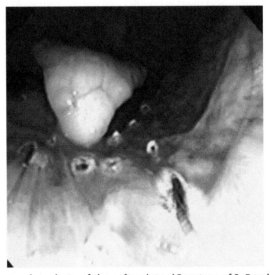

Fig. 16. Laser thermopalatoplasty of the soft palate. (*Courtesy of* S. Barakzai, Sileby, Leicestershire, UK.)

Advantages and disadvantages

This procedure is relatively simple and can be performed quickly. When combined with a sternothyroid tenectomy, a success rate of 90% has been reported.[17] However, this seems very optimistic, and the laser thermopalatoplasty was part of a combined treatment plan. As a stand-alone treatment, this procedure is unlikely to be successful and should therefore be regarded as an adjunct to other treatments.

Complications

Complications associated with this procedure are rare. However, care must be taken not to deliver too much energy to one area, as perforation of the soft palate can occur and adhesions between the soft palate and ventral epiglottis may develop.

Laser Staphylectomy

Disease treated

(Permanent) dorsal displacement of the soft palate.

Procedure

Once the soft palate has been desensitized with topically applied local anesthetic solution, a pair of bronchoesophageal forceps is used to grasp the caudal border of the soft palate. The caudal margin of the soft palate is lifted up and gentle caudal traction is applied to it. A diode or Nd:YAG laser is then used in contact fashion to remove a crescent-shaped piece of the soft palate. Not more than 1 cm of the free margin should be resected. Postoperatively, the patient is maintained on phenylbutazone for 10 days and throat spray for 5 days. Removal of the free margin of the soft palate (staphylectomy) is supposed to lead to scar formation that will increase the stability of the caudal edge of the soft palate. This procedure can be used in addition to a laryngeal tie-forward procedure, or combined with a sternothyroid tenectomy, in cases of permanent dorsal displacement of the soft palate.[13]

Advantages and disadvantages

This relatively simple procedure allows horses to return to full work after 10 to 14 days. However, a successful outcome can be expected in only up to 60% of cases.[18]

Complications

Resection of too much of the free margin will disturb the seal between the oropharynx and the nasopharynx and can result in serious complications, including dysphagia and aspiration pneumonia. An excessively shortened soft palate can also become even more prone to dorsal displacement, as the epiglottis is unable to keep the palate in its normal position. Because of these potential serious complications, this procedure should be considered only for permanently displaced soft palates or following a laryngeal tie-forward.

Videoendoscopy-Assisted Laser Resection of the Aryepiglottic Folds

Disease treated

Axial deviation of the aryepiglottic fold(s) (AEFs) (**Figs. 17** and **18**).

Axial deviation of the AEFs occurs mostly bilaterally, but unilateral (right) AEF collapse has been observed in horses with complete immobility of the left arytenoid cartilage and vocal fold (grade IV recurrent laryngeal neuropathy).[19] It also can occur following laryngoplasty when there has been incomplete abduction of the arytenoid cartilage.[20] Axial deviation of the AEFs cannot be accurately diagnosed in the standing horse at rest and requires overground/high-speed treadmill endoscopy. Transendoscopic laser resection of the right AEF can be used to treat this condition and

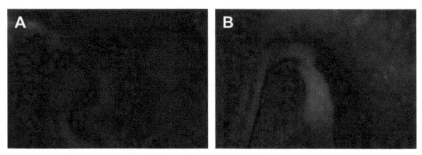

Fig. 17. (*A*) Right aryepiglottic fold collapse associated with grade 4 recurrent laryngeal neuropathy viewed using an overground endoscope with the horse galloping. (*B*) Right aryepiglottic fold collapse associated with a poor degree of left arytenoid cartilage abduction following left-sided laryngoplasty and unilateral left vocal cordectomy and bilateral ventriculectomy.

performed at the same time as the laryngoplasty and ventriculocordectomy procedure for treatment of recurrent laryngeal neuropathy (see **Fig. 17**).

Procedure

Following topical application of 60 mL of local anesthetic solution to the larynx, a videoendoscope is passed up the nostril ipsilateral to the AEF that is to be resected. The bronchoesophageal forceps are introduced into the opposite nasal passage and the center of the AEF is grasped by the bronchoesophageal forceps. Care must be taken to ensure that *only* the AEF and not the AEF along with the axial aspect of the pharyngeal mucosa is grasped. The AEF is then pulled axially across the rima glottides. This provides sufficient tension to resect the AEF by tracing a diode or Nd:YAG laser fiber (contact fashion) in a straight line from dorsal to ventral. Using this technique, an

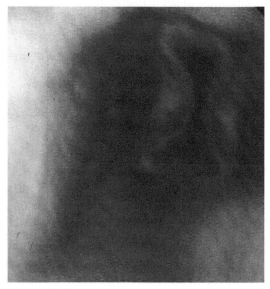

Fig. 18. Bilateral aryepiglottic fold collapse viewed with the horse undergoing high-speed treadmill examination.

approximately 2-cm wide crescent/triangle is removed from the AEF. After this, it is often necessary to resect more of the remaining ventral aspect of the AEF by elevating this part with the bronchoesophageal forceps and remove it with small horizontal passes of the laser fiber. After swapping over the nostril that the videoendoscope and bronchoesophageal forceps have been placed into, the same procedure is performed on the other side, by swapping nostrils for placement of the videoendoscope and bronchoesophageal forceps.

Advantages and disadvantages

Direct visualization allows for accurate resection, which is significantly more difficult to perform via a laryngotomy under general anesthesia. The reported success rate following AEF resection in this manner is 75%.[21]

Complications

Although no complications have been reported with this technique,[15] the first author has seen a horse that developed DDSP after excessive resection of an AEF.

Videoendoscopy-Assisted Unilateral Laser Vocal Cordectomy and Bilateral Ventriculocordectomy ("Hobday")

Diseases treated

Recurrent laryngeal neuropathy (RLN) and vocal cord collapse.

Removal of both laryngeal ventricles (saccules) as well as the left leading edge of the vocal cord does lead to a small increase of the cross-sectional area of the rima glottides. However, it is mainly used as an adjunct procedure following laryngoplasty[22–24] or as a sole treatment to reduce abnormal respiratory noise in sport and draft horses.[23,25–27] Vocal cordectomy can also be performed bilaterally, and although there is no evidence to support bilateral ventriculocordectomy over unilateral ventriculocordectomy for the treatment of RLN, some surgeons will perform the surgery bilaterally. However, there is a significant risk of laryngeal webbing occurring in inexperienced hands and, as a result, most surgeons will perform a unilateral left-sided vocal cordectomy with a bilateral ventriculectomy for RLN and if the right vocal cord needs to be removed, this can be performed 6 weeks later.

Procedure

A videoendoscope is passed up one nostril and 60 mL of local anesthetic solution is topically applied to the laryngeal mucosa and nasal passages. After a few minutes, a pair of bronchoesophageal forceps is passed up the contralateral nasal passage and used to grasp the left vocal cord at the midpoint. The forceps are rotated to apply axial traction on the dorsal part of the vocal fold. The laser fiber (Nd:YAG or diode) is passed down the biopsy channel of the endoscope until 2 cm of free fiber are protruding from the end of the endoscope. The laser is used in contact fashion to transect the vocal cord in a straight line from dorsal to ventral. Once this cut has been made, the vocal fold is pushed caudally into the airway to place tension on the ventral and cranial aspect of the remaining attachment. The laser fiber is used to make a horizontal cut starting rostrad and moving caudad to sever the remaining ventral attachment of the vocal cord. A blood vessel that runs through the ventral aspect of the vocal cord and is nearly always transected, will cause enough hemorrhage to obscure the vision of the operator. Therefore, the most ventral cut is made at the end of the procedure instead of at the beginning. Next, the laryngeal ventricles are removed. This can be performed by grasping and exteriorizing the mucosa of the ventricle with bronchoesophageal forceps or by use of a transnasal burr (**Fig. 19**).[26] In both cases, the everted mucosa is then excised with the laser. The first author prefers a third method

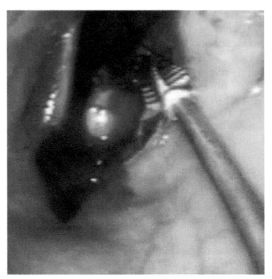

Fig. 19. Transnasal roaring burr used to exteriorize the laryngeal ventricles before laser resection. (*Courtesy of* Robinson P, Hong Kong Jockey Club, Hong Kong.)

of placing the laser fiber into the ventricle and using the laser energy to ablate the mucosal lining. This same procedure is performed on both ventricles. Postoperative care consists of administering throat spray and phenylbutazone for up to 10 days.

Advantages and disadvantages
Laser ventriculocordectomy avoids a surgical approach to the larynx and allows horses to return to work within 4 to 6 weeks. This is substantially quicker than the 3 months that are required after a conventional surgery. However, this surgery is challenging and it is recommended that only a surgeon with significant experience in the area of upper airway and laser surgery attempt this procedure in clinical cases.

Complications
Latent thermal necrosis can cause damage to the cartilages and surrounding soft tissue structures (intrinsic laryngeal muscles and mucosa). Occasionally, mucoceles may form in the ventricles following the noncontact laser ventriculectomy procedure.[28] Webbing between the 2 vocal cords is a concern when performing a bilateral vocal cordectomy in a single session. Therefore, this procedure is often performed unilaterally or in split into 2 stages.

Standing Laser Facilitated Ankylosis of the Thyroepiglottic Joint

Disease treated
Epiglottic retroversion (**Fig. 20**).

Procedure
A slightly bent 18-gauge 3-inch spinal needle is inserted through the skin at the level of the rostral aspect of the cricothyroid membrane. Using ultrasound, the needle is passed dorsal to the thyroid cartilage and advanced rostrally between the laryngeal mucosa and the cricoid without penetrating the airway. Transnasal videoendoscopy is useful to apply local anesthetic to the laryngeal mucosa and epiglottis. It also allows visualization of the needle passage and ensures that it has not penetrated the

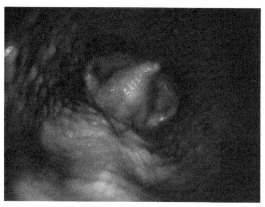

Fig. 20. Epiglottic retroversion.

laryngeal mucosa. Once the needle makes contact with the epiglottis, it's tip is slightly withdrawn, the stylet is replaced with a laser fiber (this author has only ever used a diode laser to do this at a setting of 18 W). Once the laser fiber touches the epiglottis, 3 linear passes of the laser fiber are made along the midline and the left and right aspects of the thyroepiglottic joint to deliver a total of 3000 J (N. Ducharme personal communication). The horse is rested for 30 days and reassessed; if the problem is still present, then the procedure is repeated.

Advantages and disadvantages
There are no highly successful therapeutic options for epiglottic retroversion. However, laser-facilitated ankylosis of the thyroepiglottic joint potentially provides a successful treatment. Further validation is required before the advantages and disadvantages can be fully understood.

Complications
One complication from this procedure is adhesion formation that sticks the epiglottis downward, resulting in dysphagia and aspiration (N. Ducharme personal communication). A single case that this author has performed resulted in the epiglottis being in a fixed position but at an approximate 45° angle. The result was that although the horse was less exercise intolerant, a significant, loud, and abnormal respiratory noise was still present. Further information on this technique will likely appear in the literature in due course and validation is required before it can be recommended as a suitable treatment.

Complications of Laser Surgery of the Upper Respiratory Tract
A significant complication that is often overlooked is damage to the endoscope. This risk to the endoscope can certainly increase in the standing horse. The user should always ensure that the tip of fiber is well beyond the end of the endoscope when discharged, but also that the protective lining surrounding the laser fiber is within the biopsy channel. The most common complication is collateral thermal damage, which is best avoided by using the lowest amount of energy required to complete the procedure. Taking great care to visualize the tip of the laser fiber before discharging the laser is also crucial to avoid injury to surrounding structures. Even though the laser coagulates small vessels, hemorrhage can occur during the procedure and make proper visualization impossible. Using the laser energy to stop bleeding vessels is possible but incurs the risk of additional thermal damage and inflammation. Postoperative swelling

of the surgery site(s) is a concern but rarely leads to clinically relevant complications. The administration of a dose of dexamethasone perioperatively can be used to mitigate this risk, and the authors recommend having an emergency tracheotomy kit on hand any time a laser-facilitated upper respiratory tract surgery is performed.

Standing Ventriculocordectomy

Diseases treated
Bilateral/unilateral vocal cord collapse and RLN.

Procedure
Standing ventriculocordectomy provides an alternative method to that using the laser, which has already been described. It is performed with the horse standing in stocks and the head in an extended position (**Fig. 21**). A 20-mL amount of local anesthetic is infiltrated into the subcutaneous tissues along a 10-cm line on the ventral aspect of the throatlatch, centered over the vertical ramus of the mandible (**Fig. 22**). A video-endoscope is passed up one nostril and local anesthetic (60 mL) is topical applied to the laryngeal mucosa. The videoendoscope is left in place to help with visualization of the procedure and act as the light source. The skin is incised and Metzenbaum scissors are used to part the 2 bellies of the paired sternothyroideus muscles. The muscles are separated by a small pair of Weitlander retractors, allowing exposure of the ventral cricothyroid membrane. Using a #10 scalpel blade, the membrane is opened on its entire length, cutting on midline from the cricoid cartilage to the "V" of the thyroid cartilage (**Fig. 23**). Under direct and videoendoscopic visualization, a roaring burr is placed into the ventricle, rotated until the mucosa is engaged tightly, and then moved in a ventral and medial direction to evert the mucosa. The mucosa is grasped with a pair of large forceps (Carmalt, Lahey Gall), traction is applied, and a second pair of forceps is applied behind the first pair, immediately adjacent to the vocal fold (**Fig. 24**).

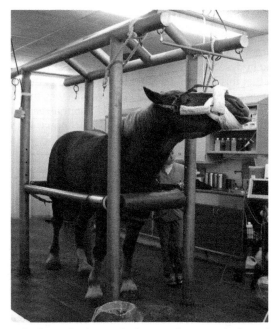

Fig. 21. Positioning of a horse in the stocks for standing ventriculocordectomy.

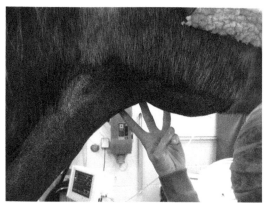

Fig. 22. Site of infiltration of local anesthesia before making a laryngotomy incision for a standing ventriculocordectomy.

The everted mucosa is transected with a pair of Metzenbaum scissors. The same procedure is repeated on the contralateral side. Now, a pair of Lahey Gall forceps is used to grasp the center of the leading edge of the vocal cord. Tension is applied to "tent" the vocal cord and a curved cut is made with a pair of Metzenbaum scissors, removing a crescent-shaped piece of vocal cord. It is important to leave approximately 1 cm of the ventral cord intact and to ensure that the corniculate process of the arytenoid

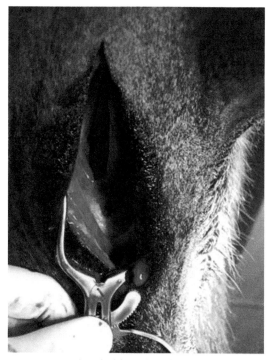

Fig. 23. Weitlander retractors in place holding the 2 bellies of the sternothryoideus muscles and the skin out of the way to facilitate the laryngotomy.

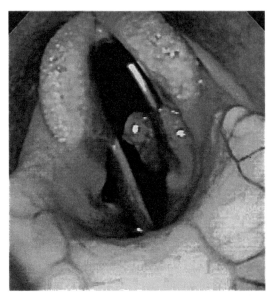

Fig. 24. The ventricle has been everted and then grasped with a pair of Carmalt forceps before transection.

cartilage is not damaged. The same procedure can, but does not have to be performed on the contralateral vocal cord (**Fig. 25**). A swab is used to clean the site of blood and the incisions are left to heal by second intention. Phenylbutazone is administered for 10 days and the use of throat spray is optional.

Advantages and disadvantages

The main advantage is that a bilateral vocal cordectomy can be performed using this technique without a significant risk of laryngeal webbing occurring. Bilateral ventriculocordectomy is an effective method of reducing abnormal respiratory noise caused by RLN and/or vocal cord collapse.[25] Furthermore, this procedure is quick, simple,

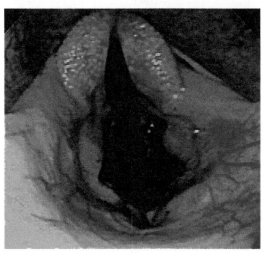

Fig. 25. A completed bilateral ventriculocordectomy.

and cost-effective and does not require any specialized equipment, and can be performed stall side if needed. The authors have commonly performed this procedure in heavy-muscled draft horses to avoid potential complications of general anesthesia. The main disadvantage is that the laryngotomy incision will produce discharge for up to 3 weeks and poses a possible risk of infection to a laryngoplasty incision, if a tieback has been performed at the same time. The laryngotomy incision usually heals without complications, but it is possible to close it partially or completely.[19]

Complications

Postoperative swelling around the ventriculocordectomy sites is a low risk, but it might be necessary to insert a tracheostomy tube into the laryngotomy to ensure a sufficient airway until the inflammation subsides. Even though bilateral ventriculocordectomy carries the risk of laryngeal webbing, it is unlikely to occur as long as the ventral 1 cm of each vocal cord is left intact. Postoperative hemorrhage can be significant, especially if the patient is left sedated with its head dropped. Therefore, it is recommended to keep the head in an elevated position for 10 to 15 minutes after completion of the procedure.

Standing Laryngoplasty

More information is due to be published on this in the near future, but the technique has been developed and is performed under local anesthesia in the same way as when performed in lateral recumbency under general anesthesia (**Fig. 26**) (N. Ducharme & F Rossignol personal communication).

Disease treated

Grade 3 and/or 4 RLN.

Advantages and disadvantages

It is reported that when performed in the standing position, a more appropriate assessment of the degree of abduction of the arytenoid cartilage is provided, which

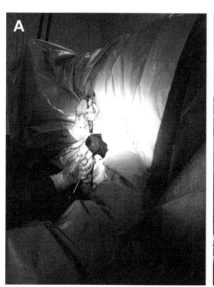
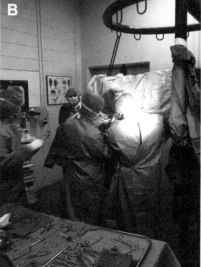

Fig. 26. (*A, B*) A standing laryngoplasty being performed. (*Courtesy of* JT Easley, Shelbyville, KY.)

hopefully reduces complications and improves success rates (N. Ducharme & F Rossignol personal communication).

TRACHEAL SURGERY
Standing Permanent Tracheostomy

Diseases treated
Any disease that has resulted in permanent upper respiratory tract obstructions, such as chondritis, bilateral laryngeal hemiplegia, and laryngeal cicatrix.

Procedure
The surgery is performed with the head of the horse in a moderately extended to "normal" position. A total of 30 mL of local anesthetic solution is placed subcutaneously in an inverted-U pattern, dorsal and lateral to the second through the fifth tracheal rings.[29] A 6-cm-long to 10-cm-long incision is made on midline, beginning 3 cm distal to the cricoid cartilage in the proximal third of the neck. Dissection is continued to the paired sternothyrohyoideus muscles, which are separated and retracted laterally. A 3-cm-wide wedge of muscle is removed from the medial aspect of each belly, the use of a diode laser or electrocautery to perform this resection aids hemostasis. The trachea is then exposed and desensitized with injection of 30 mL into the lumen of the trachea, using a 1-inch, 23-gauge needle.[29] A ventral midline incision is made through the second through to the fifth tracheal rings. This is followed by 2 paramedian incisions (1.5 cm from the midline) that are also made through each tracheal ring ensuring that the mucosa is left intact. The cartilage of each tracheal ring is then carefully dissected clear from the mucosa beneath, making sure to not penetrate or damage the mucosa. Then, the tracheal mucosa is transected in a double-ended "Y" pattern and carefully sutured to the surrounding skin, using a 2-0 monofilament suture in a simple interrupted pattern. Perioperative broad-spectrum antibiotics and phenylbutazone for 5 to 10 days are recommended. Postoperative care consists of cleaning the stoma twice daily until the sutures are removed in 2 weeks.

Advantages and disadvantages
This surgery provides a permanent and functional stoma that has a good cosmetic outcome. An advantage of doing the procedure standing is that the skin incision and the tracheostomy incision remain in the same location during and after the surgical procedure. This can be a little more difficult when the procedure is performed under general anesthesia, because it is performed in dorsal recumbency and the head and neck are extended. Furthermore, avoiding general anesthesia and endotracheal intubation in these cases with significant upper airway obstruction makes the procedure less complicated. Overall, 89% of horses return to their previous use and the 1-year survival rate is 97%, with an average survival time of 9.7 years.[30] Standing permanent tracheostomy can be safely performed and provides a viable alternative with a good prognosis for horses with permanent upper airway obstructions.

Complications
If too much of the tracheal rings is removed or if the removed segment is off-center, the trachea can collapse or become twisted.[29] Excessive shrinking of the stoma and inversion of the skin can occur, especially if there is too much tension on the incision. Excessive swelling and partial dehiscence are common complications in the immediate postoperative period.[30] Because the tracheostomy bypasses the upper airway, a significant element of the horse's natural respiratory defense mechanism is lost. This can result in an increased risk of lower airway disease.

MISCELLANEOUS SURGERIES
Standing Ceratohyoidectomy

Disease treated
Temporohyoid osteoarthropathy.

Procedure
Although this is not an upper respiratory tract procedure, it is worthy of mention.

The procedure is performed with the horse sedated and the head in an extended position. The throatlatch region aseptically is prepared. A 10-cm line extending rostrally from 2 cm caudal to the basihyoid bone and approximately half-way between the midline and the ramus of the mandible is infiltrated with local anesthetic. The skin is incised, followed by infiltration of the deeper tissues with local anesthetic solution. Next, the sternohyoideus and omohyoideus muscle fibers are bluntly separated to expose the basihyoid bone and its articulation with the ceratohyoid bone (**Fig. 27**). Dissection is continued rostrad to expose the entire ceratohyoid bone. The ceratohyoid-basihyoid bone articulation is sharply incised and the ceratohyoid bone is grasped with towel clamps (**Fig. 28**). It is then manipulated rostrad and ventrad, facilitating disarticulation from the stylohyoid bone. The area is lavaged and the incision is left to heal by second intention.

Advantages and disadvantages
The main advantage of performing this procedure in the standing horse is the ability to avoid general anesthesia in patients that are suffering from a disease that commonly leads to signs of neurologic dysfunction.

Complications
The only reported complication is the occurrence of intraoperative hemorrhage from iatrogenic damage to a branch of the linguofacial vein. This was treated successfully with ligation of the affected vessel. However, the only study that assessed this procedure was limited to 6 healthy horses and no clinical cases were included. Consequently, it remains unclear whether or not clinically affected horses would tolerate this surgery standing.[31]

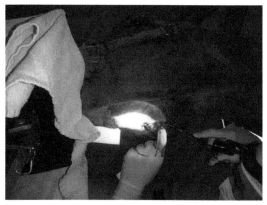

Fig. 27. Dissection of the soft tissues to expose the ceratohyoid bone in the standing horse. (*Courtesy of* T. O'Brien, Fethard, Tipperary, Ireland.)

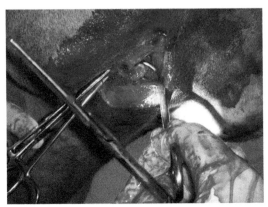

Fig. 28. Caudal end of the ceratohyoid bone disarticulated and grasped by a pair of towel clamps. (*Courtesy of* T. O'Brien, Fethard, Tipperary, Ireland.)

REFERENCES

1. Schumacher J, Dixon PM. Diseases of the nasal cavities. In: McGorum BC, Dixon PM, Robinson NE, et al, editors. Equine respiratory medicine and surgery. Philadelphia: Elsevier; 2007. p. 369–92.
2. Frankeny RL. Intralesional administration of formalin for treatment of epidermal inclusion cysts in five horses. J Am Vet Med Assoc 2003;223:221–2.
3. Tate LP, Blikslager AT, Little ED. Transendoscopic laser treatment of guttural pouch tumpany in eight foals. Vet Surg 1995;24(5):367–72.
4. Blazyczek I, Hamann H, Deegan E. Retrospective analysis of 50 cases of guttural pouch tympany. Vet Rec 2004;154:261–4.
5. Benredouane K, Lepage O. Trans-arterial coil embolization of the internal carotid artery in standing horses. Vet Surg 2012;41:404–9.
6. Judy CE, Chaffin MK, Cohen ND. Empyema of the guttural pouch (auditory tube diverticulum) in horses: 91 cases (1977–1997). J Am Vet Med Assoc 1999; 215(11):1666–70.
7. Perkins JD, Schumacher J, Kelly G, et al. Standing surgical removal of inspissated guttural pouch exudate (chondroids) in ten horses. Vet Surg 2006;35(7): 658–62.
8. Muñoz JA, Stephen J, Baptiste KE, et al. A surgical approach to the lateral compartment of the equine guttural pouch in the standing horse: modification of the forgotten "Garm technique". Vet J 2008;177:260–5.
9. Hawkins JF, Frank N, Sojka JE, et al. Fistulation of the auditory tube diverticulum (guttural pouch) with a neodymium: yttrium-aluminum-garnet laser for treatment of chronic empyema in two horses. J Am Vet Med Assoc 2001;218:405–7.
10. Gehlen H, Ohnesorge B. Laser fenestration of the mesial septum for treatment of guttural pouch chondroids in a pony. Vet Surg 2005;34(4):383–6.
11. Freeman DE. Complications of surgery for diseases of the guttural pouch. Vet Clin North Am 2009;24:485–97.
12. Perkins JD, Hughes TK, Brain B. Endoscope-guided, transoral axial division of an entrapping epiglottic fold in fifteen standing horses. Vet Surg 2007;36(8): 800–3.
13. Ducharme NG. Pharynx. In: Auer JA, Stick JA, editors. Equine surgery. Philadelphia: Elsevier; 2012. p. 569–91.

14. Lacourt M, Marcoux M. Treatment of epiglottic entrapment by transnasal axial division in standing sedated horses using a shielded hook bistoury. Vet Surg 2011;40(3):299–304.
15. Parente EJ. Laser surgery of the upper respiratory tract. In: McGorum BC, Dixon PM, Robinson NE, et al, editors. Equine respiratory medicine and surgery. Philadelphia: Elsevier; 2007. p. 533–41.
16. Rakesh V, Ducharme NG, Datta AK, et al. Development of equine upper airway fluid mechanics model for Thoroughbred racehorses. Equine Vet J 2008;40: 272–9.
17. Hogan PM, Palmer SE, Congelosi M. Transendoscopic laser cauterisation of the soft palate as an adjunctive treatment for dorsal displacement in the racehorse. In: Proceedings of the 48th Annual Convention of the American Association of Equine Practitioners. Orlando (FL): 2002. p. 228–30.
18. Anderson JD, Tullleners EP, Johnston JK, et al. Sternothyrohyoideus myectomy or staphylectomy for treatment of intermittent dorsal displacement of the soft palate in race horses: 209 cases (1986–1991). J Am Vet Med Assoc 1995;206:1909–12.
19. Beroza GA. Partial closure of laryngotomies in horses. J Am Vet Med Assoc 1994; 204:1227–9.
20. Dixon PM, Robinson NE, Wade JF, editors. Proc havemeyer workshop on equine recurrent laryngeal neuropathy. Newmarket (United Kingdom): R & W Publications; 2004. p. 96.
21. King DS, Tulleners EP, Martin BB Jr, et al. Clinical experiences with axial deviation of the aryepliglottic folds in 52 racehorses. Vet Surg 2001;30(2):151–60.
22. Rakestraw PC, Hackett RP, Ducharme NG, et al. Arytenoid cartilage movement in resting and exercising horses. Vet Surg 1991;20(2):122–7.
23. Fulton IC, Anderson BH, Stick JA, et al. Larynx. In: Auer JA, Stick JA, editors. Equine surgery. Philadelphia: Elsevier; 2012. p. 592–622.
24. Brown JA, Derksen FJ, Stick JA, et al. Laser vocal cordectomy fails to effectively reduce respiratory noise in horses with laryngeal hemiplegia. Vet Surg 2005; 34(3):247–52.
25. Cramp P, Derksen FJ, Stick JA, et al. Effect of ventriculectomy versus ventriculocordectomy in upper airway noise in draught horses with recurrent laryngeal neuropathy. Equine Vet J 2009;41:729–34.
26. Henderson CE, Sullins KE, Brown JA. Transendoscopic, laser-assisted ventriculocordectomy for treatment of left recurrent laryngeal hemiplegia in horses: 22 cases (1999–2005). J Am Vet Med Assoc 2007;231:1868–72.
27. Taylor SE, Barakzai SZ, Dixon P. Ventriculocordectomy as the sole treatment for recurrent laryngeal neuropathy: long-term results from ninety-two horses. Vet Surg 2006;35(7):653–7.
28. Hawkins JF. Neodymium: yttrium aluminum garnet laser ventriculocordectomy in standing horses. Am J Vet Res 2001;62(4):531–7.
29. Stick JA. Trachea. In: Auer JA, Stick JA, editors. Equine surgery. Philadelphia: Elsevier; 2006. p. 608–23.
30. Chesen AB, Rakestraw PC. Indications for and short- and long-term outcome of permanent tracheostomy performed in standing horses: 82 cases (1995–2005). J Am Vet Med Assoc 2008;232(9):1352–6.
31. O'Brien T, Rodgerson D, Livesey M. Surgical excision of the equine ceratohyoid bone in conscious sedated horses. Presented at the ACVS Conference. Chicago, May 1, 2011.

Standing Diagnostic and Therapeutic Equine Abdominal Surgery

Sarah Graham, DVM[a],*, David Freeman, MVB, PhD[b]

KEYWORDS

- Standing • Abdomen • Colic • Urolith • Laparoscopy • Uterus • Rectum

KEY POINTS

- The widespread use of laparoscopy in equine surgery has increased interest in the standing approach to a wide range of procedures typically regarded as feasible only through a ventral midline incision.
- Although a commonly cited benefit of standing surgery relates to avoiding costs of general anesthesia and risks associated with it, some procedures and horses are not suitable candidates for standing abdominal procedures.
- Some procedures, such as nephrectomy, colostomy, and closure of the nephrosplenic space, are not only suitable for standing surgery but are performed more easily and more safely through this approach than with general anesthesia.

STANDING FLANK LAPAROTOMY

Indications

A surgical approach to the abdomen via flank laparotomy in the standing horse is a useful technique under specific conditions. Historically, the most common indications for a standing flank approach are ovariectomy in the mare and correction of uterine torsion. Other indications that have been described include abdominal exploration, biopsy procedures, nephrosplenic entrapment of the large colon, closure of the nephrosplenic space (NSS), colostomy procedure for treatment of a rectal tear, nephrectomy, and ureterotomy. The standing flank approach in a horse with acute onset colic or anything greater than mild colic pain is not recommended because of limited exposure of the gastrointestinal tract and increased probability that the horse will be unable to remain standing for the entire procedure. Left, right, or bilateral approaches are feasible, and choice of laterality depends on the suspected diagnosis and desired exposure.

[a] Large Animal Clinical Sciences, University of Florida, Gainesville, FL, USA; [b] Large Animal Clinical Sciences, College of Veterinary Medicine, University of Florida, Gainesville, FL, USA
* Corresponding author.
E-mail address: sarahgraham@ufl.edu

Vet Clin Equine 30 (2014) 143–168
http://dx.doi.org/10.1016/j.cveq.2013.11.010
0749-0739/14/$ – see front matter © 2014 Elsevier Inc. All rights reserved.

Anatomy/Landmarks

The lateral wall of the abdomen is made up of the abdominal tunic (tunica flava abdominus), the external abdominal oblique muscle, the internal abdominal oblique muscle, the transverse abdominus muscle, transverse fascia, and peritoneum.[1] The paralumbar fossa in the horse is a triangular depression on the dorsolateral aspect of the abdomen. The boundaries of the fossa are the aponeurosis of the internal abdominal oblique muscle, the eighteenth rib, and the longissimus dorsi muscle. Surgical access to the abdomen though the paralumbar fossa is limited by its relatively small size (compared with cattle, which have a larger fossa and bigger space between the last rib and the tuber coxae).[2]

Patient Preparation

The horse is brought to the stocks area for surgery. The horse should be given a bath before surgery if it has a long and dirty hair coat. An intravenous (IV) catheter is placed in the jugular vein to allow rapid and easy access for administration of sedation or to allow administration of a continuous rate infusion (CRI). The stocks should be in a clean, quiet area with nonslip footing. The sides of the stocks should be removable in case the horse goes down. If possible, the sidebar that is on the side of the operator should be lowered to expose the entire flank region. A knowledgeable handler should be positioned at the head of the horse and should have access to the catheter and sedation. The flank region is clipped from the 15th rib to 10 cm caudal to the tuber coxae and from the fold of the flank to the dorsal midline. The tail is wrapped and secured so that it cannot be swished and contaminate the surgical site. A standard surgical preparation of the skin is performed. Local anesthesia is performed using sterile technique. An inverted L block may be performed; however, we find that local infiltration (superficially and deep) tends to provide more reliable anesthesia. Draping of the flank can be problematic, depending on the size of the horse and the configuration of the stocks. Generally, we place a large iodophor incise drape (Ioban, 3M) over the area of the intended incision. The iodophor drape provides a good surface for the adhesive backing on the large laparotomy drape, which is placed next. This large drape is passed over the dorsum of the horse and should cover the sidebar of the stocks. The closest vertical bar of the stocks can also be covered with a drape to prevent inadvertent contamination of the surgeon or assistant surgeon. We have found that with this draping technique, towel clamps are not generally required. If a towel clamp is needed to secure the drape, local infiltration of anesthetic should be performed before placement of the clamp.

Abdominal Exploration Through Standing Flank Approach

Exploration of the abdomen through a flank incision is performed largely through manual examination, because visibility is relatively poor. Exploration on the left side includes systematic palpation of the stomach, spleen, left kidney, nephrosplenic ligament, jejunum, left dorsal and ventral colons, mesenteric root, the pelvic flexure, small colon, rectum, uterus, bladder, and the left inguinal ring. For a right flank incision, palpation of the liver, duodenum, right kidney, jejunum, cecum, right dorsal and ventral colons, small colon, rectum, uterus, bladder, and the right inguinal ring should be performed. If the cecum is full of ingesta, exploration of the abdomen on the right side may be impossible.[2] Only a few structures may be safely brought to or exteriorized through the incision, and these include the jejunum, proximal ileum, left or right uterine horns, midsection of the small colon, pelvic flexure, and the apex of the cecum.

STANDING FLANK INCISION

A flank laparotomy is performed through a 12-cm to 15-cm vertical skin incision between the last rib and tuber coxae, below the tuber coxae at the dorsal border of the internal abdominal oblique muscle (**Fig. 1**). The incision should start 3 to 6 cm higher if the retroperitoneal space is to be opened. The external abdominal oblique muscle and fascia are incised sharply along the direction of the skin incision and the internal abdominal oblique is bluntly divided along its muscle fibers. In this way, a modified grid incision is made. The transversus abdominis muscle is divided bluntly along its muscle fibers, and the retroperitoneal space and peritoneal cavity are opened by blunt dissection, usually with the tips of Mayo scissors. It can be completely opened by digital separation of the tissues from dorsal to ventral. All layers of the incision can be opened as needed to allow insertion of the surgeon's hand, and the fibers of the internal abdominal oblique can be incised vertically for 2 to 3 cm for additional space.

The peritoneum and transversus abdominis muscle are closed as 1 layer with size 0 or 1 polyglactin 910 in a simple continuous pattern, and size 2 polyglactin 910 is used in a simple continuous pattern in the internal abdominal oblique muscle. The same suture material can be used in a simple continuous pattern to close the external abdominal oblique muscle, and the subcutaneous layer is closed in simple continuous fashion with size 2-0 polyglactin 910. Skin is closed with size 2-0 poliglecaprone 25 in simple continuous fashion or with a Ford interlocking pattern. The last 5 cm or so can be closed with 3 or 4 simple interrupted sutures, which can be removed as needed to facilitate drainage of a seroma or abscess, leaving the more dorsal suture line intact.

Flank incisions in horses are more prone to forming seromas or becoming infected than most incisions in this species, although this is not common enough to discourage use of this abdominal approach. This complication can probably be attributed to the

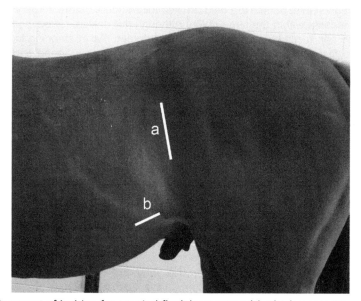

Fig. 1. Placement of incision for a typical flank laparotomy (a). The lower incision (b) is the site for placement of the stoma for a loop colostomy created with the double-incision technique.

muscle and tissue trauma associated with the incision and the depth of layers penetrated to enter the abdomen. In addition, the tight space in the horse's flank can contribute to the incisional trauma as the surgeon's hand and arm are repeatedly inserted and withdrawn.

STANDING FLANK LAPAROSCOPY
Indications

Laparoscopic evaluation of the abdomen in a standing horse is less commonly used than exploratory celiotomy under general anesthesia. The requirements for successful evaluation of a horse with colic signs are similar to those of standing laparotomy, the most important factor is that the horse is comfortable and healthy enough to remain standing for the procedure. Additionally, horses with acute onset or severe colic signs are poor candidates for laparoscopic exploration, because of increased likelihood of distended viscera, and therefore have an increased risk of iatrogenic injury. Conversely, some horses may be better suited for standing laparoscopic exploration, because of weakness from chronic disease, old age, or concomitant lameness, because the risks of anesthesia and recovery are mitigated. In some cases, laparoscopic evaluation may be used to confirm a diagnosis that indicates immediate surgical intervention (under general anesthesia) or euthanasia. However, the benefits of having a definitive diagnosis must be weighed against the cost of lost time and increased expense to the owner. Laparoscopic evaluation of the abdomen is therefore most commonly used for cases with chronic or recurrent colic after routine diagnostics have failed to result in a diagnosis. It can also be used to diagnose periparturient problems, such as postfoaling trauma to the uterus[3] or small colon,[4] hemorrhage into the broad ligament,[5] splenic trauma,[6] neoplasia, diaphragmatic hernia, abdominal abscesses,[5] and intestinal rupture.[5]

Patient Preparation

Whenever reasonable, horses are held off feed for 24 hours before surgery to reduce the bulk of ingesta within the large colon. Although not universally advocated, withholding feed can facilitate exploration of the abdomen. As in standing laparotomy, the horse is first restrained in standing stocks and the tail wrapped and secured. The preferred sedation protocol is generally initiated at this time. Left and right flank regions should be clipped, aseptically prepared, and draped to expose the paralumbar fossae. It is recommended that introduction of instruments is first performed on the left side of the horse to avoid unintended puncture of the cecum.[7] Use of disposable, guarded trocar and cannula[8] or use of an optical trocar (Covidian Medical) may also reduce the risk of organ penetration.

The laparoscope is introduced into the abdomen at a point that is halfway between the tuber coxae and the last rib, just dorsal to the crus of the internal abdominal oblique muscle. That site is blocked using infiltration of local anesthetic. A 1.5-cm-long skin incision is made with a number 10 scalpel blade. The laparoscopic trocar and cannula are then introduced through the muscle and into the abdomen by aiming toward the opposite coxofemoral joint. The trocar is removed and replaced with the laparoscope once a loss of resistance is perceived. Confirmation that the abdominal cavity has been entered is important before beginning insufflation; the abdomen is insufflated to a pressure of 10 to 15 mm Hg. Alternatively, some surgeons elect to insufflate the abdomen before introduction of the laparoscope to further reduce the potential for inadvertent puncture of bowel. A long teat cannula or Veress needle is inserted through the musculature and into the peritoneal cavity. Kolata and colleagues[9] described several ways to ensure that the Veress needle or cannula has penetrated the peritoneum: (1) a small hissing noise may be heard on penetration of the abdomen; (2) if the insufflation tubing is connected to the needle on penetration, a negative pressure may read on the insufflator; (3) aspirate from the needle to ensure no intestinal contents or blood from splenic puncture before injecting saline (no resistance should be appreciated on injection, and no saline recovered after injection); (4) when insufflating, the pressure within the abdomen should increase slowly and should not increase higher than 5 to 8 mm Hg within the first liter; (5) observation and ballottement of the abdominal cavity as it is filling may confirm insufflation. If asymmetric swelling, crepitus, or emphysema is noted near the cannula, or the horse becomes uncomfortable soon after insufflation has started, then the cannula is not within the abdomen. Alternatively, if a hand-assisted procedure is to be performed, the flank incision is made first (as described earlier). The surgeon's hand is then introduced into the abdomen and used to protect the viscera as the trocar and cannula are inserted into the abdomen.

The laparoscopic anatomy of the abdomen in the standing horse has been well described.[7] Evaluation of the left side is performed first, followed by the right. The laparoscope is passed up the left body wall, dorsal to the spleen to reach the left cranial abdomen. From the dorsal aspect, the diaphragm, left lobe of the liver, greater curvature and fundus of the stomach, gastrophrenic, phrenicosplenic, gastrosplenic, and nephrosplenic ligaments, the left kidney, and the spleen can be seen.[7] Ventrally, the spleen, stomach, and the left lateral lobe of the liver can be seen. The jejunum, small colon, left dorsal colon and pelvic flexure can be observed by directing the laparoscope more caudally.[7] The urinary bladder, left ovary and uterine horn or mesorchium and ductus deferens (depending on the sex of the patient) can be identified in the left pelvic region.[7] The laparoscope must be removed and inserted on the right side for evaluation of that portion of the abdomen. On the right side, left lateral, right lateral, caudate and quadrate lobes of the liver, pylorus, diaphragmatic flexure of the colons, hepatoduodenal and hepatorenal ligaments, descending and ascending duodenum, epiploic foramen, right lobe of the pancreas, right dorsal colon, transverse colon, base of the cecum, jejunum, small colon, rectum, right ovary and uterine horn or mesorchium and ductus deferens, and urinary bladder can be observed.[7] Other structures of lesser clinical importance may also be identified.[7]

BIOPSY TECHNIQUES

Intestinal biopsy may be indicated in cases of chronic weight loss or colic in order to diagnose neoplasia, eosinophilic or lymphocytic-plasmocytic enteritis, and primarily in Europe, grass sickness. If the affected bowel is exteriorizable, such as jejunum or pelvic flexure, then standard surgical biopsy techniques may be used. Often, the affected bowel cannot be accessed or exteriorized through a standard flank incision, and therefore, the surgeon must consider midline celiotomy or standing laparoscopic techniques. A full-thickness laparoscopic biopsy technique used in standing, experimental horses has been described.[10] This technique, although elegant, is technically challenging and requires good intracorporeal suturing skills.[10] Alternatively, another technique using an endoscopic linear stapler for obtaining small intestinal biopsies has been developed.[11] Use of either of these techniques in clinical cases has not yet been reported.

RECTAL TEARS

Rectal tears are usually caused by palpation per rectum. Noniatrogenic tears have been reported but are extremely rare.[12] Once a rectal tear is suspected, it should be evaluated for severity, the owner informed about the nature of the problem, first aid given if possible,[13] and the horse should then be referred to a veterinary hospital. Rectal tears are graded by severity of the tear and associated risk of peritonitis from I to IV.[13] Grade I (torn mucosa) and grade II (torn muscle layers) have the best prognosis, and grade III (torn mucosa and muscle layers) and grade IV (full thickness) have the poorest prognosis and require the most aggressive treatment.[13] Most tears are dorsolateral and a forearm's length from the anus, and the true extent and depth can be assessed by careful digital palpation after epidural anesthesia.[13–15]

All affected horses receive flunixin meglumine (1.1 mg/kg every 24 hours IV) and broad-spectrum antibiotics, such as sodium or potassium penicillin (22,000 IU/kg of body weight every 6 hours IV), gentamicin (6.6 mg/kg every 24 hours IV), and metronidazole (15 mg/kg every 6 hours or 20 mg/kg every 12 hours by mouth) until signs of peritonitis have resolved. IV fluids are required to treat shock initially. Antibiotics and laxatives are usually sufficient treatment of grade I, II, and some grade III tears, combined with daily inspection and careful manual removal of feces.

Colostomy

The preferred method for surgical treatment is loop colostomy, occasionally for grade III tears and mostly grade IV, with the goal of diverting feces away from these injuries so they do not become contaminated and impacted, enlarged, or in the case of grade III tears, converted to grade IV tears.[16] Colostomy can be combined with direct suture repair,[17] because it protects the suture line during healing. The loop colostomy technique is preferred over others, because it is easier and quicker to establish and to reverse later.[16] Concerns about incomplete diversion of feces do not apply to a loop colostomy in horse, because gravity, combined with correct construction of the stoma, prevents feces from entering the distal small colon and rectum.[16]

A double-incision colostomy involves a standard incision in the left flank below the tuber coxae and a separate lower flank incision for the stoma (see **Fig. 1**). The principle behind this approach is that it allows creation of a snug fit for the colon in the body wall in the lower incision, where the colon can empty readily and feces can fall away from the stoma with minimal contact with the skin.[16] Alternatively, a single incision can be placed low in the left flank for the stoma, but this is difficult as a standing procedure, because the incision must be large enough to correctly locate and place the colon.[16] Because this procedure involves a large flank incision, the body wall must be closed around the colon, and this creates a weaker body wall repair and makes the ventrally placed stoma prone to prolapse and herniation. With the double-incision technique, the stoma is placed in a low and snug flank incision, so that it is surrounded by intact body wall, and the risks of prolapse and herniation are reduced.

A standing approach is ideal for colostomy because: (1) muscle layers and landmarks are not distorted as they would be in the recumbent horse, so the colon can be placed more accurately through all layers; (2) the cost of general anesthesia is eliminated; and (3) dehiscence of the stoma during a rough anesthetic recovery is avoided. With the double-incision technique, a standard flank incision is used to prepare the distal loop of small colon and guide it into a separate low flank incision, midway between the fold of the stifle and the costal arch. Draping is optional for this procedure, because it can interfere with accurate location of landmarks, but a large iodophor adhesive drape should be used to protect the upper incision. The distal incision is approximately 8 cm long and is almost parallel with the flank fold, angled upwards at its caudal end by 20° to 30°. Deep dissection is guided by a hand through the flank incision. Small transverse incisions are made in muscles and fascia as needed to create an even and continuous opening through all layers, without bands that could obstruct fecal passage. The stoma should not be large but should fit snugly in the body wall. These guidelines should reduce the risk of stomal obstruction, prolapse, and herniation.[16]

The stoma is made in the small colon at least 1 m from the rectum, so that the small colon can be easily exteriorized for colostomy reversal.[16] The selected segment of small colon is folded to form a loop, and the 2 arms of the loop are sutured together side to side for 8 to 10 cm. For this, an absorbable material such as 2-0 polydioxanone is used in a continuous Lembert pattern that runs longitudinally midway between the mesentery and the antimesenteric band of each segment.[16] This suture line approaches the mesentery at the folded end to turn the antimesenteric tenia outward. The adhesion along this suture line creates a complete mucosal separation between the proximal and distal segments of small colon to ensure complete fecal diversion. The adhesion can also stabilize the loop and reduce the risk of prolapse. The loop of small colon is then inserted into the flank incision so that the proximal part is in the cranial end of the incision, the distal part is in the caudal end, and the antimesenteric tenia projects 3 to 4 cm beyond the skin.

The seromuscular layer of the colon is sutured to the abdominal muscles, fascia, and subcutaneous tissues using several interrupted sutures of 0 or 2-0 absorbable material, taking care not to penetrate the lumen or occlude or puncture mesenteric vessels.[16] To form the stoma, an 8-cm incision is made along the exposed antimesenteric tenia of the colon, and the cut edges are folded back and sutured to skin with simple interrupted sutures of 2-0 polydioxanone. The resulting stoma is approximately the same size as the small colon lumen. Because fecal balls are eliminated individually through the small colon, without accumulating as in the rectum, the risk of obstruction is low.

In the first 5 to 7 days after surgery, the mucosal protrusion of the stoma becomes markedly congested and slowly sloughs, to be replaced with healthy tissue.[16] The associated peristomal swelling resolves with time. Antibiotics and laxatives are continued for 3 to 5 days, and horses are fed hay at half the usual amounts for the first 2 to 3 days after surgery. A petrolatum-based ointment is applied to the skin around the stoma to protect it from scalding and a cradle is applied to prevent the horse from rubbing the colostomy.

When the rectal tear has started to granulate, usually after 5 to 7 days, the bypassed small colon and rectum are flushed daily in normograde fashion with approximately 20 L of warm water through a garden hose to exercise these segments. This procedure keeps the lumen as large as possible to facilitate end-to-end anastomosis at reversal.[16] For colostomy reversal, usually after 6 weeks or more, the horse is anesthetized in right lateral recumbency, the stoma is resected en bloc, and an end-to-end colocolostomy is performed through the resulting flank incision. This procedure could also be performed with the horse standing, but closure of the body wall defect created by removal of the stoma is difficult and must be secure. However, a standing closure is not jeopardized by a rough anesthetic recovery.

The most common complications of colostomy are dehiscence, abscessation, peristomal herniation, prolapse, and stomal obstruction before reversal, and anastomotic impaction and flank incisional dehiscence after reversal.

RECTAL PROLAPSE

Surgical treatment of rectal prolapse is a standing surgery on an abdominal organ that is performed with the organ in the prolapsed state. Causes of rectal prolapse are straining from diarrhea, dystocia, intestinal parasitism, colic, and rectal tumors.[18,19]

In many cases, a cause cannot be identified. Types of rectal prolapse are I to IV, with the first 3 types involving progressively greater amounts of rectal mucosa and submucosa projecting through the anus and including a variable amount of small colon in type III.[19] In a type IV prolapse, the peritoneal rectum and a variable length of the small colon form an intussusception through the rectum and anus.[19] This type of prolapse occurs during dystocia in mares and is evident as a tubular projection of a mucosa-lined organ, even reaching the point of the hock in severe cases.

Surgery

Most early type I and II prolapses respond to reduction and treatment of the primary problem. A submucosal resection may be indicated for type III and IV prolapses if the prolapsed tissues are devitalized or the prolapse recurs after conservative treatment.[18] After epidural anesthesia and gentle cleaning of the prolapsed tissues, 2 14-gauge, 13-cm-long (5.25 in) catheters with the stylet in place are inserted at right angles to each other through the external anal sphincter and healthy mucosa to maintain the prolapse during dissection.[18] Starting at the 12 o'clock position, circumferential incisions are made in healthy tissue for one-third of the prolapse circumference, combined with deep dissection to elevate a strip of edematous and necrotic mucosa and submucosa.[18] Remaining healthy proximal and distal edges of the mucosa and submucosa are apposed with size 1 polydioxanone in an interrupted, horizontal mattress pattern.[18] These steps are repeated for each of the remaining thirds of the circumference until all necrotic tissue has been removed.[18] Mucosal edges are subsequently apposed with 2-0 polydioxanone in a simple continuous pattern interrupted at 3 equidistant points around the circumference.[18] The retaining catheters are removed and the tissues allowed to return to their normal positions. Postoperative management includes laxatives, a laxative diet, and, if necessary, careful digital removal of impacted feces from the rectum.

Resection and anastomosis may be indicated for type IV prolapse if the prolapsed tissues are devitalized or too much is involved to allow reduction.[18] The procedure can be performed as for submucosal resection, except that full-thickness circumferential incisions are made in healthy tissue through the inner and outer walls of the intussusceptum.[18] The concentric edges thus created are apposed with size 1 polydioxanone in an interrupted, full-thickness, horizontal mattress pattern. These steps are repeated for each of the remaining thirds of the circumference until all necrotic tissue has been removed. Care must be taken during resection to identify and ligate any mesenteric vessels in the prolapse. Mucosal edges are then apposed in a simple continuous pattern with 2-0 polydioxanone, interrupted at 3 equidistant points around the circumference. The transfixing cross-needles and the weight of the necrotic tissue maintain the line of anastomosis outside the rectum during surgery, and removal of the needles allows it to return to the abdomen afterward. Postoperative management is the same as for submucosal resection.[18] The prognosis is favorable if there is no associated vascular damage or mesenteric disruption. However, such changes are unlikely if viable and healthy margins are evident along the line of resection.

UTERINE TORSION

Uterine torsion causes low-grade abdominal pain in mares during late pregnancy and can account for 5% to 10% of total dystocias in mares.[20,21] In 1 study of 26 cases, torsion occurred at a mean of 9.6 months (288 days) of gestation, and in a study of 103 mares, stage of pregnancy at presentation was 236 to 368 days, with 4 mares (3.9%) presenting at parturition.[22] The direction of rotation is almost equally distributed between counterclockwise and clockwise,[22–24] and the degree of torsion ranges from 180° to 540°.[20,21] The uterus can rupture secondary to torsion, but this is uncommon. Diagnosis is not always straightforward, although it can be made if the twist in the uterus can be palpated per rectum, cranial to the cervix, and 1 or both broad ligaments can be felt following the direction of rotation.

Treatment

The choice of treatment is determined largely by the condition of the mare and fetus, the stage of gestation, and expense. Correction through a flank approach with the mare standing is a widely used and successful method. In 1 multicenter study, foal survival was significantly better if uterine torsion was corrected by standing flank laparotomy than by ventral midline celiotomy.[24] No reason for this finding was apparent except that maybe general anesthesia itself was harmful to these foals.[24] Also, large mares in advanced pregnancy are an anesthetic challenge[25] and are at increased risk of long bone fracture and incisional dehiscence during recovery. Therefore, the midline approach should be reserved for those mares that are unsuitable for other methods or have a concurrent gastrointestinal tract disease. Rolling is a cost-saving option, but not always successful, especially in late pregnancy.[24] It is imperative that the direction of rotation is accurately diagnosed for rolling to be successful.

Flank Approach

Flank laparotomy is used on the standing mare with local anesthetic infiltrated along the proposed incision site, and with a CRI of detomidine to keep the mare sedated and comfortable. Although epidural anesthesia may be used in conjunction with a local anesthetic, this is unnecessary and might be contraindicated, because it could induce hindlimb weakness, frequent weight shifting, and recumbency.

Vandeplassche and colleagues[20,21] recommended that the abdomen be entered from the side to which the torsion is directed (eg, left flank if the torsion is counterclockwise, right if it is clockwise as viewed from behind the mare). A 15-cm to 20-cm incision is placed high on the flank, with the top of the incision at the level of the ventral aspect of the tuber coxae. A vertical incision is made through all layers except the internal abdominal oblique muscle, which is divided along its fibers. The direction of torsion is confirmed. Generally, the uterus is not compromised, and some discoloration and edema do not signify a poor prognosis for continued pregnancy. If working from the side to which the rotation is directed (eg, right flank if the torsion is clockwise, left flank if counterclockwise), the uterus overlying a prominent part of the foal is gently rocked up and down through short arcs (25–30 cm) to gain some momentum. The rotation is then completed by lifting and pushing the uterus to its correct position. Care must be used to avoid tension on the wall, which could rupture the uterus, especially if it is edematous and friable. This procedure can be facilitated by alternating between pulling up on the uterus and pushing against its dorsal edge.

If the abdomen is entered on the side opposite that to which the torsion is directed (eg, left flank if the torsion is clockwise, right flank if counterclockwise), the hand is passed dorsally above the uterus to find a prominent part of the foal, which is then pulled toward the operator. Once rotation is started, the weight of the fetus and uterus may help to draw them around completely to a normal position. An alternative is to push the ventral aspect of the uterus from the operator, instead of pulling on the dorsal aspect of the uterus. Both methods can be alternated as needed to correct the torsion.

Correction of a uterine torsion close to term is difficult through a flank approach, because of the weight and size of the foal and uterus. Torsions of 240° or less are easiest to correct and are associated with less uterine edema than more severe torsions. If it proves impossible to correct the torsion through a flank approach, the incision can be closed, and the mare is then anesthetized for a ventral midline celiotomy. In some cases, 2 surgeons might have to work simultaneously through right and left flank incisions to correct the torsion.[22]

The main concern after successful correction of uterine torsion is abortion, and progesterone therapy (respositol progesterone, 1000 mg intramuscularly every 4 days, or progesterone in oil, 300 mg daily) is considered by some to be of value. Preoperative treatment is the same as for an adult horse with colic, but might need to be more aggressive after surgery when complicated by shock, uterine congestion, or rupture. Mares should be confined to a stall for 3 weeks to reduce stress on the suture line.

Prognosis

In a recent retrospective study that combined cases from 4 equine referral hospitals,[24] the stage of gestation at which uterine torsion developed was a risk factor for survival of mare and foal. Although overall mare survival was 53 of 63 (84%), survival was 97% when uterine torsion developed at less than 320 days' gestation, compared with 65% survival rate when uterine torsion developed at 320 days' gestation or more.[24] Although overall foal survival was 54% (29/54) in the same study, it was 72% when uterine torsion developed at less than 320 days' gestation, compared with 32% when uterine torsion developed at 320 days' gestation or more.[24] The prognosis for delivery of a live foal was good if the mares were discharged from the hospital with a viable fetus, with 25 of 30 mares (83%) in this group delivering live foals that survived beyond the neonatal period.

The prospects for subsequent fertility seem to be good in mares that have had a uterine torsion.[22] A chronic form of uterine torsion has been described as a result of failure to diagnose the disease in its early stages, and can cause weight loss, anemia, fever, and mild colic.[26] This condition be treated only by ovariohysterectomy, which can save the mare, but obviously terminates her reproductive career.[26]

NSS CLOSURE

Ablation or closure of the NSS is a commonly performed laparoscopic surgery intended to reduce recurrent entrapment of the left dorsal and ventral colons over the nephrosplenic ligament (left dorsal displacement of the large colon [LDDLC]).[27–30] In a report of 44 horses with laparoscopic surgery and of 4852 horses treated for colic over 16 years,[27] 6% had LDDLC, and 21% of this group of horses had recurrence of the displacement. Hand-assisted laparoscopic ablation of the NSS is the technique with which we are most familiar and is described in some detail, and other methods are described briefly.

Case Selection

In our hospital, horses that are typical candidates for hand-assisted laparoscopic closure of the NSS fall into 3 main categories: (1) horses in which recurrent LDDLC has been confirmed at a surgery after a previous surgical treatment of LDDLC; (2) horses in which recurrent LDDLC is strongly suspected based on a favorable response to nonsurgical treatment (phenylephrine, rolling) at a subsequent admission after a previous successful treatment of LDDLC (surgical or nonsurgical); and (3) horses that have recurrent episodes of colic attributed on clinical examination to recurrent colonic displacement, but without confirmation of LDDLC as the cause.

Many horses with recurrent LDDLC in the first category would be candidates for a colopexy or large colon resection at the same surgery that confirmed recurrence, if planned in advance by the owner and surgeon and depending on surgeon preference. Although ultrasonography can be used to confirm or refute recurrence in the third group, it has limitations, and colic can resolve in some horses with this disease before they arrive at a hospital where ultrasonography can be performed. In such cases, the owner is informed that other problems could cause recurrent colic, and closure of the space prevents only one of them, which may not be the cause. Once recurrent LDDLC is diagnosed at surgery or suspected based on response to nonsurgical treatment, and a decision is made to close the NSS, the surgery should be performed as soon as the horse is stabilized after correction of LDDLC and within the same hospitalization period.

Surgical Preparation

NSS ablation can be performed standing through the left paralumbar fossa using a traditional surgical flank incision combined with laparoscopy. Feed is withheld for 12 to 24 hours preoperatively to reduce intestinal contents and thereby improve access and laparoscopic view of the NSS. The horse is sedated with detomidine hydrochloride CRI in stocks and the left flank is prepared for sterile surgery. Local anesthesia of the skin and body wall can be accomplished with an inverted L in the paralumbar fossa, a paravertebral block, or by direct injection along each proposed incision.[31] A 20-gauge or 18-gauge 3.81-cm (1.5-in) needle is used to inject 2% lidocaine or 2% mepivacaine at each site, making sure that the skin blebs are visible. Large volumes of local anesthetic are required, including additional intraoperative injections if needed, but usually less than 200 mL per 500 kg horse.[31] Separate sites for towel clamps are injected with local anesthetic through 20-gauge needles and marked by leaving the needles in place until clamps are applied. Drapes are applied to cover the dorsum and left side of the horse.

Surgery

After a 12-cm to 15-cm flank incision is made below the tuber coxae and behind the last rib, the laparoscope is inserted dorsocranial to it through a 2-cm to 2.5-cm incision, with abdominal insertion guided by a hand in the abdomen (**Fig. 2**). Abdominal insufflation is not possible nor necessary for this procedure. The spleen, NSS, and stomach should be visible cranial to the incision, and some intestine, small or large, might need to be swept manually from the NSS. Needle holders for this surgery should be robust enough to handle the large needle that is required, and 2 are optimal, so the needle can be passed through the tissue by one and then retrieved as it exits by the other. The preferred needle holders have a 40-cm working length (Surgical Direct, Deland, FL). The preferred suture is size 2 Vicryl (Polyglactin 910, Ethicon, Summerville, NJ), which provides an ideal length of 135 cm (54 in) and has a large taper point needle, which can span 2 to 4 cm of tissue.

The needle is first passed through 2 to 4 cm of the most cranial aspect of the perirenal fascia in a dorsal to ventral direction, with the point of insertion level with or slightly below the dorsal edge of the spleen. This placement ensures that the line of traction on the dorsal rim of the spleen is horizontal from lateral to medial and not dorsomedial to ventrolateral, which could impose too much upward traction on the spleen and cause the suture to pull through the capsule. The next bite is in a ventral to dorsal direction from the medial side of the splenic rim to emerge through the dorsal edge. The needle is then exteriorized and passed through a small loop at the end of the suture or through a modified Roeder knot (more secure), and this is tightened by using a laparoscopic Babcock forceps to push the knot (**Fig 3**A). This procedure

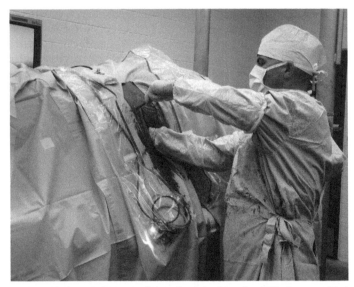

Fig. 2. Laparoscope inserted dorsocranial to flank incision for NSS closure with hand in the abdominal incision to guide safe cannula insertion.

should roll the dorsal edge of the spleen medially to contact the perirenal fascia (see **Fig 3**B).

Subsequent bites continue in the same fashion, using hand assistance as needed, to create a continuous suture line from cranial to caudal, with each successive set of bites at 1 to 2 cm apart (**Fig. 4**). As each bite through spleen and capsule is completed, it is manually drawn, so as to maintain snug apposition between spleen and perirenal fascia. As the line of closure continues, the space between the kidney and spleen becomes progressively narrower, which can impede needle placement. Some hemorrhage is inevitable and can be removed with a laparotomy sponge introduced with a grasping forceps and then rotated as it is drawn from cranial to caudal along the trough between the spleen and kidney. The NSS is closed entirely when the caudal extent of the nephrosplenic ligament is reached, and a hand tie is then used to secure the needle end of the suture to the last loop on the suture line. The flank incision and laparoscopy portal are closed routinely.

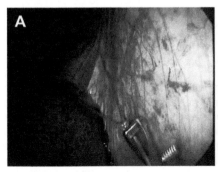
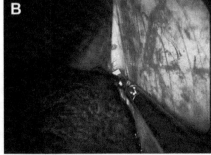

Fig. 3. Intraoperative view of the use of the modified Roeder knot. Using laparoscopic Babcock forceps to tighten the knot (*A*). The dorsal edge of the spleen moves medially to contact the perirenal fascia, once the knot once is tightened (*B*).

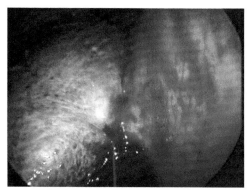

Fig. 4. Intraoperative view of continuous suture line from cranial to caudal for NSS closure.

Outcomes and Comments

The advantages of hand-assisted laparoscopic ablation of the NSS include an easier procedure than surgery performed completely by laparoscopy, avoidance of general anesthesia and associated expense, and manual suture tightening, which allows the appropriate degree of tension to be applied without risk of a loose attachment or cutting through the splenic capsule. The same approach can also be used to correct entrapment if present at the time of surgery and then close the NSS by laparoscopy.[32]

With all methods designed to close the NSS, horses can develop other forms of colic not prevented by this procedure.[28] Nonetheless, laparoscopic NSS closure can decrease the overall prevalence of colic and need for colic surgery.[28] Although recurrence of LDDLC after any method of NSS closure is rare, it has been reported at 6.5 years after laparoscopic space ablation in 1 horse.[33] This finding was attributed to the horse's young age at the time of surgery or inadequate suture bites or spacing in the perirenal fascia and splenic capsule.[33] Complications of laparoscopic closure of the NSS are rare, but a delayed bout of intra-abdominal hemorrhage was tentatively attributed to this procedure in 1 horse, presumably because the suture tore through part of the splenic capsule. Therefore, these horses should be kept quiet in a stall during the first 3 weeks after surgery. The line of closure of the NSS usually heals completely and is free of adhesions to other abdominal structures.

Other Methods for NSS Closure

A laparoscopic method to close the NSS, which requires laparoscopic instruments only (not hand assisted) and uses a custom cannula, was shown to prevent LDDLC over a 22-month follow-up period.[28] A method of laparoscopic closure with mesh was evaluated in 5 healthy mature horses.[29] A polypropylene mesh measured to fit the NSS was inserted and attached to the dorsolateral splenic capsule and perirenal fascia with helical titanium coils.[29] This method requires 1 laparoscopic and 2 instrument portals in the left flank.[29] At repeat laparoscopy 4 weeks later and necropsy at intervals of 4 to 14 weeks after surgery, all mesh implants were covered by fibrous tissue, and the mesh adhered to itself and drew the splenic capsule and perirenal fascia into apposition.[29] Each mesh implant was firmly adhered to the spleen, nephrosplenic ligament, and perirenal fascia, but 1 horse had an adhesion from the mesh to the small colon mesentery.[29] No horse developed colic.[29] In another laparoscopic method, etilefrin-induced splenic contraction facilitated suture placement and closure of the NSS.[27] LDDLC did not recur, although 5 horses had subsequent episodes of colic; 4 horses had displacement of the ascending colon between the spleen and body wall.[27] Others have also reported displacement of the colon between the spleen and body wall.[32]

STANDING LAPAROSCOPIC NEPHRECTOMY

In the horse, nephrectomy by a hand-assisted laparoscopic approach on the standing horse seems to be considerably safer and easier than the open approach on an anesthetized horse.[34–39] The procedure can avoid the long and expensive anesthesia associated with the open method. Rib resections are not necessary, and therefore, the risk of pneumothorax is avoided.[34] The most common indications for nephrectomy in the horse include unilateral diseases, such as hydronephrosis, nephrolithiasis, pyelonephritis, abscessation, neoplasia, and ectopic ureter.[34–39]

The horse is fasted for 12 to 24 hours before surgery to reduce the volume of ingesta within the digestive tract and is then prepared for a standing surgery as described earlier for closure of the NSS.[34] A 10-cm to 12-cm vertical skin incision is made in the middle of the paralumbar fossa, beginning at the dorsal border of the internal abdominal oblique muscle, and a modified grid technique is used to expose the peritoneum. The peritoneum is then bluntly penetrated and the peritoneal opening is enlarged. A hand in the abdomen guards against trauma to adjacent viscera (see **Fig. 2**) as a trocar-cannula unit is inserted through the flank musculature just dorsal to the most dorsal margin of the skin incision (**Fig. 5**).[34] The trocar is removed and a 320-mm, 0° laparoscope is inserted through the cannula. An instrument portal is made 4 to 6 cm cranial to and 2 to 3 cm dorsal to the laparoscope portal (see **Fig. 5**). The left and right kidneys can be located but cannot be seen behind the perirenal fat and fascia that encloses them in the retroperitoneal space.

A laparoscopic injection needle is inserted through the flank incision to infiltrate the retroperitoneal space between the kidney and peritoneum with 20 to 50 mL of 2% mepivacaine. The perirenal peritoneum is lacerated with the tip of the needle

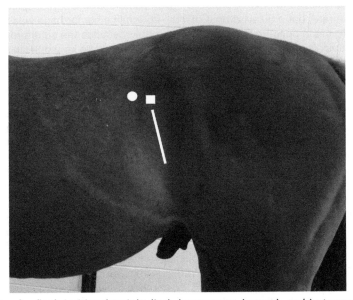

Fig. 5. Sites for flank incision (*straight line*), laparoscope (*square*), and instrument portals (*circle*) for left standing laparoscopic nephrectomy.

before removal.[34] The peritoneum around the kidney is massaged to distribute the local anesthetic throughout the retroperitoneal space. The peritoneal laceration is digitally enlarged and the kidney is dissected free from surrounding retroperitoneal fat to expose the ureter and renal vein and artery.

Careful digital dissection is used to expose the renal pedicle and ureter so that they can be viewed through the endoscope. The artery is identified and separated by careful digital dissection and a loop of size 2 polyglactin 910, 135 cm (54 in) long, is placed around it by digital insertion and retrieved with a laparoscopic instrument. Alternatively, a Deschamps needle is used to place the suture around the artery so that it can be digitally retrieved. Alternatively, the suture can be passed from a laparoscopic needle holder around the cranial edge of the artery to be retrieved by another needle holder passed dorsal to the vessel. The tips of the needle holders are angled slightly (Surgical Direct, Deland, FL), and this feature can be used to direct the suture end around the cranioventral edge of the vessel so it comes into view dorsal to the vessel. The suture is then tied through the flank incision with a sliding half hitch or Roeder knot, and the knot is digitally tightened until the surgeon is satisfied that it is secure. At least 2 more ligatures are applied in the same manner, so the artery is occluded distal to the line of transection with 1 ligature and about 1 cm proximal to it by 2 ligatures. The artery is then transected between the distal 2 ligatures. The artery is ligated before the vein, because venous occlusion as the first step would cause blood to pool in the kidney and possibly enlarge it.

These steps are repeated for the vein, and then the ureter is freed up by blunt dissection, and the kidney is drawn through the flank incision (**Fig. 6**). The ureter is double-ligated distal to the proposed line of transection and is then cut with laparoscopic scissors. Transecting the ureter before the vessels is another option that allows easy identification of both the renal artery and vein.[34] Also, care should be taken to ensure there are no accessory arterial branches to the kidney that require ligation.[34] If the kidney has an abscess or is enlarged with pyelonephritis, special care must be taken to ensure that septic contents are not released into the abdomen or into the incision. Placement of the kidney in a sterile plastic bag within the abdomen before it is drawn through the incision might be indicated in these cases.[34] The incisions are closed in a routine manner.

Outcomes and Comments

Although the preceding description applies to left-sided nephrectomy, a similar method can be used for the right kidney.[35] Intraoperative hemorrhage has been

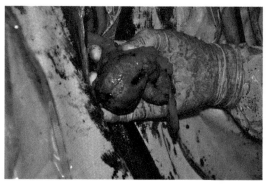

Fig. 6. After the ureter is freed up by blunt dissection, the kidney can be drawn through the flank incision, with the ureter as the only remaining attachment.

reported during this procedure,[35] but it can be controlled with Carmalt or Rochester Pean forceps. Back bleeding from the kidney can be substantial if the vein is cut before adequately ligated and before the artery is ligated. Some horses might be mildly uncomfortable after surgery, but this is manageable.[35] Obviously, health of the remaining kidney is critical to outcome, and some diseases, such as nephrolithiasis, are bilateral to some degree.[40–42] Therefore, function of the remaining kidney needs to be monitored frequently, and phenylbutazone, other nonsteroidal antiinflammatory drugs, and potentially nephrotoxic drugs should be avoided or used with care. Although a recent report described nephrectomy through a ventral midline approach in equids,[43] this method was not tested on large adult horses, which is the group most suited to a standing nephrectomy. However, the ventral midline approach allows excellent access for nephrectomy in foals and is the method of choice for foals with ureteral defects and ectopia that are unresponsive to other surgical treatments.

OTHER STANDING LAPAROSCOPIC PROCEDURES

Standing laparoscopy has also been used to investigate causes of colic in horses,[6] but it is most suitable for diseases without abdominal distention or pain at the time of surgery. Suitable candidates are horses with a history of chronic, recurrent colic with mild or no pain at surgery, or horses with weight loss. In some cases, standing laparoscopy is useful to confirm or refute a tentative diagnosis that has evolved from other diagnostic procedures, such as abdominal radiographs, abdominal ultrasonographic examination, gastroscopy, rectal examination, and peritoneal fluid analysis. It might be an easier and less expensive alternative to a ventral midline celiotomy for horses suspected of having untreatable lesions, such as ruptured viscus or neoplasia, when the owner wants absolute confirmation before granting permission for euthanasia. It can also be used for intestinal biopsy (see earlier discussion).

Laparoscopic adhesiolysis (**Fig. 7**) has been described in the horse,[44–47] and a standing approach could be used when the adhesions are strongly suspected to be in the dorsal abdomen. Adhesion prevention after adhesiolysis is improved by the addition of 0.5% ferric hyaluronate gel to the affected serosal surfaces.[44] An intra-abdominal abscess and cyst can also be evaluated and drained by standing laparoscopic surgery.[48,49] Experimentally induced rectal tears have been successfully repaired by standing laparoscopy.[50] In a broodmare that underwent a ventral midline

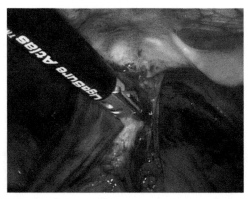

Fig. 7. Adhesiolysis using the Ligasure. (*Courtesy of* Dean Hendrickson, DVM, Fort Collins, CO.)

correction of a small intestinal strangulation in a rent in the mesenteric duodenum, the most dorsal aspect of the rent was inaccessible at surgery.[51] Subsequently, a standing right flank laparoscopic approach allowed excellent access and complete closure of the defect.[51]

A method for inguinal hernioplasty has been described as a standing laparoscopic procedure on stallions that were previously treated for strangulating inguinal herniation without castration.[52] Three portals in the flank were used to approach the vaginal rings.[52] A large inverted U-shaped peritoneal flap was then dissected and elevated proximal and cranial to the vaginal ring, and was reflected caudally over it.[52] The flap was secured to the abdominal wall with laparoscopic staples.[52] Inguinal herniation recurred in a few horses if only the cranial and middle thirds of the vaginal ring were covered but was completely prevented if the flap sealed the entire vaginal ring.[52] Major complications were not encountered, and all stallions were successfully used for breeding after surgery.[52] Although standing laparoscopy seems well suited for repair of dorsal diaphragmatic hernia in horses, access can be restricted by curvature of the diaphragm away from the surgeon and by viscera overlying the defect.[53] Instead, thoracoscopy and intrathoracic suture can be used in the standing sedated horse.[53]

STANDING FLANK APPROACH TO REMOVE URETEROLITHS

Nephroliths and ureteroliths are well-recognized causes of proximal urinary tract obstruction in horses, and induce an insidious and progressive disease, which can be characterized by varying severities of lethargy, depression, anorexia, and weight loss.[40–42] By the time diagnosis is usually made, renal disease from the obstruction has progressed to the point that renal damage is irreversible, and residual function in the affected kidney is minimal. Also, proximal urinary tract obstruction from uroliths or nephroliths can be bilateral, which reduces the chances for complete recovery.[40,41] Ureteral calculi can also be rare incidental findings on palpation per rectum for other reasons,[42] and nephroliths can be incidental findings at necropsy (**Fig. 8**). In these cases, a functional contralateral kidney is presumed to be responsible for the lack of clinical signs and absence of azotemia.[42] In all horses in which a urolith is found in any part of the urinary tract, other segments should be examined for involvement.[54]

Laboratory evidence of upper urinary tract obstruction is reflected in serum biochemical changes, such as elevated blood urea nitrogen, creatinine, and

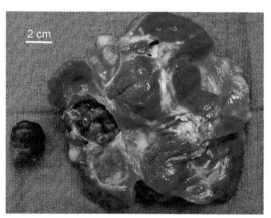

Fig. 8. Nephroliths as incidental findings at necropsy in a horse without renal disease. Note several small stones in the renal pelvis after the 1 large stone was removed.

potassium levels. On examination per rectum, when the hand is swept dorsally for a short distance from the brim of the pelvis, a ureteral stone can usually be found approximately 10 cm from the neck of the bladder. The distended and thickened ureter can be palpated in the retroperitoneal space cranial to that point. Both sides of the abdomen should be checked.

An ultrasonographic examination of both kidneys and ureters is usually diagnostic. Transrectal ultrasonographic examination with a 7.5-mHz linear array transducer can show a distended ureter proximal to a variable-sized ureteral calculus, which shadows as a mineral opacity.[42] The kidneys are closely examined by transabdominal ultrasonographic examination with a 3.5-mHz curved array transducer, and obstructed kidneys can range in size from smaller to larger than normal and have abnormal renal architecture and cystic cavities, which indicates some degree of hydronephrosis. A careful search for shadows from mineral opacities is needed to find nephroliths, which could be obstructing outflow from the pelvis in the absence of any evidence of ureteral obstruction. Cystoscopy can be used to subjectively compare and assess urine flow from the ureteral openings into the bladder and can show a large mucous plug in the opening on the obstructed side.[42]

A renal biopsy can be taken to assess renal damage, if it would contribute meaningfully to available information, but this procedure carries risks.[40]

Surgery

Obstructive ureteroliths approximately 10 cm from the bladder were removed from 2 mature geldings through a standing flank approach, which allowed simultaneous access to the peritoneal cavity and the retroperitoneal space (**Fig. 9**).[42] Goals of the surgery were to allow excretion of urine and mucus from the affected kidney so that it might regain some function and not undergo further deterioration or develop pyelonephritis.

The obstructed ureter is usually thick walled, dilated to approximately 2.5 cm in diameter, and tortuous, all of which makes it more amenable to surgical access and ureterotomy closure through this approach.[42] The added length gained through distention and associated tortuosity allows approximately 10 to 12 cm of ureter to be freed up in proximal and distal directions so that a 6-cm segment can be elevated to the level of the skin (see **Fig. 9**). A hand inserted into the peritoneal cavity can palpate a ureterolith distal to the isolated segment but cannot massage it away from there in either direction, because of the degree of ureteral constriction around the calculus and the adhesion of ureteral lining to its rough surface. Removal by manual massage toward the ureterotomy might be easier for a recent obstruction, but most are likely to be long-standing by the time of surgery.

Two 2.54-cm-wide (1 in) Penrose drains are used to retain the ureter at skin level, so it can be incised longitudinally for 3 cm (see **Fig. 9**). Some mucus can drain through the incision, and this can be removed by suction and submitted for culture. A 56.5-cm-long uterine biopsy forceps (Eppendorfer Uterine Biopsy Forceps, Miltex, Bethpage, NY) is introduced through the ureterotomy, approximately 25 cm proximal to the calculus (**Fig. 10**). When it reaches the calculus, the jaws of the instrument are opened, and a hand in the abdomen manipulates the calculus into the jaws to be crushed into fragments, which can be removed in piecemeal fashion (**Fig. 11**).

After the stone is removed, a 6.6-mm × 137-cm stallion catheter (Jorgensen Laboratories, Loveland, CO) is inserted distally into the ureter, and sterile saline is injected through this to assess patency and flush any loose fragments into the bladder. A urethrostomy can be made beforehand in geldings to create an egress for the lavage fluid and to place an indwelling urinary catheter as a stent to maintain patency if the ureter

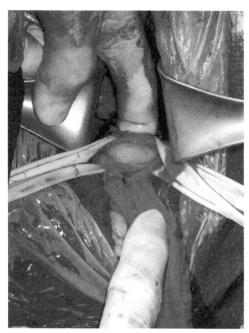

Fig. 9. Flank approach that allows simultaneous access to the peritoneal cavity and the retroperitoneal space so the ureter can be exposed. Two 2.54-cm-wide (1-in) Penrose drains are used to retain the ureter at skin level so it can be incised. Note the sponge in the incision to catch any fragments that could drop off the instrument as it is removed.

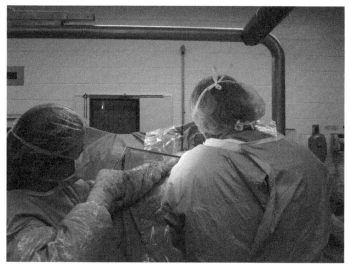

Fig. 10. Insertion of a long uterine biopsy forceps (Eppendorfer Uterine Biopsy Forceps, Miltex, Bethpage, NY) through the ureterotomy, proximal to the calculus and directed distally toward it.

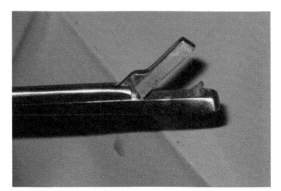

Fig. 11. Jaws of the uterine biopsy forceps containing part of ureterolith removed and showing the shape of the jaws, which allows them to elevate the fragment from the mucosa (*bottom jaw*) and crush it (*upper jaw*).

swells.[42] However, the latter is not essential and can cause an ascending pyelonephritis if left in for long periods.[42] The ureterotomy is then closed in a simple continuous pattern with size 2-0 polydioxanone, taking care to avoid mucosal penetration, and the flank incision is closed in routine manner.

Aftercare

Perioperative care involves IV polyionic fluids at maintenance rates until biochemical measures of renal function return to normal (**Fig. 12**). Preoperative antibiotics such as potassium penicillin (22,000 U/kg [10,000 U/lb], IV, every 6 hours) are given and need be continued in the postoperative period only if an indwelling stent is left in

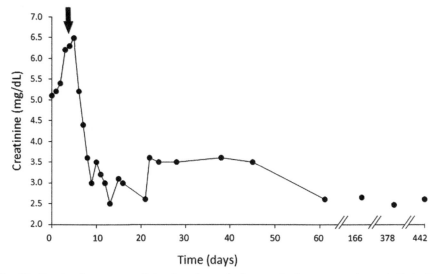

Fig. 12. Graph of serum creatinine in a horse before and after surgery (*arrow*). Note the marked improvement after the left kidney was unobstructed, but failure to regain normal values (reference range, 0.8–2.2 mg/dL), because this horse had bilateral renal disease. It was subsequently killed because of bilateral obstructive renal disease.

the ureter. Such tubes and contents as well as any fluid removed from the ureter at surgery should be cultured and sensitivity tested in case the horse subsequently develops an ascending urinary tract infection.[42] Flunixin meglumine can be given for pain control, if IV fluids are given concurrently. Cecal impaction can develop in hospitalized horses that have undergone a variety of surgical procedures, including surgery for ureteral obstructions,[42,54,55] and therefore motility modifying drugs, such as butorphanol, should be used sparingly if at all.

Urine acidifiers such as ammonium chloride and ascorbic acid are recommended but have not proved to prevent recurrence of calculi in horses.[56,57] Ascorbic acid must be given daily by stomach tube, because it is not consumed willingly in the dose required.[56,58] Ammonium chloride (Ammonium chloride USP granular, Fisher Scientific, Pittsburgh, PA) can be given by dose syringe in syrup at 28.3 g (1 oz) by mouth every 12 hours to acidify the urine and prevent recurrence, but can fail in this purpose and also cause inappetance.[42] It can increase urinary fractional excretion of calcium in goats and thereby increase the risk of calcium-based uroliths.[59] Dietary measures to consider are diets low in cation-anion balance to decrease urinary pH,[60] grass hay to reduce urinary calcium excretion, and a concentrate diet to lower urinary pH.[40,56]

Outcomes and Comments

The technique used for ureterolith removal was successful in both horses in which it was reported, and did not require sophisticated equipment. The uterine biopsy forceps is superior to shorter grasping instruments, such as arthroscopic forceps, because of its length and robust design.[42] Despite successful removal of the urolith, 1 horse developed pyelonephritis in the affected kidney and died of complications from subsequent nephrectomy. The other horse was killed, because it developed obstructive nephroliths in the contralateral kidney. These deaths underscore the importance of bilateral renal involvement in such cases, the need for early intervention whenever possible, the need for continued monitoring of renal function (see **Fig. 12**), and the importance of nephrectomy as first-line of treatment in horses with advanced renal disease[40] (see earlier discussion for description). Therefore, owners should be advised that removal of a ureterolith might not resolve renal failure, even if it does resolve hydronephrosis on the affected side.[42]

Other methods for urolith removal require retrieval baskets (Segura Basket, Cook Urological, Spencer, IN), laser technology (see later discussion), or various instruments for lithotripsy that cannot be easily inserted into the ureter of geldings.[58,61–67] Although ureteral entry with such instruments is possible in mares,[40,68] a perineal urethrostomy in male horses would not provide the same degree of access without a rigid endoscope.[58] A ventral midline celiotomy in the anesthetized horse might not allow adequate access for ureterotomy closure[68] and might necessitate an additional paralumbar incision and exteriorization of much of the large and small intestines to improve access.[55]

SURGICAL REMOVAL OF CYSTIC CALCULI

Horses with cystic calculi usually have a history of dysuria, hematuria, frequent urination, low-grade colic, urine scalding of the hind legs, stilted hind leg gait, prolonged penile protrusion, and passage of dark, cloudy urine. Geldings seem to be affected more so than mares, possibly because mares can pass the calculus before they reach a certain size. Although cystic calculi can be removed through a caudal ventral midline celiotomy, access to them in the caudal abdomen can be gained through a standing perineal urethrostomy[69] or through a standing pararectal cystotomy (Gokel procedure).[70] Uroliths can range in size from 3 to 10 cm, with mean and median diameters of 6.37 and 6 cm, respectively.[70] Usually, these uroliths are solitary, but multiple calculi have been reported.[70] Most are formed from calcium carbonate and have a rough, spiculated surface.

Surgery

For the pararectal approach, the neck of the bladder is approached through a vertical incision lateral to the rectum, followed by blunt dissection.[70] The bladder is entered through a retroperitoneal cystotomy, and the calculus is removed intact. A perineal urethrostomy is performed through a 6-cm vertical skin incision, which starts proximally 10 cm ventral to the anus and extends distally to the ischial arch.[69] A stay suture is placed on both sides of the urethrostomy through the urethral mucosa, corpus spongiosum penis, bulbospongiosus muscle, and retractor penis muscle, and then sutured to the adjacent skin to retract the urethrostomy edges. Before removal through a perineal urethrostomy, the typical cystic calculus in a horse must be broken into several small fragments by lithotripsy, which can be time consuming.

For lithotripsy, the calculus is stabilized in the neck of the bladder by a hand in the rectum. An osteotome or a long screwdriver with a wide slotted head is placed against the calculus and is rotated into the center of it with some force until the surface starts to crumble. The process is repeated at different sites on the calculus until more fragments progressively break off around the edges. A lithotrite can be used instead for lithotripsy, but these are not readily available (**Fig. 13**). A uterine biopsy forceps or a sponge forceps is used to grasp and remove fragments, and most of the remaining sediment is syphoned from the bladder through a sterile stomach tube.

The perineal urethrostomy is left open to heal by second intention (**Fig. 14**). Within a few days after surgery, the bladder should be free of any sediment and the mucosal inflammation should be reduced. Other instruments developed specifically for lithotripsy can also be used, such as electrohydraulic,[61,62] ballistic shock wave,[63] radial extracorporeal shock wave,[64] pulsed dye laser,[65,66] and holmium:yttrium aluminum garnet laser.[67] These lasers require specialized and expensive equipment and expertise with their use.[58]

Perioperative treatment involves antibiotics (optional; see earlier discussion for ureterotomy) and flunixin meglumine for pain control (1.1 mg/kg [0.5 mg/lb], IV, every 12 hours). Urinary tract acidifiers are also recommended, although these have some limitations that influence efficacy (see earlier discussion for ureterotomy). In general, urethrostomy has a low complication rate, and usually the incision is fully healed within 3 weeks in horses.[54,69]

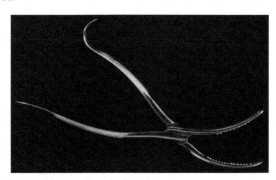

Fig. 13. Lithotrite for crushing cystic calculi in horses.

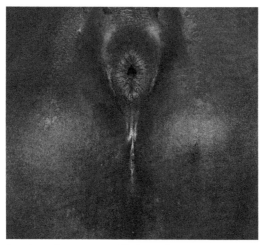

Fig. 14. Healing perineal urethrostomy at 10 days after surgery.

REFERENCES

1. Sisson S. Equine myology. In: Getty R, editor. Sisson and Grossman's the anatomy of domestic animals. 5th edition. Philadelphia: WB Saunders; 1975. p. 407–12.
2. Ross MW. Standing abdominal surgery. Vet Clin North Am Equine Pract 1991; 7(3):627–39.
3. Hassel DM, Ragle CA. Laparoscopic diagnosis and conservative treatment of uterine tear in a mare. J Am Vet Med Assoc 1994;205:1531.
4. Ragle CA, Southwood LL, Galuppo LD, et al. Laparoscopic diagnosis of ischemic necrosis of the descending colon after rectal prolapse and rupture of the mesocolon in two post-partum mares. J Am Vet Med Assoc 1997;210:1646.
5. Fischer AT. Laparoscopic evaluation of horses with acute and chronic colic. In: Fischer AT, editor. Equine diagnostic and surgical laparoscopy. Philadelphia: WB Saunders; 2002. p. 131–42.
6. Mehl ML, Ragle CA, Mealey RH, et al. Laparoscopic diagnosis of subcapsular splenic hematoma in a horse. J Am Vet Med Assoc 1998;213(8):1171–3.
7. Galuppo L. Laparoscopic anatomy. In: Fischer AT, editor. Equine diagnostic and surgical laparoscopy. Philadelphia: WB Saunders; 2002. p. 7–28.
8. Walmsley JP. Review of equine laparoscopy and an analysis of 156 laparoscopies in the horse. Equine Vet J 1999;31:456.
9. Kolata RJ, Freeman LJ. Access, port placement and basic endoscopic skills. In: Freeman LJ, editor. Veterinary endosurgery. St Louis (MO): Mosby; 1999.
10. Schambourg MM, Marcoux M. Laparoscopic intestinal exploration and full-thickness biopsy in standing horses: a pilot study. Vet Surg 2006;35:689–96.
11. Bracamonte JL, Bouré LP, Geor RJ, et al. Evaluation of laparoscopic technique for collection of serial full-thickness small intestinal biopsy specimens in standing sedated horses. Am J Vet Res 2008;69(3):431–9.
12. Slone DE, Humburg JM, Jagar JE, et al. Noniatrogenic rectal tears in three horses. J Am Vet Med Assoc 1982;180(7):750–1.
13. Baird AN, Taylor TS, Watkins JP. Rectal packing as initial management of grade 3 rectal tears. Equine Vet J Suppl 1989;7:121–3.

14. Arnold S, Meagher D, Lohse C. Rectal tears in the horse. J Equine Med Surg 1978;2:55–63.
15. Arnold J, Meagher D. Management of rectal tears in the horse. J Equine Med Surg 1978;2:64.
16. Freeman DE, Richardson DW, Tulleners EP, et al. Loop colostomy for management of rectal tears and small colon injuries in horses: 10 cases (1976–1989). J Am Vet Med Assoc 1992;200(9):1365–71.
17. Eastman TG, Taylor TS, Hooper RN, et al. Treatment of grade 3 rectal tears in horses by direct suturing per rectum. Equine Vet Educ 2000;63.
18. Turner TA, Fessler JF. Rectal prolapse in the horse. J Am Vet Med Assoc 1980; 177(10):1028–32.
19. Turner TA. Rectal prolapse. In: Robinson NE, editor. Current therapy in equine medicine. 2nd edition. Philadelphia: WB Saunders; 1987.
20. Vandeplassche M. Obstetrician's view of the physiology of equine parturition and dystocia. Equine Vet J 1980;12:45–9.
21. Vandeplassche M, Spincemaille L, Bouters R, et al. Some aspects of equine obstetrics. Equine Vet J 1972;4:105–13.
22. van der Weijden B. Proceedings of foal and fertility congress, Zwolle International, Zwolle, Netherlands, 2007. p. 1–10.
23. Pascoe JR, Meagher OM, Wheat JD. Surgical management of uterine torsion in the mare: a review of 26 cases. J Am Vet Med Assoc 1981;179:351–4.
24. Chaney KP, Holcombe SJ, LeBlanc MM, et al. The effect of uterine torsion on mare and foal survival: a retrospective study, 1985–2005. Equine Vet J 2007;39:33–6.
25. Maney JK, Quandt JE. Anesthesia case of the month. J Am Vet Med Assoc 2012;241:562–5.
26. Doyle AJ, Freeman DE, Sauberli DS, et al. Clinical signs and treatment of chronic uterine torsion in two mares. J Am Vet Med Assoc 2002;220:349–53.
27. Röcken M, Schubert C, Mosel G, et al. Indications, surgical technique, and long-term experience with laparoscopic closure of the nephrosplenic space in standing horses. Vet Surg 2005;34:637–41.
28. Farstvedt E, Hendrickson D. Laparoscopic closure of the nephrosplenic space for prevention of recurrent nephrosplenic entrapment of the ascending colon. Vet Surg 2005;34:642–5.
29. Epstein KL, Parente EJ. Laparoscopic obliteration of the nephrosplenic space using polypropylene mesh in five horses. Vet Surg 2006;35(5):431–7.
30. Mariën T, Adriaenssen A, Hoeck FV, et al. Laparoscopic closure of the renosplenic space in standing horses. Vet Surg 2001;30(6):559–63.
31. Hendrickson DA. A review of equine laparoscopy. ISRN Vet Sci 2012;492650: 1–17. http://dx.doi.org/10.5402/2012/492650.
32. Muñoz J, Bussy C. Standing hand-assisted laparoscopic treatment of left dorsal displacement of the large colon and closure of the nephrosplenic space. Vet Surg 2013;42:595–9.
33. Barrell EA, Kamm JL, Hendrickson DA. Recurrence of renosplenic entrapment after renosplenic space ablation in a seven-year-old stallion. J Am Vet Med Assoc 2011;239:504–7.
34. Rodgerson DH. Laparoscopic assisted nephrectomy and nephrosplenic space ablation. In: Proceedings of American College of Veterinary Surgeons. 2008. p. 60–2.
35. Röcken M, Mosel G, Stehle C, et al. Left- and right-sided laparoscopic-assisted nephrectomy in standing horses with unilateral renal disease. Vet Surg 2007; 36(6):568–72.

36. Keoughan CG, Rodgerson DH, Brown MP. Hand-assisted laparoscopic left nephrectomy in standing horses. Vet Surg 2003;32(3):206–12.
37. Cokelaere SM, Martens A, Vanschandevijl K, et al. Hand- assisted laparoscopic nephrectomy after initial ureterocystostomy in a shire filly with left ureteral ectopia. Vet Rec 2007;161(12):424–7.
38. Romero A, Rodgerson DH, Fontaine GL. Hand assisted laparoscopic removal of a nephroblastoma in a horse. Can Vet J 2010;51(6):637–9.
39. Mariën T. Laparoscopic nephrectomy in the standing horse. In: Fischer AT, editor. Equine diagnostic surgical laparoscopy. Philadelphia: Saunders; 2002. p. 273–81.
40. Schott HC. Obstructive disease of the urinary tract. In: Reed SM, Bayly WM, Sellon DC, editors. Equine internal medicine. 3rd edition. St Louis (MO): Saunders Elsevier; 2010. p. 1201–43.
41. Ehnen SJ, Divers TJ, Gillette D, et al. Obstructive nephrolithiasis and ureterolithiasis associated with chronic renal failure in horses: eight cases (1981-1987). J Am Vet Med Assoc 1990;197:249–53.
42. Frederick J, Freeman DE, MacKay RJ, et al. Removal of ureteral calculi in two geldings via a standing flank approach. J Am Vet Med Assoc 2012;241(9): 1214–20.
43. Arnold CE, Taylor T, Chaffin MK, et al. Nephrectomy via ventral median celiotomy in equids. Vet Surg 2013;42(3):275–9.
44. Lansdowne JL, Bouré LP, Pearce SG, et al. Comparison of two laparoscopic treatments for experimentally induced abdominal adhesions in pony foals. Am J Vet Res 2004;65(5):681–6.
45. Bleyaert HF, Brown MP, Bonenclark G, et al. Laparoscopic adhesiolysis in a horse. Vet Surg 1997;26(6):492–6.
46. Bouré L, Pearce SG, Kerr CL, et al. Evaluation of laparoscopic adhesiolysis for the treatment of experimentally induced adhesions in pony foals. Am J Vet Res 2002;63(2):289–94.
47. Bouré L, Marcoux M, Lavoie JP, et al. Use of laparoscopic equipment to divide abdominal adhesions in a filly. J Am Vet Med Assoc 1998;212(6):845–7.
48. Mair TS, Sherlock CE. Surgical drainage and postoperative lavage of large abdominal abscesses in six mature horses. Equine Vet J Suppl 2011;43(39):123–7.
49. Scheffer CJ, Drijfhout PN, Boerma S. Subperitoneal cyst in a Friesian mare. Tijdschr Diergeneeskd 2004;129(14–15):468–70.
50. Brugmans F, Deegen E. Laparoscopic surgical technique for repair of rectal and colonic tears in horses: an experimental study. Vet Surg 2001;30(5):409–16.
51. Sutter WW, Hardy J. Laparoscopic repair of a small intestinal mesenteric rent in a broodmare. Vet Surg 2004;33(1):92–5.
52. Wilderjans H, Meulyzer M, Simon O. Standing laparoscopic peritoneal flap hernioplasty technique for preventing recurrence of acquired strangulating inguinal herniation in stallions. Vet Surg 2012;41(2):292–9.
53. Röcken M, Mosel G, Barske K, et al. Thoracoscopic diaphragmatic hernia repair in a warmblood mare. Vet Surg 2013;42(5):591–4.
54. Laverty S, Pascoe JR, Ling GV, et al. Urolithiasis in 68 horses. Vet Surg 1992;21: 56–62.
55. Byars TD, Simpson JS, Divers TJ, et al. Percutaneous nephrostomy in short-term management of ureterolithiasis and renal dysfunction in a filly. J Am Vet Med Assoc 1989;195:499–501.
56. Wood T, Weckman TJ, Henry PA, et al. Equine urine pH: normal population distributions and methods of acidification. Equine Vet J 1990;22:118–21.

57. Reimillard RL, Modransky PD, Welker FH, et al. Dietary management of cystic calculi in a horse. J Eq Vet Sci 1992;12:359–63.

58. Rodger LD, Carlson GP, Moran ME, et al. Resolution of a left ureteral stone using electrohydraulic lithotripsy in a thoroughbred colt. J Vet Intern Med 1995;9: 280–2.

59. Mavangira V, Cornish JM, Angelos JA. Effect of ammonium chloride supplementation on urine pH and urinary fractional excretion of electrolytes in goats. J Am Vet Med Assoc 2010;237:1299–304.

60. McKenzie EC, Valberg SJ, Godden SM, et al. Plasma and urine electrolyte and mineral concentrations in thoroughbred horses with recurrent exertional rhabdomyolysis after consumption of diets varying in cation-anion balance. Am J Vet Res 2002;63:1053–60.

61. MacHarg MA, Foerner JJ, Phillips TN, et al. Electrohydraulic lithotripsy for treatment of cystic calculus in a mare. Vet Surg 1985;14:325–7.

62. Eustace RA, Hunt JM. Electrohydraulic lithotripsy for the treatment of cystic calculus in two geldings. Equine Vet J 1988;20:221–3.

63. Koenig J, Hurtig M, Pearce S, et al. Ballistic shock wave lithotripsy in an 18-year-old thoroughbred gelding. Can Vet J 1999;40:185–6.

64. Verwilghen D, Ponthier J, Van Galen G, et al. The use of radial extracorporeal shockwave therapy in the treatment of urethral urolithiasis in the horse: a preliminary study. J Vet Intern Med 2008;22:1449–51.

65. Howard RD, Pleasant RS, May KA. Pulsed dye lithotripsy for treatment of urolithiasis in two geldings. J Am Vet Med Assoc 1998;212:1600–3.

66. May KA, Pleasant RS, Howard RD, et al. Failure of holmium:yttrium-aluminum-garnet laser lithotripsy in two horses with calculi in the urinary bladder. J Am Vet Med Assoc 2001;219:957–61.

67. Judy CE, Galuppo LD. Endoscopic-assisted disruption of urinary calculi using a holmium:YAG laser in standing horses. Vet Surg 2002;31:245–50.

68. Macharg MA, Foerner JJ, Phillips TN, et al. Two methods for the treatment of ureterolithiasis in a mare. Vet Surg 1984;13:95–8.

69. Lillich JD, DeBowes RM. Urethra. In: Auer JA, Stick JA, editors. Equine surgery. 3rd edition. St Louis (MO): Elsevier; 2006. p. 887–93.

70. Abuja GA, García-López JM, Doran R, et al. Pararectal cystotomy for urolith removal in nine horses. Vet Surg 2010;39(5):654–9.

Standing Male Equine Urogenital Surgery

Aric Adams, DVM[a],*, Dean A. Hendrickson, DVM, MS[b]

KEYWORDS

- Standing ● Male ● Equine ● Urogenital surgery ● Cryptorchid ● Inguinal hernioplasty
- Phallectomy

KEY POINTS

- Standing laparoscopic cryptorchidectomy provides exceptional visualization of inguinal anatomy of horses and allows for consistent identification of retained testicles.
- Laparoscopic inguinal herniorrhaphy or hernioplasty should be considered after correction of acquired inguinal hernias to prevent recurrence in stallions that are to be breeding animals.
- Standing castration is safe to perform and avoids the time, cost, and complications associated with general anesthesia.
- The standing modified Vinsot partial phallectomy technique[54] is a safe and simple surgery that is particularly suited for debilitated or very large horses.

Given that male urogenital surgeries are among the most common soft tissue surgeries performed in horses, it is beneficial for the equine practitioner to be familiar with a variety of standing techniques. The advantages of performing standing male urogenital surgeries are often numerous when compared with performing the same surgery in the anesthetized animal. Some traditional standing male urogenital surgeries, such as castrations, may be faster to perform and can be performed with less expense, because general anesthesia is avoided. Laparoscopic standing male urogenital surgeries may allow for improved visualization of the surgical field, decreased hemorrhage, and decreased morbidity and convalescence. Limitations of standing procedures may include increased danger to the surgeon because of fractious behavior of the patient, and increased expense and training associated with instrumentation for specialized procedures such as laparoscopy.

STANDING LAPAROSCOPIC CRYPTORCHIDECTOMY

Laparoscopic cryptorchidectomy has become one of the most common laparoscopic procedures performed in equine hospitals, because of the high prevalence

[a] Equine Medical Center of Ocala, 7107 W Hwy 326, Ocala, FL 34482, USA; [b] Professional Veterinary Medicine, 1601 Campus Delivery, Colorado State University, Fort Collins, CO 80523, USA
* Corresponding author.
E-mail address: aadams@emcocala.com

Vet Clin Equine 30 (2014) 169–190
http://dx.doi.org/10.1016/j.cveq.2013.11.005
0749-0739/14/$ – see front matter © 2014 Elsevier Inc. All rights reserved.

> **Key points**
>
> - Standing laparoscopic cryptorchidectomy provides exceptional visualization of inguinal anatomy of horses and allows for consistent identification of retained testicles.
> - Transabdominal ultrasonography and hormonal assays help identify cryptorchid horses if the history of castration is uncertain.
> - Initial trocar cannula placement with or without prior insufflation of the abdomen is one of the most important steps of the procedure.
> - Suture loop placement, extracorporeal emasculation, and electrosurgical methods are all safe and effective techniques that are used to remove retained testicles.

of cryptorchidism in horses.[1] Cryptorchidism is the failure of 1 or both testicles to normally descend into the scrotum, resulting in abdominal or inguinal retention of the testicle. Surgical removal of cryptorchid testicles can be performed using a variety of traditional techniques, including inguinal, parainguinal, and flank laparotomy. These traditional techniques can often be performed more quickly than the standing laparoscopic technique, but the surgeon's inability to visualize the abdominal testicle using these techniques can lead to frustration and prolonged surgery time on occasion. The main surgical advantage of performing standing laparoscopic cryptorchidectomies compared with traditional techniques is superior observation of the surgical field, leading to repeatable identification of the testicle. Avoiding the complications associated with general anesthesia and the surgeon's ability to make smaller incisions while performing the laparoscopic technique may also decrease the likelihood of postoperative morbidity compared with traditional techniques.

Diagnosis

Cryptorchid testicles are capable of producing testosterone, so these horses continue to have undesirable stallionlike behavior, even without a normal scrotal testicle. Identification of cryptorchid stallions can be challenging, because many of these horses have inaccurate histories regarding previous castration.

Diagnostic techniques

- Inguinal or transrectal palpation: easy to perform but may be inaccurate or dangerous in young and fractious horses.
- Transabdominal ultrasonography: can be accurate and easy to perform[2] but, in our experience, can be time consuming and less reliable than previously described. If you find a testicle you can be confident one is there, if you do not find a testicle, it does not rule out the presence of a testicle.
- Hormonal assays: accurate and easy to perform but can be expensive.
  - Basal testosterone: geldings are generally less than 40 pg/mL. Cryptorchid horses are generally greater than 100 pg/mL.[3] Wide variations in basal testosterone levels in both geldings and stallions may lead to inaccurate interpretation of the results.[4]
  - Human chorionic gonadotropin (hCG) stimulation test: an hCG stimulation test improves the accuracy of using testosterone to identify retained testicular tissue to about 95%.[5] This test helps identify the false-negative horses that the basal testosterone test alone misses. A baseline serum sample is obtained, and then the horse is given 6000 to 12,000 IU of hCG intravenously. A second serum sample is taken 30 to 120 minutes later. Horses are considered geldings if the testosterone levels are less than 40 pg/mL and cryptorchids if the levels are greater than

100 pg/mL.[5] If the initial testosterone level is low but then increases greater than 2-fold after the administration of hCG, the horse is likely a cryptorchid as well.
   ○ Estrone sulfate: in horses greater than 3 years of age, serum estrone sulfate levels greater than 400 pg/mL indicate a retained testicle with 96% accuracy.[5]

Preoperative Preparation

The first consideration for this surgery is choosing an appropriate patient for the standing technique. The horse must be willing to stand in stocks to safely perform the surgery. If the horse is too small or is too fractious, then it may be more appropriate to choose a technique performed under general anesthesia. Consideration should also be made regarding the location of the retained testicle or testicles. If the history of previous castration of a horse is uncertain, a cryptorchid stallion may have been unilaterally castrated or may have 1 or 2 inguinal or abdominal testicles.[6] As previously discussed, transabdominal ultrasonography or transrectal and inguinal palpation may identify the location of the testicle. If these diagnostic modalities are unable to identify the location of the testis, then it may be helpful to remember that retained left testicles are abdominal about 75% of the time and retained right testicles are abdominal about 42% of the time.[5] Although inguinal testicles can be removed using standing laparoscopic techniques by pulling the testicle back into the abdomen, some surgeons recommend removal of inguinal testicles using traditional techniques under general anesthesia to avoid disruption of the vaginal ring.[7]

The horse should be fasted for 24 to 36 hours to help decrease the volume of ingesta present within the bowel and provide for improved observation of the abdomen during laparoscopic surgery.

Box 1
Sedative choices for standing cryptorchidectomy

- Repeated intravenous (IV) bolus of xylazine (0.5 mg/kg IV) or detomidine (0.01–0.02 mg/kg IV) either alone or in combination with butorphanol (0.01 mg/kg IV). Resedation is given as needed.

- Caudal epidural of detomidine (0.03–0.06 mg/kg) diluted to 10 mL with 0.9% saline with no concurrent IV sedation.[8] Sedation lasts up to 2.5 hours. This method may occasionally cause the horse to collapse, so caution should be used.[9]

- Constant rate infusion of detomidine (20 mg/L) and butorphanol (10 mg/L) in saline given IV titrated to effect.[10] Given after initial sedation with detomidine and butorphanol mentioned earlier.

Preoperative antibiotics, nonsteroidal antiinflammatories, and tetanus toxoid vaccination may be given. Providing appropriate sedation is crucial in safely and successfully performing a standing cryptorchidectomy (**Box 1**). The tail is wrapped and secured with a rope and the head is stabilized by an assistant. It may be useful to secure the head with side snaps or provide a small table to allow the horse to rest its head to stabilize itself. The flank is clipped on the affected side or both flanks are clipped if the horse has bilaterally retained testis or if the affected side is unknown. The flank or flanks are aseptically prepared and then the horse is draped. The left flank is approached first if it is unknown which testicle is retained, because of the increased likelihood that a retained testicle on the left is more frequently abdominal.[5] The surgeon then blocks the corners of the draped opening using about 5 mL of 2% lidocaine or mepivacaine at the location at which each towel clamp will be placed. Some surgeons prefer to use skin staples to secure the drape without the use of local anesthetic. The drape is then secured with towel clamps and the intended surgical site is blocked using 2% lidocaine or mepivacaine. It may be blocked using a variety of techniques, including a line block over the intended surgical site, direct infiltration into the intended site for each trocar/cannula unit, or using an inverted L block. A paravertebral thoracolumbar block can also be performed in horses[11] but can be technically challenging and can cause motor deficiency in the ipsilateral hind limb. Typically, each portal site is infused with about 10 mL of local anesthetic, or about 60 to 100 mL is used for either a line block or inverted L block.

Surgical Considerations

Insufflation techniques

Insufflation of the abdomen with carbon dioxide allows for abdominal distention, which improves visualization of the surgical field. The first consideration that the surgeon must make is whether to insufflate the abdomen before or after insertion of the laparoscope. This is an important consideration, because placement of the first portal is considered to be the most dangerous part of the procedure.[12]

Insertion of the trocar cannula before insufflation The laparoscopic trocar cannula can be inserted before insufflation by making a 15-mm incision through the skin, and the outer fascia of the external abdominal oblique muscle in the paralumbar fossa midway between the last rib and the tuber coxae at the dorsal margin of the internal abdominal oblique muscle. A sharp pyramidal trocar cannula is inserted by using a twisting motion and pushing the instrument in a slight caudoventral direction. Insertion of the trocar cannula on the left side may decrease the risk of inadvertent trauma to bowel because of the presence of the spleen. Care is taken on the left side to avoid the injury to the spleen and on the right side to avoid perforation of the cecum. The 3-way stopcock is left open so that negative pressure can be heard when the instrument enters the abdominal cavity. The trocar cannula should be at least 15 cm long to make sure that it is long enough to penetrate the peritoneum to avoid retroperitoneal insufflation.[7] The trocar is then removed, and the laparoscope is inserted into the abdomen to ensure correct placement and decrease the risk of retroperitoneal insufflation. The abdomen is then insufflated to 15 mm Hg with a carbon dioxide insufflator. To decrease the risk of accidental perforation of intestine or trauma to the spleen, some surgeons advocate the use of a guarded trocar or they replace the sharp trocar with a blunt-tip trocar before insertion in the abdominal cavity, or use only a blunt-tip trochar.[13,14] This strategy may increase the risk of retroperitoneal insufflation, by causing peritoneal detachment during insertion of the trocar cannula.[15]

Insufflation using a trocar catheter or Veress needle Insufflation of the abdomen before insertion of the laparoscopic cannula/trocar can be accomplished by using a 12-French trocar catheter or by using a Veress needle (**Fig. 1**), which may reduce the risk of trauma to viscera during insertion of the laparoscopic cannula.[8] Placement of a 12-French trocar catheter allows for more rapid insufflation of the abdomen than the Veress needle. A small stab incision is made just ventral to the crus of the internal abdominal oblique muscle midway between the last rib and the tuber coxae. The 12-French trocar catheter is then directed caudally and ventrally toward the opposite coxofemoral joint (**Fig. 2**). Confirmation of correct positioning is noted with the sound of air being pulled into the abdomen. The abdomen is then insufflated as previously described. The Veress needle has a spring-loaded mechanism, which slides forward on entry into the abdomen to protect bowel, but its small lumen restricts flow rates, preventing rapid insufflation of the large volumes required in equine laparoscopy.[12] Some Veress needles are too short for horses with thick body walls.

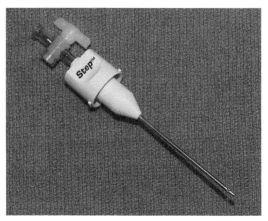

Fig. 1. Veress needle.

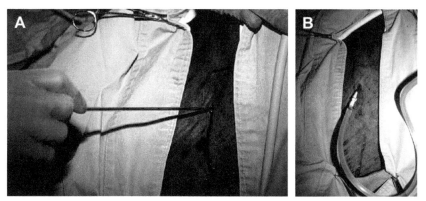

Fig. 2. (*A*) Placement of 12-French trocar catheter. (*B*) Insufflation after placement of the catheter.

Insertion of an optical trocar Some surgeons advocate the use of an optical trocar to allow for a more controlled insertion of the trocar cannula.[15] These optical trocars allow the laparoscope to be inserted so that the surgeon can visualize the insertion of the cannula (**Fig. 3**). This strategy may help prevent inadvertent damage to organs and retroperitoneal insufflation, because of more controlled placement and sharp transection of the peritoneum on its insertion.[15] The trocars are typically 10 to 15 cm long, which may pose a problem in large or fat horses, because the trocars may be too short to easily penetrate the abdominal cavity. The optical trocar must be directed perpendicular to the abdominal wall because of its short length, because it may not penetrate the peritoneum if it is directed ventrally. An Endo TIP (endoscopic threaded imaging port Karl Storz, El Segundo, CA, USA) is another type of laparoscopic cannula, which may decrease the risk of inadvertent trauma to abdominal viscera. It consists of a threaded cannula (**Fig. 4**), which is inserted into the abdomen using a rotating motion without the use of a trocar. The laparoscope can be inserted into the cannula for direct visualization of its placement into the abdomen.[12]

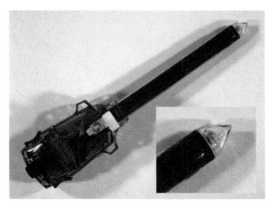

Fig. 3. Optical trocar allows for direct visualization of the cannula during placement.

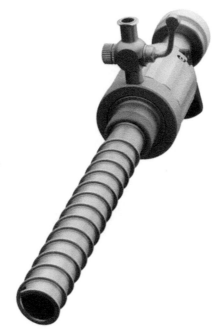

Fig. 4. Threaded EndoTIP cannula. (*Courtesy of* Karl Storz Endoscopy-America, El Segundo, CA; with permission.)

Laparoscopic exploration of the inguinal region

Once the abdomen is insufflated properly and the laparoscope has been placed as described earlier, a thorough examination of the inguinal region should be performed. The surgeon may use a standard 10-mm, 33-cm-long laparoscope, because they are sufficiently long for this procedure, unless trying to examine the contralateral inguinal region in a large horse. In that case, a 10-mm, 57-cm-long laparoscope may be needed (**Fig. 5**). The ipsilateral inguinal region should be examined first. At times, the abdominal testicle can be found adjacent to the vaginal ring without the aid of instruments to retract mesorchium or manipulate bowel (**Fig. 6**).

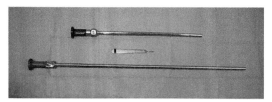

Fig. 5. 10-mm × 33-cm laparoscope and 10-mm × 57-cm laparoscope.

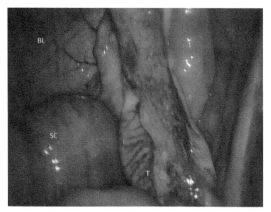

Fig. 6. Abdominal testicle (T) with adjacent bladder (BL) and small colon (SC).

Either 1 or 2 instrument portals are then placed in a similar fashion to the placement of the scope portal, with the first instrument portal being about 6 to 8 cm ventral to the scope portal. If necessary, the second instrument portal is then about 4 to 6 cm to the first instrument portal (**Fig. 7**). If the surgeon is using a laparoscope with a 30°

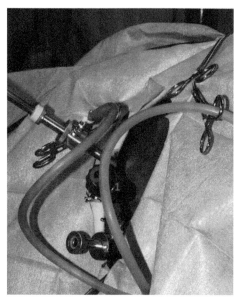

Fig. 7. Placement of laparoscope portal (L) and instrument portals 1 and 2 in the left paralumbar fossa.

angled viewing field, they may visualize the penetration of the trocar through the peritoneum, thus minimizing injury to bowel or the spleen. Babcock forceps may be used to gently manipulate intestine that obstructs the viewing field. If the ductus deferens and spermatic vasculature can be seen coursing into the vaginal ring, then the testicle has either been previously removed or is within the inguinal canal. The mesorchium can be grasped and elevated with Babcock grasping forceps to determine if the testicle is present within the inguinal canal. Inguinal testicles can be seen bulging into the vaginal ring when traction is applied to the spermatic cord. If the horse has an uncertain castration history or is a bilateral cryptorchid, the laparoscope can then be manipulated under the small colon to examine the contralateral inguinal region. A small defect can also be made in the mesocolon, and the scope can be passed to the other side.[16] This technique may require closure of the defect if it becomes enlarged during manipulation of the scope.

Techniques for ligation and removal of the abdominal testicle

After identification of the testicle, the surgeon can use one of several techniques for ligation and removal of the testicle. The main factors that determine the technique that a surgeon chooses are often the instrumentation available and their familiarity with a specific technique.

Loop ligation technique The use of a suture loop for ligation of the spermatic cord within the abdominal cavity is a technique that has been well proved and frequently used[16,17] to provide reliable and inexpensive hemostasis before transection of the spermatic cord. It allows for ligation and transection of both testicles within the abdomen without loss of insufflation, which is useful in removing bilaterally retained testicles. Traumatic grasping forceps are introduced through one of the instrument portals and the testicle is grasped and examined to verify that the entire testicle and its associated structures are within the abdomen. It is then released and a premanufactured (Endoloop ligature, Ethicon Endo-Surgery, Cincinnati, OH, USA) or hand-tied slip knot is placed through the second instrument portal. The traumatic grasping forceps are placed through the loop, and the testicle is grasped. The loop is then manipulated over the testicle and around the spermatic cord (**Fig. 8**). It is tightened using a knot push rod, and the long end of the suture is transected with laparoscopic scissors. The spermatic cord is then transected and inspected for hemorrhage (**Fig. 9**). A second suture loop is applied if bleeding is noted.

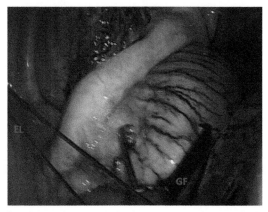

Fig. 8. Placement of Endoloop ligature (EL) after grasping the testicle (T) using laparoscopic traumatic grasping forceps (GF).

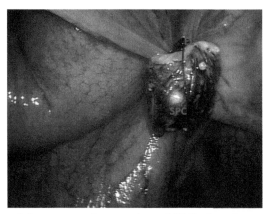

Fig. 9. Examination of the transected spermatic cord (SPC) after placement and transection of Endoloop ligature.

Extracorporeal emasculation If the horse is a unilateral cryptorchid, then extracorporeal emasculation of the spermatic cord is a safe and effective technique for transecting the cord and providing hemostasis.[18] The testicle is secured with traumatic grasping forceps, exteriorized through a low flank instrument portal (**Fig. 10**A), and the cord can be emasculated or ligated and transected (see **Fig. 10**B). Infiltration of local anesthetic into the testicle may aid in exteriorization of the testicle without eliciting a painful response. This technique is unique in that only 1 instrument portal is necessary for securing and exteriorizing the testicle, and it does not require additional instrumentation other than standard emasculators. A disadvantage is that abdominal insufflation is lost when the testicle is exteriorized to emasculate, so this technique does not work well for bilateral cryptorchids. Horses can also become agitated with this technique, so patient selection is important.

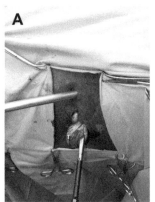
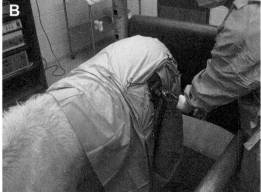

Fig. 10. Exteriorization of an abdominal testicle (T) through the flank (*A*) and extracorporeal emasculation (*B*) of spermatic cord through the flank incision. (*Courtesy of* Jeremiah Easley, DVM.)

Electrosurgical Bipolar electrosurgery has been proved to be safe and effective at achieving adequate hemostasis before transection of the spermatic cord for removal of cryptorchid testicles.[19] Bipolar electrosurgery forceps are inserted through the most dorsal instrument portal, and grasping forceps are placed through the ventral portal. The forceps are used to grasp the vasculature within the cranial aspect of the mesorchium about 2 cm dorsal to the testicle. The forceps are activated until the tissue is blanched and shrinks. This process is repeated 1 to 2 cm dorsal to the first site and at a third site if needed. The bipolar forceps are removed and replaced with 5-mm grasping forceps. Laparoscopic scissors are placed through the ventral portal, and the mesorchium, underlying vessels, and ductus deferens are transected. Additional application of the electrosurgery forceps can be used if hemorrhage is noted. The use of a LigaSure vessel sealing device (Covidien, Mansfield, MA, USA) (**Fig. 11**) has also been described for achieving hemostasis in removal of normal testicles in stallions[20] and can be similarly used in laparoscopic removal of cryptorchid testicles.

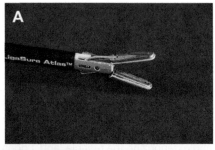

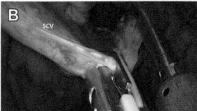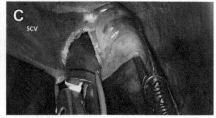

Fig. 11. (*A*) LigaSure vessel sealing device handpiece; (*B*) Spermatic cord vasculature (SCV) being grasped with the LigaSure laparoscopic handpiece (LS); (*C*) Transection of the spermatic cord vasculature (SCV) after activation and sealing using the LigaSure (LS). (*Courtesy of* Jeremiah Easley, DVM.)

Laparoscopic removal of the inguinal testicle

If the retained testicle is found to be inguinally retained during exploration, the surgeon must make a decision whether to remove the testicle laparoscopically or to anesthetize the horse and remove it making an inguinal incision. Small inguinal testicles may be retracted into the abdomen by applying steady gentle traction on the spermatic cord and can often be performed without enlarging the vaginal ring. If the testicle is too large to be pulled through the vaginal ring, then the vaginal ring must be enlarged with laparoscopic scissors to allow the testicle to be pulled through. The vaginal ring can be closed using a laparoscopic stapler if it has been excessively enlarged.[21]

Removal of bilateral abdominally retained testicles

When considering removal of bilateral testicles, the surgeon must decide if they will be performing the ligation and transection of the spermatic cord of each testicle from 1 side or on each side of the horse. As discussed earlier, the laparoscope should be inserted on the left side first in horses that have an uncertain history of castration and horses that are bilateral cryptorchids. After examination of the left inguinal region, the right inguinal region can be examined by passing the laparoscope ventral to the small colon. This examination typically requires the use of a 57-cm-long laparoscope, because the standard 33-cm-long laparoscope is marginally long enough even in average sized horses (see **Fig. 5**). Once the testicle has been identified, the surgeon must decide if they want to attempt to ligate and transect the spermatic cord of the right testicle from the left side. Although this procedure can be accomplished and can decrease surgical time by negating the need for inserting the laparoscope and instrument portals on the right, it can also be technically challenging because the small colon obscures complete visualization of the surgical field. Alternatively, the surgeon can ligate and transect the spermatic cord of the left testicle and keep the testicle secured by locking traumatic grasping forceps and leaving them in place. Abdominal insufflation can be maintained if the laparoscopic cannulas are left in place on the left side. A second set of laparoscopic cannulas are then inserted on the right side, and the right spermatic cord is ligated and transected. The right testicle can then be passed under the small colon and grasped on the left side. Both testicles can then be removed through 1 enlarged flank incision on the left side.[17]

Postoperative Care

Horses are kept in a stall for 24 hours to monitor manure production and appetite. They can return to light work in 3 days and full work in 5 days.

STANDING LAPAROSCOPIC CASTRATION

Laparoscopic castration techniques have been described in both standing and dorsally recumbent, anesthetized horses.[21] Standing laparoscopic castration can be performed in a similar fashion to standing cryptorchidectomy, with the main difference being in situ destruction of the testis, which is left in the scrotum, by ligation and transection of the spermatic vessels and ductus deferens within the abdomen. The testes then undergo avascular necrosis and atrophy over time. This procedure has not gained widespread acceptance, mainly because of concerns regarding continued viability of inguinal or scrotal testicles after completion of the surgery because of alternative blood supply from the cremasteric or external pudendal arteries.[22,23]

STANDING LAPAROSCOPIC INGUINAL HERNIOPLASTY

Key points

- Laparoscopic inguinal herniorrhaphy or hernioplasty should be considered after correction of acquired inguinal hernias to prevent recurrence in stallions that are to be breeding animals.

- The surgical technique should be carefully chosen based on testicular viability, the horse's temperament, available surgical instrumentation, and the surgeon's laparoscopic skill level.

- Standing laparoscopic testicle-sparing hernioplasty techniques include peritoneal flap hernioplasty, cylindrical mesh prosthesis implantation, hernioplasty with barbed suture, and hernioplasty with cyanoacrylate glue.

Inguinal Hernia Overview

Inguinal hernias in mature stallions almost always constitute a medical emergency, because there is usually strangulated small intestine incarcerated through the internal inguinal ring.[24] Acquired inguinal hernias are more common among certain breeds, such as warmbloods, standardbreds, Andalusians, and draft breeds, and are believed to be related to an enlarged or flaccid vaginal ring.[25] Although acquired inguinal hernias in mature stallions are usually nonreducible in the standing horse, they may be resolved successfully in the anesthetized horse while in dorsal recumbency with external manipulation of the scrotum.[26] This procedure can be performed in conjunction with laparoscopic traction of the small intestine to aid in both reduction of the hernia and evaluation of intestinal viability. Conventional techniques for treatment of acquired inguinal hernias include correction through a ventral midline celiotomy with or without intestinal resection, depending on intestinal viability.[24,27] At that time, a unilateral or bilateral castration with external inguinal ring closure may be performed to reduce the risk of reherniation. If the testicle remains viable, a conventional testicle-sparing inguinal herniorrhaphy (or hernioplasty) may be performed, in which the external inguinal ring is sutured around the spermatic cord while under general anesthesia to reduce the risk of reherniation in intact stallions.[28] Laparoscopic techniques that reduce the size of the internal inguinal ring are believed to be more reliable in preventing recurrence of inguinal hernia formation than the conventional inguinal herniorrhaphy technique. Several laparoscopic techniques that are performed under general anesthesia include transabdominal preperitoneal mesh insertion,[29] a peritoneal flap technique,[30] and direct laparoscopic suturing of the vaginal ring.[31]

Standing Laparoscopic Testicle-Sparing Hernioplasty Techniques

- Developed to allow for improved observation of the surgical field and avoid the cost and risks associated with general anesthesia.
- These techniques include peritoneal flap hernioplasty,[25] placement of a mesh cylinder into the inguinal canal,[32] closure of the inguinal canal with cyanoacrylate glue,[33] and possibly closure of the internal inguinal ring with barbed suture.[34]

Preoperative Preparation

Factors to consider when choosing a laparoscopic hernioplasty technique

1. The testicle must be viable if a testicle-sparing hernioplasty technique is used.
2. The patient must be willing to stand in stocks safely if a standing technique is used.
3. The surgeon must have sufficient laparoscopic skills and must have appropriate instrumentation to perform the technique.
4. The technique must provide adequate security in closing the internal inguinal ring to prevent recurrence of hernia formation. Some laparoscopic techniques have been believed to be superior to others because they provide a more secure inguinal ring closure, especially if the internal inguinal ring is particularly large or there is an inguinal rupture.[12] This theory has not been proved to date, and the techniques that seem to provide less secure closure of the internal inguinal ring seem to prevent recurrence in clinical cases.

Patient preparation for standing inguinal hernioplasty is similar to the patient preparation discussed for standing laparoscopic cryptorchidectomy. The horse is fasted for 24 to 36 hours and is given preoperative antibiotics, nonsteroidal antiinflammatories, and tetanus toxoid vaccination at the surgeon's discretion. The tail is wrapped and secured with a rope, and the head is stabilized by an assistant. The horse is placed in stocks and sedated using previously discussed protocols for standing cryptorchidectomy. Both flanks are clipped, aseptically prepared, and draped. Local anesthetic is infiltrated at the proposed sites of the laparoscopic portals.

Surgical Considerations

Laparoscopic insufflation and laparoscopic exploration of the inguinal region for standing inguinal hernioplasty are performed as described for laparoscopic cryptorchidectomy. If a bilateral inguinal hernioplasty is to be performed, the laparoscope and instrument portals must be placed in the ipsilateral paralumbar fossa on each side.

Standing peritoneal flap hernioplasty

This is the most technically demanding standing laparoscopic technique for inguinal hernioplasty. An inverted U-shaped 10-cm-long by 6-cm-wide peritoneal flap dorsal and cranial to the internal inguinal ring is dissected using laparoscopic instruments (**Fig. 12**A).[25] A subperitoneal block with local anesthetic and a laparoscopic injection needle are necessary to reduce movement during dissection. The volume of block should be limited to 30 mL or less to prevent inadvertent femoral nerve paresis. Electrocoagulation may be required to achieve hemostasis during the dissection of larger vessels adjacent to the flap. The flap is then rotated over the internal inguinal ring (see **Fig. 12**B) and secured with a 12-mm, 30-cm-long endohernia roticulator (Endo Universal 65°, Covidien, Belgium) containing 10 4.8-mm stainless steel staples (see **Fig. 12**C).

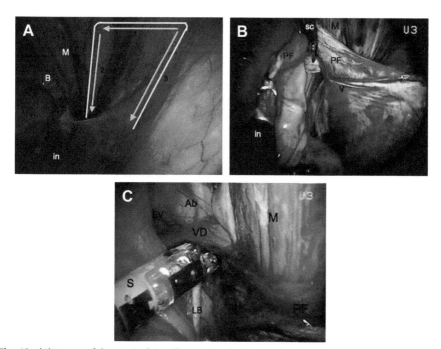

Fig. 12. (*A*) Image of the vaginal ring illustrating the inverted U-shaped peritoneal flap with the numbers and arrows indicating the sequence and direction of dissection; (*B*) Dissection of the peritoneal flap using endoscopic scissors followed by rotation of the flap; (*C*) Secure the peritoneal flap with a 12-mm 30-cm long endohernia roticulator (Endo Universal 65°, Covidien, Belgium) containing 10 4.8-mm stainless steel staples. Ab, Abdomen; B, Bladder; EV, epigastric vein; In, instrument; Lb, lateral ligament of bladder; M, Mesorchium; PF, peritoneal flap; S, stapler; Sc, scissors; V, vaginal ring; VD, Vas deferens. (*Courtesy of* Hans Wilderjans, DVM.)

Although postoperative adhesions were not identified in a recent study,[25] they remain a concern because of the large subperitoneal area that is left open to heal by second intention.

Standing cylindrical mesh prosthesis technique

This technique is less technical to perform and is faster than the peritoneal flap technique. It provides closure of the internal inguinal ring by placing a cylinder of polypropylene mesh (Ethicon Endo-Surgery, Cincinnati, OH, USA) into the inguinal canal.[32] A 6-cm × 8-cm section of Prolene mesh is rolled into a cylinder and secured with 1 or 2 circumferential absorbable sutures. This cylinder is then grasped with Babcock laparoscopic forceps and carried through a laparoscopic instrument cannula in the paralumbar fossa. It is placed partially into the internal inguinal ring, and the circumferential sutures are cut with laparoscopic scissors. The cylinder of mesh is then pushed into the inguinal canal with the laparoscopic forceps and secured with 3 laparoscopic staples to the parietal wall. The mesh is believed to elicit an inflammatory response that causes tissue ingrowth, which blocks the opening of the inguinal canal. Potential concerns with this technique include possible migration of the mesh, inadvertent damage to the spermatic cord caused by adhesions from the mesh, and a recurrence rate of up to 25%.[25]

Standing hernioplasty with barbed suture

A case report was recently published using this technique to close the internal inguinal rings of a gelding with a reducible inguinal hernia.[34] The cranial portion of the internal inguinal ring is sutured using a continuous suture pattern created with unidirectional barbed suture (Covidien, Mansfield, MA, USA) connected to a mechanical suturing instrument. This procedure can be performed quickly and easily, because it avoids the use of intracorporeal knots. Only 1 instrument portal is necessary with this technique, so it avoids the interference often associated with using multiple instruments in the paralumbar fossa. Obviously, this technique needs to be used in more horses to evaluate its efficacy in preventing recurrence of inguinal hernias. The use of this technique as a testicular-sparing method to prevent reherniation is not well proved and needs to be researched further before it can be recommended. Some surgeons advocate that direct suturing of the cranial portion of the vaginal ring may be inadequate as a testicle-sparing technique, because of reherniation of intestine at the caudal margin of the vaginal ring.

Standing hernioplasty with cyanoacrylate glue

Closure of the internal inguinal ring and inguinal canal with cyanoacrylate glue has recently been report in a few cases.[33] This technique is fast and is not expensive, because laparoscopic stapling devices are not used. It is also simple to perform and does not require extensive laparoscopic training compared with the peritoneal flap technique. Babcock forceps are placed through a ventral instrument portal and used to retract the spermatic cord caudally. If the inguinal ring is very large, a cruciate suture of 0 USP Polysorb (Covidien, Mansfield, MA, USA) may be placed at the cranial portion of the ring using an Endo Stitch device (Covidien, Mansfield, MA, USA). A laparoscopic needle sheath with 2-mm-diameter polyethylene extension tubing is then placed through a second instrument portal, and the tubing is placed in the craniolateral part of the vaginal ring. About 2 mL of cyanoacrylate glue is injected into the inguinal canal, and the Babcock forceps are used to compress the craniolateral vaginal ring together, taking care not to get glue on the forceps or any viscera. It is unclear if adhesions from cyanoacrylate glue contacting the spermatic cord affects testicular viability.

STANDING ROUTINE CASTRATION

> **Key points**
>
> - With appropriate sedation and local analgesia, standing castrations are safe to perform in a wide range of horses.
> - The time, cost, and complications associated with general anesthesia are avoided by performing standing castrations.

Historically, one of the most common surgical procedures performed in the horse is castration.[35] Standing castrations are usually performed based on the surgeon's preference derived from previous experiences. Some veterinarians elect to perform most of their castrations on standing horses and anesthetize only dangerous, small, or young horses. Other practitioners perform most of their castrations with the horse under general anesthesia and perform standing castrations only on horses for which recovery from anesthesia is of particular concern, such as large draft breeds, horses with serious musculoskeletal injuries, or horses with neurologic disease. Advocates of performing standing castrations often argue that they can be performed more safely, faster, and with less assistance compared with horses that are castrated under general anesthesia.

Surgical Considerations

The horse is sedated with xylazine (0.5 mg/kg IV) or detomidine (0.02 mg/kg IV) either alone or in combination with butorphanol (0.05 mg/kg IV). Preoperative antibiotics, nonsteroidal antiinflammatories, and tetanus toxoid vaccination may be given. The scrotum should be palpated to ensure that both testicles can be palpated and are of adequate size to be removed standing. The horse's tail should be wrapped and secured to prevent contamination of the surgical site. The scrotum is then briefly prepared with chlorhexadine or povoiodine scrub and wiped clean. The scrotum is blocked on each side of the median raphae from the cranial to the caudal pole of the testicle by using lidocaine or bupivacaine locally. Each spermatic cord is also blocked with 15 to 30 mL of local anesthetic. This procedure can cause a hematoma, which can impede emasculation, so instead, the testicle can be directly injected with 25 mL of local anesthetic and be allowed to diffuse proximally. In addition, the scrotum can then be scrubbed if needed.

The surgeon and handler should then both be positioned on the same side of the horse before making an incision. A right-handed surgeon is on the left side of the horse. Their left hand grasps the scrotum and forces the testicles ventrally, and the scalpel blade is grasped in their right hand (**Fig. 13**). Two incisions are made

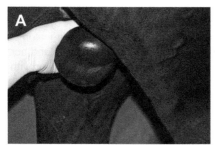 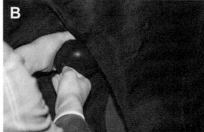

Fig. 13. Grasping the scrotum with the left hand (*A*) and scalpel blade with the right hand (*B*) for standing castration.

about 1 cm on either side of the median raphe, parallel to it. Conversely, the scrotum can be grasped with the left hand and pulled ventrally, and the bottom of the scrotum can be excised with 1 incision. The parietal tunic can then either be left in place and stripped of surrounding fascia (closed technique) or opened, after which the testicle and epididymis are freed (open technique).[36] The spermatic cord is then either ligated and emasculated or only emasculated. The spermatic cord is secured with hemostatic forceps before opening the emasculators so that it can be examined for hemorrhage before being released. The scrotal incisions are stretched to ensure adequate drainage. Some surgeons remove the median raphe before completion if the 2 incision technique is performed.

Complications

Complications of standing castrations are similar to those of castrations under general anesthesia and include hemorrhage, evisceration/eventration, edema, hydrocele formation, septic peritonitis, septic funiculitis, and continued stallionlike behavior.[35–40] One study identified that there was a higher complication rate with the standing castration of thoroughbred racehorses with scrotal incisions that were left open when compared with castrations that were performed in a hospital and closed primarily.[41] However, none of the complications associated with the standing castrations was fatal, although 1 of the 96 horses that were anesthetized for castration suffered a fatal fracture during recovery from anesthesia. This study also determined that the total cost of the group of standing castrations (even including the cost of treatment of complications) was significantly less than the group that was primarily closed. Many practitioners perform open castrations while performing a standing castration. For some time, it was believed that open castrations increased the risk of hydrocele formation and the occurrence of septic funiculitis,[36] because of the amount of redundant parietal tunic that is often left behind, although a retrospective study[37] failed to show that there is a difference between the 2 techniques. A more recent study found that there was a higher incidence of complications with a semiclosed technique versus a closed technique. However, it could be argued that there is little difference in the surgical technique of the 2 types of castrations and that the higher incidence might have been related to the disparity in age of the semiclosed group (mean age of 46.6 months) versus the closed group (mean age of 18.6 months).[42]

Perineal Urethrotomy

Perineal urethrotomy is a useful surgery performed in the standing male horse to allow for treatment of a variety of urogenital problems. It allows for temporary urine diversion to aid in the treatment of urethral obstructions caused by trauma, soft tissue masses, and urethrolithiasis.[43–46] A perineal urethrotomy (also called a subischial perineal urethrotomy) provides access to the bladder for treatment of cystic calculi by mechanical fragmentation, or fragmentation with a holmium:yttrium aluminum garnet laser or with various types of lithotripsy.[47–51] Hematuria in geldings and hemospermia in stallions can also be treated using a perineal urethrotomy with or without entering the urethral lumen at the site of the urethral defect.[52,53] A permanent urethrostomy may be necessary for permanent urine diversion if a partial phallectomy is being performed.[54]

Surgical Considerations

The horse is placed in stocks and is sedated with xylazine (0.5 mg/kg IV) or detomidine (0.01–0.02 mg/kg IV) either alone or in combination with butorphanol (0.05 mg/kg IV).

Preoperative antibiotics, nonsteroidal antiinflammatories, and tetanus toxoid vaccination may be given at the surgeon's discretion. A caudal epidural is placed using a combination of xylazine (0.17 mg/kg) and 2% lidocaine (0.22 mg/kg) diluted to 10 mL with 0.9% sodium chloride. If the surgeon opts to not use a caudal epidural, adequate desensitization may be achieved with local infusion of lidocaine in an inverted V pattern in the region of the proposed incision. The perineal region is then clipped and aseptically prepared. A stallion catheter is placed to aid in identification of the urethra for more accurate dissection. For the treatment of terminal hematuria or hemospermia, an endoscope can be passed until the urethral defect is visualized for more accurate placement.[52]

A 4-cm-long to 6-cm-long incision is then made, starting about 4 cm ventral to the anus and extending distally to the ischial arch (**Fig. 14**). The subcutaneous tissues, bulbospongiosus muscle, and corpus spongiosum (CSP) muscle are divided and retracted to expose the urethral mucosa.

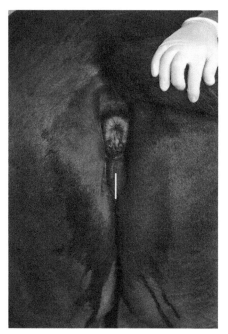

Fig. 14. Line indicating the location of the incision for perineal urethrotomy or urethrostomy. (*Courtesy of* Carolyn Arnold, DVM.)

- For urethral defects causing terminal hematuria or hemospermia: the urethral mucosa may be left intact, because the defect made in the CSP directs bleeding away from the mucosal defect and aids in healing.[52,53]
- For perineal urethrotomy: the urethral mucosa is transected longitudinally and left open. This incision usually closes in about 2 to 3 weeks.
- For placement of a permanent urethrostomy: the muscles are apposed using a simple continuous pattern with 3-0 absorbable monofilament suture. The skin and urethral mucosa are apposed using a simple continuous or simple interrupted pattern with the same suture.

Complications

Postoperative complications after performing a perineal urethrotomy include hemorrhage, incisional dehiscence, urine scalding of the hind legs, and urethral stricture formation.[55] However, serious complications, including urethral stricture formation, are rare, according to several retrospective studies.[52–54]

STANDING PARTIAL PHALLECTOMY

> **Key points**
>
> - Standing partial phallectomy allows for the surgical treatment of horses with penile neoplasia, paraphimosis, and priapism that have not responded to medical treatment.
> - The standing modified Vinsot technique[54] is a safe and simple surgery that is particularly suited for debilitated or very large horses in which general anesthesia is a concern or in cases with financial limitations.

Partial phallectomy or penile amputation is a common urogenital surgery in horses, because of the high incidence of penile squamous carcinoma.[56,57] Chronic paraphimosis caused by genital trauma, extensive edema, neurologic disease, severe debilitation, and drug-induced paralysis may also require partial phallectomy if retraction of the penis does not improve with medical treatment.[58–60] Priapism in stallions may also require partial phallectomy. Well-accepted partial phallectomy techniques such as the Williams, Vinsot, and Scott techniques are typically performed under general anesthesia because of the extensive dissection and suturing that are required to successfully perform the procedure.[60–64] More recently, a modified Vinsot technique was described in the standing horse.[54] Because this technique is performed with the horse standing, it is safer to perform on debilitated horses and large or draft breed horses. This technique is also easier and faster to perform, so it is a good surgical option in cases that have significant financial limitations.

Surgical Considerations

The horse is sedated with xylazine (0.5 mg/kg IV) or detomidine (0.01–0.02 mg/kg IV) either alone or in combination with butorphanol (0.05 mg/kg IV). Preoperative antibiotics, nonsteroidal antiinflammatories, and tetanus toxoid vaccination may be given at the surgeon's discretion. The urethral orifice of the penis is then aseptically prepared, and a stallion catheter is placed through the urethral orifice into the bladder to aid in identification of the urethra for formation of the urethrostomy.

The standing modified Vinsot technique[54] is simple to perform, because it involves formation of a urethrostomy, and then application of a penile tourniquet using a cattle bander castration tool (Callicrate Bander, No-Bull Enterprises, St Francis, KS) and specialized latex tubing (ES-10, No-Bull Enterprises, St Francis, KS). The specific site for placement of both the urethrostomy and the penile tourniquet is dependent on the location of the penile lesion.

Two possible surgical scenarios for standing modified Vinsot partial phallectomy

1. Most of the penis must be removed: perform a subischial urethrostomy using the same approach that was described earlier. The permanent stoma is made by suturing the urethral mucosa to the skin with a simple interrupted pattern using 2-0 or 3-0 monofilament absorbable suture. Perform a ring block around the penis near the prepucial opening with 20 mL of 2% lidocaine. Remove the stallion

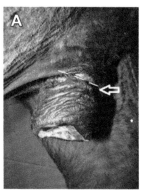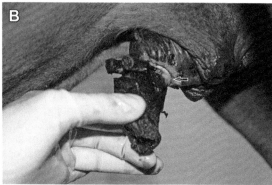

Fig. 15. Appearance of penile stump after tourniquet application and transection of the penis using the modified Vinsot partial phallectomy immediately after surgery (*A*) and 7 days postoperatively (*B*). Both *arrows* indicate location of the tourniquet band. (*Courtesy of* Carolyn Arnold, DVM.)

catheter. Apply the tourniquet to the penis just distal to the penile ring block and transect the penis about 2 cm distal to the tourniquet (**Fig. 15**).
2. Glans or distal half of the penis must be removed: perform a penile ring block near the prepucial opening, as described earlier. Perform a ventral penile urethrostomy between the prepucial ring and prepucial opening in the same fashion as the subischial urethrostomy described earlier. Remove the stallion catheter. Apply the penile tourniquet about 1 cm to the ventral urethrostomy and transect the penis about 2 cm distal to the tourniquet.

A standing castration should be performed in all stallions after the penile amputation. Antibiotics and antiinflammatories can be given at the surgeon's discretion. The penile tourniquet is left in place and sloughs off along with the necrotic tissue distal to it about 3 to 4 weeks after surgery.

Complications

Mild hemorrhage may be noted initially after surgery, especially during urination. Horses with subischial urethrostomies usually have some degree of urine scalding on their hind legs. This complication may persist for an indefinite period. Urethral stricture has been reported as a complication of the Vinsot technique. Adhesions of the distal amputation site of the penis may form to the sheath during the healing process, thus preventing the remaining portion of the penis from dropping.[54]

REFERENCES

1. Hayes HM. Epidemiological features of 5009 cases of equine cryptorchidism. Equine Vet J 1986;18:467.
2. Schambourg MA, Farley JA, Marcoux M, et al. Use of transabdominal ultrasonography to determine the location of cryptorchid testes in the horse. Equine Vet J 2006;38(3):242–5.
3. Cox JE. Cryptorchid castration. In: McKinnon AO, Voss JL, editors. Equine reproduction. Philadelphia: Lea & Febiger; 1993. p. 915–20.
4. Cox JE, Redhead PH, Dawson FE. Comparisons of the measurement of plasma testosterone and plasma oestrogens for the diagnosis of cryptorchidism in the horse. Equine Vet J 1986;18:179.

5. Rodgerson DH, Hanson RR. Cryptorchidism in horses. Part I. Anatomy, causes and diagnosis. Compend Contin Educ Pract Vet 1997;19:1280–8.

6. Marshall JF, Moorman VJ, Moll HD. Comparison of the diagnosis and management of unilaterally castrated and cryptorchid horses at a referral hospital: 60 cases (2002-2006). J Am Vet Med Assoc 2007;231(6):931–4.

7. Rodgerson DH. Cryptorchidectomy. In: Ragle CA, editor. Advances in equine laparoscopy. West Sussex (UK): John Wiley; 2012. p. 140.

8. Trumble TN, Hendrickson DA. Standing male equine urogenital endoscopic surgery. Vet Clin North Am Equine Pract 2000;16(2):269–84.

9. Wittern C, Hendrickson DA, Trumble TN, et al. Complications associated with administration of detomidine into the caudal epidural space in a horse. J Am Vet Med Assoc 1998;213:516–8.

10. Seabaugh KA, Goodrich LR, Morley PS. Comparison of peritoneal fluid values after laparoscopic cryptorchidectomy using a vessel-sealing device(LigaSure™) versus a ligating loop and removal of the descended testis. Vet Surg 2013;42(5):600–6.

11. Moon PF, Suter CM. Paravertebral thoracolumbar anaesthesia in 10 horses. Equine Vet J 1993;25:304–8.

12. Fischer AT. Equine diagnostic and surgical laparoscopy. Philadelphia: WB Saunders; 2002.

13. Hanson CA, Galuppo LD. Bilateral laparoscopic ovariectomy in standing mares: 22 cases. Vet Surg 1999;28:106–12.

14. Palmer SE. Fundamentals of standing equine laparoscopy. Proc Am Assoc Equine Practnr 1993;39:241–2.

15. Desmaizières LM, Martinot S, Lepage OM, et al. Complications associated with cannula insertion techniques used for laparoscopy in standing horses. Vet Surg 2003;32:501–6.

16. Hendrickson DA, Wilson DG. Laparoscopic cryptorchidectomy in standing horses. Proc Am Assoc Equine Pract 1996;42:184–5.

17. Hendrickson DA, Wilson DG. Instrumentation and techniques for laparoscopic and thoracoscopic surgery in the horse. Vet Clin North Am Equine Pract 1996;12:235–59.

18. Davis EW. Laparoscopic cryptorchidectomy in standing horses. Vet Surg 1997; 26(4):326–31.

19. Hanrath M, Rodgerson DH. Laparoscopic cryptorchidectomy using electrosurgical instrumentation in standing horses. Vet Surg 2002;31(2):117–24.

20. Gracia-Calvo LA, Martín-Cuervo M, Jiménez J, et al. Intra and postoperative assessment of resterilised LigaSure Atlas for orchidectomies in horses. Vet Rec 2012;171(4):98.

21. Wilson DG, Hendrickson DA, Cooley AJ, et al. Laparoscopic methods for castration of equids. J Am Vet Med Assoc 1996;209:112–4.

22. Voermans M, Rijkenhuizen AB, van der Velden MA. The complex blood supply to the equine testis as a cause of failure in laparoscopic castration. Equine Vet J 2006;38(1):35–9.

23. Bergeron JA, Hendrickson DA, McCue PM. Viability of an inguinal testis after laparoscopic cauterization and transection of its blood supply. J Am Vet Med Assoc 1998;213:1303–4.

24. van der Velden MA. Surgical treatment of acquired inguinal hernia in the horse: a review of 51 cases. Equine Vet J 1988;20:173–7.

25. Wilderjans H, Meulyzer M, Simon O. Standing laparoscopic peritoneal flap hernioplasty technique for preventing recurrence of acquired strangulating inguinal herniation in stallions. Vet Surg 2012;41:292–9.

26. Wilderjans H, Simon O, Boussauw B. Strangulating hernia in 63 horses–results of manual closed non-surgical reduction followed by a delayed laparoscopic closure of the vaginal ring. Proceedings of the 16th ECVS Annual Meeting. Dublin, Ireland, June 28–30th, 2007. p. 92–7.

27. Freeman DE. Small intestine. In: Auer JA, Stick JA, editors. Equine surgery. 3rd edition. St Louis (MO): Saunders; 2006. p. 401–36.

28. Vaughan JT. Surgery of the testes. In: Walker DF, Vaughan JT, editors. Bovine and equine urogenital surgery. Philadelphia: Lea & Febiger; 1980. p. 145–69.

29. Fischer AT, Vachon AM, Klein SR. Laparoscopic inguinal herniorrhaphy in two stallions. J Am Vet Med Assoc 1995;207:1599–601.

30. Rossignol F, Perrin R, Boening KJ. Laparoscopic hernioplasty in recumbent horses using transposition of a peritoneal flap. Vet Surg 2007;36:557–62.

31. Caron JP, Brakenhoff J. Intracorporeal suture closure of the internal inguinal and vaginal rings in foals and horses. Vet Surg 2008;37:126–31.

32. Marien T. Standing laparoscopic herniorrhaphy in stallions using cylindrical polypropylene mesh prosthesis. Equine Vet J 2001;33:91–6.

33. Rossignol F. Inguinal hernioplasty using cyanoacrylate. In: Ragle CA, editor. Advances in equine laparoscopy. West Sussex (UK): John Wiley; 2012. p. 161–6.

34. Ragle CA, Yiannikouris S, Tibary AA, et al. Use of a barbed suture for laparoscopic closure of the internal inguinal rings in a horse. J Am Vet Med Assoc 2013;242(2):249–53.

35. Thomas HL, Zaruby JF, Smith CL, et al. Postcastration eventration in 18 horses: the prognostic indicators for long-term survival (1985–1995). Can Vet J 1998;39:764–8.

36. Schumacher J. Testis. In: Auer JA, Stick JA, editors. Equine surgery. 3rd edition. St Louis (MO): Saunders; 2006. p. 775–810.

37. Shoemaker R, Bailey J, Janzen E, et al. Routine castration in 568 draught colts: incidence of evisceration and omental herniation. Equine Vet J 2004;36:336–40.

38. Schumacher J. Complications of castration. Equine Vet Educ 1996;8:254–9.

39. Searle D, Dart AJ, Dart CM, et al. Equine castration: review of anatomy, approaches, techniques and complications in normal, cryptorchid and monorchid horses. Aust Vet J 1999;77:428–34.

40. Nickels FA. Complications of castration and ovariectomy. Vet Clin North Am Equine Pract 1988;4:515–23.

41. Mason BJ, Newton JR, Payne RJ, et al. Costs and complications of equine castration: a UK practice-based study comparing 'standing nonsutured' and 'recumbent sutures' techniques. Equine Vet J 2005;37(5):468–72.

42. Kilcoyne I, Watson JL, Kass PH, et al. Incidence, management, and outcome of complications of castration in equids: 324 cases (1998–2008). J Am Vet Med Assoc 2013;242(6):820–5.

43. Firth EC. Dissecting hematoma of the corpus spongiosum and urinary bladder rupture in a stallion. J Am Vet Med Assoc 1976;169:800.

44. Gibbons WJ. Hematoma of the penis. Mod Vet Pract 1974;45:76.

45. Robertson JT. Conditions of the urethra. In: Robinson NE, editor. Current therapy in equine medicine 2. Philadelphia: WB Saunders; 1987. p. 719–20.

46. Trotter GW, Bennett DG, Behm RJ. Urethral calculi in five horses. Vet Surg 1981;10:159.

47. Laverty S, Pascoe JR, Ling GV, et al. Urolithiasis in 68 horses. Vet Surg 1992;21(1):56–62.

48. Carter EJ, Galuppo LD. Endoscopic-assisted disruption of urinary calculi using a holmium:YAG laser in standing horses. Vet Surg 2002;31:245–50.

49. Howard RD, Pleasant RS, May KA. Pulsed dye laser lithotripsy for treatment of urolithiasis in two geldings. J Am Vet Med Assoc 1998;212:1600–3.
50. Eustace RA, Hunt JM. Electrohydraulic lithotripsy for the treatment of cystic calculus in two geldings. Equine Vet J 1988;20:221–3.
51. Koenig J, Hurtig M, Pearce S, et al. Ballistic shock wave lithotripsy in an 18-year-old thoroughbred gelding. Can Vet J 1999;40:185–6.
52. Schumacher J, Varner DD, Schmitz DG, et al. Urethral defects in geldings with hematuria and stallions with hemospermia. Vet Surg 1995;24(3):250–4.
53. Sullins KE, Bertone JJ, Voss JL, et al. Treatment of hemospermia in stallions: a discussion of 18 cases. Compend Contin Educ Pract Vet 1988;10(12): 1396–403.
54. Arnold CE, Brinsko SP, Love CC, et al. Use of a modified Vinsot technique for partial phallectomy in 11 standing horses. J Am Vet Med Assoc 2010;237(1): 82–6.
55. Lillich JD, DeBowes RM. Urethra. In: Auer JA, Stick JA, editors. Equine surgery. 3rd edition. St Louis (MO): Saunders; 2006. p. 887–93.
56. van den Top JG, de Heer N, Klein WR, et al. Penile and preputial tumours in the horse; a retrospective study of 114 affected horses. Equine Vet J 2008;40(6): 528–32.
57. van den Top JG, de Heer N, Klein WR, et al. Penile and preputial squamous cell carcinoma in the horse: a retrospective study of treatment of 77 affected horses. Equine Vet J 2008;40(6):533–7.
58. Schumacher J, Vaughn JT. Surgery of the penis and prepuce. Vet Clin North Am Equine Pract 1988;4:473–91.
59. Van Harreveld PD, Gaughn EM. Partial phallectomy to treat priapism in a horse. Aust Vet J 1999;77:167–9.
60. Brinsko SP, Blanchard TL, Varner DD. How to treat paraphimosis. Proc Am Assoc Equine Practnr 2007;53:580–2.
61. Williams WL. The diseases of the genital organs of domestic animals. 3rd edition. Worcester (MA): Ethel Williams Plimpton; 1943. p. 201–436.
62. Frank ER. Veterinary surgery. 7th edition. Minneapolis (MN): Burgess; 1964.
63. Scott EA. A technique for amputation of the equine penis. J Am Vet Med Assoc 1976;168:1047–51.
64. Schumacher J. Penis and prepuce. In: Auer JA, Stick JA, editors. Equine surgery. 3rd edition. St Louis (MO): Saunders; 2006. p. 811–35.

Urogenital Surgery Performed with the Mare Standing

Kathryn A. Seabaugh, DVM, MS, DACVS[a],*,
Jim Schumacher, DVM, MS, DACVS, MRCVS[b]

KEYWORDS

- Urogenital tract • Surgery • Mare • Standing

KEY POINTS

- Urogenital surgery of the mare can be performed safely with the mare standing.
- Ovariectomy performed using laparoscopy is safer than ovariectomy performed using conventional methods and allows the mare to return more rapidly to its normal function.
- Reproductive abnormalities commonly corrected by reconstructive surgery performed with the mare standing include cervical lacerations, perineal injury, pneumovagina, and urovagina.
- Uteropexy is a recently reported technique that may prolong the fertility of aged, multiparous mares.

SEDATION AND LOCAL ANESTHESIA

One of the many benefits of performing surgery with the horse standing is that general anesthesia is avoided. To achieve compliance by the horse and to enhance the safety of the surgeon when performing surgical procedures with the horse standing, the horse should be sedated and the site of surgery desensitized by using local or regional anesthesia. The horse can be sedated by using a combination of an alpha-2 agonist and an opioid. This combination can be administered as needed or by continuous, intravenous infusion. Continuous intravenous infusion results in a longer, more constant level of sedation when performing long procedures. Detomidine hydrochloride (20 mg/L) and butorphanol tartrate (10 mg/L) in a 1-L bag of isotonic saline solution has provided a consistent level of sedation for standing procedures for the authors. A constant state of sedation can be maintained for most horses by administering the solution at 1 to 2 drops per second.

Caudal epidural anesthesia should be considered when performing surgery of the perineum and caudal portion of the urogenital tract with the mare standing. It not

[a] Department of Large Animal Medicine, College of Veterinary Medicine, University of Georgia, 501 DW Brooks Drive, Athens, GA 30602, USA; [b] Department of Large Animal Clinical Sciences, University of Tennessee, 2407 River Drive, Knoxville, TN 37996-4545, USA
* Corresponding author.
E-mail address: seabaugh@uga.edu

Vet Clin Equine 30 (2014) 191–209
http://dx.doi.org/10.1016/j.cveq.2013.11.007   vetequine.theclinics.com
0749-0739/14/$ – see front matter © 2014 Elsevier Inc. All rights reserved.

only provides analgesia of the perineal region, it also prevents contamination of the surgical site by preventing the horse from defecating during the procedure. An alpha-2 agonist is often combined with the local anesthetic agent to provide longer and more profound analgesia. The use of caudal epidural anesthesia is described in more detail elsewhere in this issue by Vigani and colleagues. **Table 1** represents the various drugs or drug combinations for use in epidural anesthesia for most urogenital surgeries performed with the mare standing.

PERIOPERATIVE MEDICATIONS

Mares undergoing urogenital surgery while standing should receive flunixin meglumine (1.1 mg/kg orally or intravenously) or phenylbutazone (2.2–4.4 mg/kg orally or intravenously) before surgery and every 12 to 24 hours for 2 to 4 days. The duration of administration depends on the time for which the mare is expected to be in discomfort.

Most mares undergoing urogenital surgery while standing should also receive perioperative antimicrobial therapy. Because laparoscopic procedures are minimally invasive and clean, antimicrobial therapy is not necessary if no breaks in sterility are expected. Procedures that involve the vestibule and perineum should be considered to be contaminated procedures, and therefore, when performing these procedures, perioperative antimicrobial therapy should be administered to decrease the likelihood of dehiscence of the repair from infection. Administering trimethoprim-sulfa (20–30 mg/kg) orally for 7 to 10 days may prevent delayed healing of a repair in the caudal aspect of the tubular portion of the urogenital region.

Table 1
Drugs and drug combinations that can be used for epidural anesthesia for most urogenital surgeries performed with the mare standing

Drug	Dose	Quick Dose (500-kg Horse)	Comments
Lidocaine	0.22 mg/kg	110 mg	—
Xylazine	0.17 mg/kg	85 mg	Induces analgesia sufficient for perineal surgery
Detomidine	0.03–0.06 mg/kg	15–30 mg	Can result in systemic sedation Variable degree of analgesia and sedation
Morphine[17]	0.1 mg/kg	Diluted to 6–8 mL with PSS	Pruritus
Drug Combinations			
Lidocaine + xylazine[35]	0.22 mg/kg + 0.17 mg/kg	110 mg + 85 mg (6 mL volume)	—
Morphine + detomidine[35,36]	0.2 mg/kg + 0.03 mg/kg	—	Less predictable local anesthesia; better for pain management
Neostigmine + lidocaine[37]	1.0 μg/kg + 0.2 mg/kg	—	—
Bupivacaine + morphine[38]	0.02 mg/kg + 0.1 mg/kg	—	—

Abbreviation: PSS, physiologic saline solution.
Data from Refs.[17,32,35–38]

OVARIECTOMY

Ovaries are typically removed from mares for 2 reasons: because an ovary is diseased or for managerial reasons, such as to ameliorate abnormal behavior during estrus or to resolve cycle-related episodes of colic. Bilateral ovariectomy to ameliorate abnormal behavior during estrus improved behavior in 83% of mares.[1] Multiple techniques have been described for removing 1 or both ovaries, and many of these techniques can be performed with the mare standing.

Ovariectomy via Colpotomy

Ovariectomy via colpotomy is best reserved for bilateral removal of nontumorous ovaries. This approach is inexpensive and, because the incision is usually not sutured, the technique is performed quickly. The mare can be returned to athletic function sooner with this approach than with ovariectomy performed using other approaches.

A major disadvantage of this technique is that the ovariectomy is performed blindly, making excessive intra-abdominal hemorrhage difficult to detect. A chain écraseur is used to crush and sever the mesovarian. When the procedure is performed by an inexperienced surgeon, a fecal ball can be mistaken for an ovary, resulting in lethal, septic peritonitis. Because of these disadvantages, ovariectomy is no longer commonly performed with an écraseur through a colpotomy approach. However, a laparoscopic-assisted ovariectomy performed through a colpotomy was recently reported.[2] This technique combines the benefits of both colpotomy and laparoscopy. It allows visualization of the colpotomy sites, guarantees appropriate placement of the écraseur, and provides visual monitoring of hemostasis, but use of the laparoscope increases the cost of the procedure.

To perform ovariectomy via colpotomy, the perineum and vaginal vault should be desensitized by administering caudal epidural anesthesia (discussed earlier). After thoroughly cleaning the perineum, a gloved hand holding a scalpel blade is passed into the vagina. The blade can be tethered to the hand with umbilical tape to prevent inadvertent loss of the blade. One or both ovaries can be removed through 1 incision at the 1-o'clock to 2-o'clock position. The stab incision should extend only through the submucosa. The stab incision is spread by using a hemostat, and the fascia and peritoneum are perforated with a finger. The hole into the peritoneal cavity is enlarged to accommodate a hand and arm. After the ovaries have been palpated, local anesthetic solution is applied to the mesovarium by using a long needle introduced into the abdomen through the colpotomy or by applying sterile gauze, tethered to a string and saturated with local anesthetic solution, to the mesovarium for about 5 minutes.

After the pedicles are adequately desensitized, the écraseur, the chain of which is secured over the hand of the surgeon (**Fig. 1**), is inserted into the abdomen. The ovary is grasped, and the chain is slipped over the hand of the surgeon to encircle the mesovarium. The surgeon should be certain that the structure to be removed is an ovary and that intestine has not entered the loop of chain before the chain is slowly tightened. Tightening is continued until the écraseur severs the ovarian pedicle, permitting the ovary to be extracted through the vagina. The surgeon should take care not to stretch the ovarian pedicle while the pedicle is being crushed and severed. The same procedure is performed on the contralateral ovary. The surgeon should make sure that the hand has passed beneath the colon to access the second ovary and is not grasping the ovary through the mesocolon. The incision in the vaginal wall is typically not sutured, but evisceration through the opening is a concern. Evisceration may be more likely if the mare is allowed to lie down, and consequently some surgeons recommend leaving the mare tied for 3 days to prevent the mare from becoming

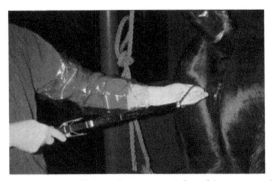

Fig. 1. Écraseur with chain secured over the surgeon's hand in preparation for an ovariectomy via colpotomy.

recumbent.[3] The mare can be returned to work after being confined to a stall for 3 to 5 days. By this time, the colpotomy should be nearly healed.

Flank Ovariectomy

The flank approach for ovariectomy should be reserved for cases in which anesthetizing the mare is a concern. This approach can be performed without laparoscopic assistance but that removing an ovary larger than 10 cm in diameter through a flank incision without laparoscopic equipment is difficult.[4] Removal of ovaries of up to 40 cm has been reported with laparoscopic assistance.[5-7] The ovarian pedicle is crushed by using a écraseur or compressed with staples (eg, using a Thoraco-abdominal stapler, 90 mm [TA 90]) or heavy ligatures (eg, no. 1 or no. 2 absorbable suture). Complications include fatal hemorrhage, septic peritonitis, and (most commonly) formation of a seroma or abscess at the incision.

The flank is prepared for surgery, and with the mare sedated, the proposed site of incision is desensitized with local anesthetic solution using an inverted L block or by infusing local anesthetic solution subcutaneously along the proposed line of incision. A modified grid technique can be used to gain access to the abdomen.[4] The flank incision is closed in 3 to 4 layers after the ovary or ovaries are removed.

The mare should be confined to a stall until skin sutures are removed at 12 to 14 days. Because flank celiotomies are prone to becoming infected, antimicrobial therapy should be administered before surgery and for at least 3 to 5 days.

Laparoscopic Ovariectomy

The use of laparoscopy for various procedures in the horse has gained in popularity during the past few decades and is especially useful for ovariectomies. It is a minimally invasive procedure that allows excellent visualization of the ovarian pedicle. Multiple methods of laparoscopic ovariectomy have been reported, with most differing primarily in the method of achieving hemostasis. Methods described to establish hemostasis of the ovarian pedicle during laparoscopic ovariectomy include placing an encircling ligature,[8-10] using a polyamide Tie-rap,[11] electrocautery,[12] ultrasonic shears,[13] a vessel-sealing device (LigaSure Atlas Laparoscopic Sealer/Divider Instrument; Covidien),[6,9,14-16] staples or clips,[6,17] electrocoagulation,[18] bipolar and monopolar laser dissection,[6,19,20] and harmonic scalpel.[21] The laparoscopic approach is similar in all these reports.

Food should be withheld from the mare for at least 24 hours before surgery to decrease abdominal fill, thereby improving visualization. The paralumbar fossae are prepared for aseptic surgery. If a unilateral ovariectomy is planned, only the ipsilateral paralumbar fossa need be prepared. A local anesthetic solution (eg, mepivacaine hydrochloride) is injected subcutaneously at the intended portal sites. Epidural anesthesia can be used to provide analgesia of the ovarian pedicle. Instilling detomidine hydrochloride into the epidural space induces hormonal responses and visual analog scores that are similar to those observed during continuous intravenous infusion of detomidine hydrochloride in response to stimuli designed to provoke pain.[22]

If both ovaries are to be removed, the left ovary should be removed first so that intra-abdominal pressure equilibrates with atmospheric pressure before the trocar/cannula assembly is inserted through the right paralumbar fossa. Equilibration of pressure causes the cecum to fall away from the right side of the body wall so that injury to the cecum is avoided when the trocar/cannula assemblies are eventually placed through the right flank. The portal locations and the order in which the portals are created vary among surgeons. All portal sites are located within the paralumbar fossa or 17th intercostal space (**Fig. 2**).

A controlled-access, laparoscopic cannula (10-mm diameter, 20 cm long; Karl Storz Veterinary Endoscopy) or a standard laparoscopic cannula (10-mm diameter, 20 cm long) and trocar are used to create the first portal. After access into the abdomen has been created, as indicated by endoscopic visualization of abdominal viscera or by observing influx of air into the abdomen through the cannula, the peritoneal cavity can be insufflated with carbon dioxide to 10 to 15 mm Hg, if necessary, to enhance visualization. Two other instrument portals are then created with standard trocar/cannula assemblies. A long (eg, $\geq$56 cm), 10-mm diameter, 30°, forward-viewing laparoscope (authors' preference) is inserted into the most cranial cannula. A shorter or 0° scope can also be used.

Mepivacaine hydrochloride (0.01–0.05 mL/kg) is injected into the mesovarium through a laparoscopic injection needle, and the ovary is grasped with a laparoscopic grasping forceps. The mesovarian is then transected using a technique that provides secure hemostasis (**Fig. 3**).[6,8–21]

When performing bilateral ovariectomy with the abdomen insufflated, the first ovary removed from its pedicle is left in the jaws of the grasper while the pedicle of the

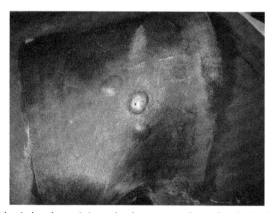

Fig. 2. Local anesthetic has been injected subcutaneously at the desired portal sites in the left paralumbar fossa. The middle portal site is level with the ventral portion of the tuber coxae and halfway between the tuber coxae and the last rib. The dorsal portal is 3 to 4 cm dorsal and 3 to 4 cm cranial to the middle portal. The ventral portal is 3 to 4 cm ventral to the middle portal. That distance may be dictated by the size of the ovary to be removed.

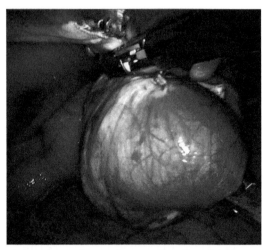

Fig. 3. Transection of the mesovarium with a vessel-sealing device.

contralateral ovary is being transected; each ovary is removed through its associated flank. Delaying removal of the first ovary from the abdomen until the second ovary has been removed from its pedicle avoids loss of insufflated gas from the abdomen. Another option for removing the ovaries from the abdomen is to pass 1 ovary to the contralateral side of the abdomen so that both are removed from 1 laparotomy. To accomplish this, 1 ovary, secured in a grasping forceps, is manipulated beneath the small colon and mesentery cranial and dorsal to the bladder. This maneuver can be challenging in large-bodied mares and requires 2 grasping forceps. The benefit is that only 1 laparotomy is needed to extract both ovaries from the abdomen.

The mare should be confined to a stall for 1 week after undergoing ovariectomy. The mare can be walked in hand after a week, provided that the laparotomy created to extract the ovary (or ovaries) was small. The mare should be confined to a stall for 2 weeks before beginning light work if the laparotomy was large or if a laparotomy was created at each flank. Moderate emphysema may develop at the portal sites of some mares after laparoscopy, and for these mares antiinflammatory therapy should be continued for 3 to 5 days to reduce the inflammation and pain associated with the emphysema.

Natural Orifice Transluminal Endoscopic Surgery

Natural orifice transluminal endoscopic surgery (NOTES) is an endoscopic approach to the abdomen through an incision in a body orifice, such as the vagina or stomach. The first report[23] of NOTES performed in the mare compared the results of exploring the abdomen using a 63 cm long, rigid laparoscope with the results of exploring the abdomen using a 2 m long, flexible endoscope. The flexible endoscope was more maneuverable, allowing better visualization of the contents of the abdomen.[23] The benefits of transvaginal NOTES included no visible scar, accessibility of both sides of the abdomen through 1 incision, and earlier return to exercise.

The mare should be starved for 24 to 48 hours before performing transvaginal NOTES. Feces should be evacuated from the rectum, and the perineum should be prepared for aseptic surgery. A dilute solution of povidone-iodine can be used to rinse the vestibule and vagina, but lavage is probably unnecessary if the mare has no evidence of pneumovagina. Placement of a urinary catheter into the bladder for the duration of the procedure is also advisable. An incision into the abdominal cavity is made just to the right or left of the cervix (ie, the 11-o'clock or 1-o'clock position). Before creating the vaginal incision, the vaginal mucosa is desensitized by holding gauze soaked with local anesthetic solution at the proposed site of incision for about 5 minutes. This local anesthetic may be the only analgesia necessary if the only procedure to be performed through the incision is exploration of the abdomen. The vaginal wall can be penetrated sharply or bluntly. Sharp dissection risks fatal hemorrhage from transection of the vaginal branch of the uterine artery.

The portal for transvaginal ovariectomy should be created with a controlled-access, laparoscopic cannula (**Fig. 4**; EndoPath Xcel Bladeless, Ethicon Endo-Surgery, Inc), which is replaced with a standard 10-mm diameter laparoscopic cannula. That portal site is then dilated by placing a 33-mm diameter EndoPath Large-Port assembly (Ethicon Endo-Surgery, Inc) into the portal. This large-bore cannula allows passage of a rigid laparoscope or a flexible endoscope and instruments throughout the procedure.

The mesovarian of the ovary or ovaries to be removed is desensitized with a local anesthetic agent using a laparoscopic injection needle inserted through the vaginal portal. The mesovarian is transected using one of a variety of techniques described earlier. The working length of the instrument used to transect the mesovarian and seal the vessels is usually longer than the instruments that are commercially available. Pader and colleagues[24] created a 60 cm long, vessel-sealing device by joining two 45-cm instruments. This longer instrument allowed easy access to the mesovarian. After the mesovarian is transected, the ovary is extracted through the 33-mm diameter EndoPath, or, if the ovary is too large to be extracted though the cannula, the cannula is removed, the vaginal portal is digitally dilated, and the ovary is extracted. If the contralateral ovary is to be removed, the EndoPath cannula is then replaced into the same colpotomy, and the procedure is repeated.

Because of its large size, the colpotomy should be sutured to minimize the risk of eventration. A single cruciate suture with no. 2 absorbable suture placed through the vaginal mucosa and muscularis provides adequate closure. The suture can be placed under endoscopic guidance using laparoscopic or long-handled needle drivers.

UTEROPEXY

Mares are normally resistant to uterine infection even though debris and bacteria are deposited in the uterus during copulation.[25] Some mares are unable to clear debris from the uterus because multiple pregnancies have caused the uterus to deviate ventrally from its normal horizontal position.[26] The strength of contractions of a ventrally positioned uterus may be inadequate to rid the uterus of debris and bacteria, resulting in an environment that is inhospitable to an embryo.[25,26] Returning a ventrally oriented uterus to a normal, horizontal orientation may improve uterine clearance and hence fertility.

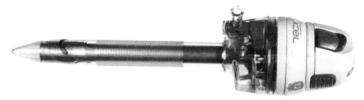

Fig. 4. Endopath Xcel Bladeless Trocar for use in the transvaginal NOTES procedure for ovariectomy. (*Courtesy of* Ethicon Endo-Surgery, Inc, Cincinnati, OH; with permission.)

A ventrally oriented uterus can be returned to a horizontal orientation by shortening the broad ligaments laparoscopically with the mare sedated in a standing position.[27]

Surgery is performed after withholding feed from the mare for about 36 hours. The left broad ligament is imbricated first. Three portals are used to access the broad ligament. The central portal site is halfway between the tuber coxae and the last rib and slightly dorsal to the dorsal aspect of the internal abdominal oblique muscle. A 25-mm diameter cannula is placed at this portal site. The cranial portal is in the 17th intercostal space 2 cm dorsal or ventral to the first portal site. The caudal portal site is 6 cm ventral and 2 cm caudal to the first portal site. Positive pressure is usually not necessary to visualize and manipulate the uterine horns, provided that the mare has been starved sufficiently. The uterine body and horn and broad ligament are desensitized by instilling local anesthetic solution into the broad ligament through a laparoscopic needle. The broad ligament is imbricated by suturing the uterine body and horn to the broad ligament using a laparoscopic needle holder or an endoscopic automated suturing device.

To imbricate the broad ligament using a needle holder, the needle holder and a 1.5-m strand of no. 6 polyglactin 910 suture swaged to a large, half-circle needle are inserted into the abdomen through a 25-mm diameter, middle cannula. The needle is inserted through the seromuscular layer of the uterus close to the attachment of the broad ligament and then through the broad ligament about 3 cm or more dorsal to its attachment on the uterus. The suture is anchored by passing the needle through a small loop created at the end of the suture. The uterus and the dorsal aspect of the broad ligament are then sutured together to the tip of the uterine horn using a simple continuous pattern, taking care to avoid incorporating the oviduct in the suture line. The suture is tied extracorporeally or intracorporeally, and the same approach and technique are then used to imbricate the right broad ligament.

As an alternative, the broad ligament can be imbricated using an endoscopic, automated suturing device (**Fig. 5**; Endo Stitch Automatic Endoscopic Suturing Device; Auto Suture Company, Division of Covidien Surgical, Norwalk, CT). This device can be inserted through a 10-mm diameter cannula, making insertion of the 25-mm diameter cannula unnecessary. The suture used to imbricate the broad ligament is a 122-cm, no. 0 suture (polyglycolide colactide, polyester, or nylon) attached to the center of a 9 mm long needle that is sharp on both ends (Endo Stitch, United States Surgical, Tyco Healthcare Group LP, Norwalk, CT). Although a heavier suture would be ideal, the 0 suture is the largest available for use with the Endo Stitch. When the surgeon squeezes the instrument's jaw closure handles and pivots the flip lever, the needle moves from one jaw to the other, through tissue interposed between the

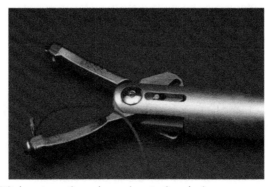

Fig. 5. The Endo Stitch automatic endoscopic suturing device.

jaws. To anchor the first stitch, the needle is passed through a small loop created on the end of the suture. The dorsal aspect of the uterus and the dorsal aspect of the broad ligament are sutured together using a simple continuous suture pattern, and the cranial end of the suture line is ended with a knot tied intracorporeally.

The mare is given a nonsteroidal antiinflammatory drug before surgery and for 1 or 2 days after surgery. The mare is confined to a stall for 2 weeks, during which time it can be walked. Mares are then allowed access to a small paddock for the next 2 weeks before being allowed unrestricted exercise at 1 month after surgery.

Postoperative complications of imbricating the broad ligament, other than mild signs of colic reported to have occurred in 1 horse, have not been observed. Enlarged uterine horns decrease in size, and some mares with chronic endometritis have experienced resolution of endometritis without other treatment.[27] Abnormal perineal conformation is improved because suspending the uterus relieves traction on the vestibule and vulva imposed by the uterus (**Fig. 6**). Even though preliminary results indicate beneficial results with little medical risk,[27] insufficient numbers of mares have undergone the surgery to determine the procedure's effectiveness in improving fertility.

CLEARING AN OBSTRUCTED OVIDUCT

Some mares with normal ovaries and tubular portion of the reproductive tract that seem to ovulate normally nevertheless fail to conceive, and the cause of this infertility may be oviducal concretions that prevent the oocyte from reaching the site of fertilization at the ampullary/isthmic junction, or passage of the embryo into the uterus.[28] The equine embryo secretes prostaglandin E2 (PGE2) on day 5 after conception,[29] and binding of PGE2 to the oviductal musculature hastens embryonic transport through the oviduct.[30] The physiologic quantities of PGE2 secreted by an embryo may not provide sufficient impulse to dislodge a blockage, but laparoscopic application of a

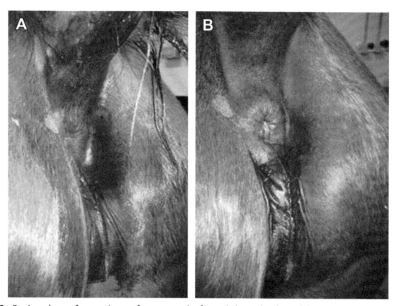

Fig. 6. Perineal conformation of a mare before (A) and after (B) uteropexy. Improved perineal conformation can be seen.

pharmacologic dose of PGE2 gel to the external surface of an occluded oviduct may help restore patency to the oviduct.

To perform this laparoscopic procedure, the mare is prepared in a manner identical to that for other laparoscopic procedures. The cranial portal for the laparoscope is at the level of the tuber coxae at the 17th intercostal space and the caudal portal is within the paralumbar fossa. Using an embryo transfer pipette, dinoprostone (Prostin E2 Vaginal Gel) is placed over the oviduct. This product is a vaginal suppository used to induce labor in women and contains 0.2 mg of PGE2 in 0.5 mL of triactin gel. Its glutinous properties cause it to adhere to tissue. The same procedure is repeated on the right side, and the portals are closed in 1 or 2 layers. As reported by Allen and colleagues[28] (2006), 14 of 15 barren mares conceived in the same (12 mares) or following breeding season (2 mares).

CAUDAL UROGENITAL TRACT

Abnormal conformation of the vulva can predispose a mare to uterine infection and subsequent infertility.[31] Mares with a conformational abnormality of the external genitalia are candidates for reproductive surgery if the results of a breeding soundness examination indicate that the procedure is likely to restore fertility. Reproductive abnormalities commonly corrected by reconstructive surgery include cervical lacerations, caused by insufficient dilatation of the cervix during parturition; perineal injury, caused by fetal malposture during foaling; pneumovagina, caused by cranial deviation of the anus and vulva; and urovagina, caused by cranioventral deviation of the vagina.

CERVICAL LACERATIONS

A cervical laceration occurs when the cervix does not dilate sufficiently to accommodate passage of the foal and is often not detected until it is discovered during routine postpartum examination or during examination to determine the cause of infertility, abortion, or repeated uterine infection. Most cervical lacerations are longitudinal and are best identified by palpating the wall of the cervix between an index finger (or thumb) inserted into the lumen of the cervix and a thumb (or index finger) placed on the vaginal aspect of the cervix.

Repair of a torn cervix may not be necessary if the cervix remains competent. Competency is best evaluated when the mare is in diestrus because during this stage of the cycle a competent cervix is closed and must be dilated to allow insertion of a finger into the uterine lumen. If the cervix appears to be incompletely closed when the mare is in diestrus, the cervix should be repaired.

A cervical tear is most easily repaired when the mare is in diestrus or anestrous because at this stage of the cycle the size of the mucosal folds projecting into the lumen is minimal. The rectum should be evacuated and the perineum aseptically prepared. A caudal epidural should be performed to provide local anesthesia (discussed earlier) and to prevent the mare from defecating during surgery. A Finochietto retractor with long blades can be used to expose the cervix. As an alternative, the labia can be retracted with stay sutures or towel clamps. Three heavy stay sutures are used to retract the cervix (**Fig. 7**). One is placed on either side of the defect and another is place directly across from it. Long-handled instruments are necessary for the repair. The edges of the tear are excised with long scissors to expose the muscular layer of the cervix, and the defect is closed in 2 or 3 layers. The mucosa lining the lumen of the cervix is sutured first with no. 00 or no. 0 absorbable, monofilament suture placed in a continuous horizontal mattress pattern so that the mucosa is inverted into the lumen of the cervix. Suturing begins at the cranial end of the defect and is

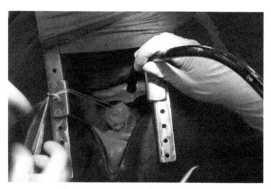

Fig. 7. Finochietto retractors placed in the vestibule allow visualization of the cervix. Stay sutures aid in caudal retraction of the cervix for cervical tear repair.

continued caudally to the external os. Good apposition of the mucosal layer is important to avoid intraluminal adhesions, which can result in pyometra (**Fig. 8**). Good apposition is most easily achieved by using the Endo Stitch (Endo Stitch Automatic Endoscopic Suturing Device; Auto Suture Company, Division of Covidien Surgical, Norwalk, CT). The suture used is a 122-cm, no. 0 polyglycolide colactide suture (Endo Stitch, United States Surgical, Tyco Healthcare Group LP, Norwalk, CT). The muscular layer is sutured cranially to caudally with no. 0 absorbable, monofilament suture inserted in a simple continuous pattern. The outer (ie, vaginal) mucosal layer is sutured cranially to caudally using no. 0 monofilament, absorbable suture material inserted in a continuous horizontal mattress pattern so that the mucosa is everted into the lumen of the vagina.

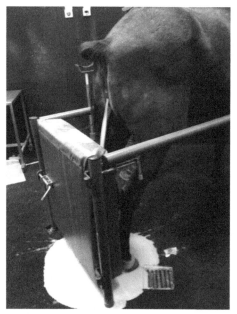

Fig. 8. This mare developed intraluminal mucosal adhesions after repair of a cervical laceration, and these adhesions resulted in pyometra.

The mare should receive sexual rest for 1 month, and its cervix should be examined for competency and patency before the mare is bred. Seventy-five percent of mares in one study population became pregnant after surgery.[32] Before the cervix is repaired, the owner should be warned that scar tissue at the site of repair is often torn during the subsequent parturition because the repaired cervix is incapable of dilating completely.

RECTOVESTIBULAR LACERATIONS AND FISTULAE

A perineal laceration or fistula occurs at parturition when the foal's forefoot or nose catches the annular fold of the hymen at the vaginovestibular junction. This injury occurs predominately in primiparous mares because the annular fold of these mares is more prominent than that of pluriparous mares. A first-degree perineal laceration involves only the skin and mucous membrane of the dorsum of the vestibule, whereas a second-degree perineal laceration is characterized by disruption of the constrictor vulvae muscle, compromising the ability of the perineal musculature to constrict the vestibule. A third-degree perineal laceration, or rectovestibular laceration, is charac-terized by a complete disruption of tissue between the rectum and vestibule, resulting in a common rectal and vestibular vault. The vaginovestibular seal is usually disrupted, but the vagina is seldom involved in the injury. A rectovestibular fistula occurs when the tissue between the rectum and vestibule is perforated by the foal, but the nose or limb of the foal is retracted into the vestibule before the foal is delivered, preserving at least a portion of the perineal body. A rectovestibular laceration or fistula allows fecal contamination of the mare's vestibule, which results in bacterial infection of the vagina and endometrium. Mares with a first-degree perineal laceration can be treated with a Caslick vulvoplasty, but mares with a second-degree perineal laceration require vestibuloplasty because the constrictor vulvae muscle is disrupted, causing the perineum to shift cranially and ventrally, predisposing the mare to pneumovagina and urovagina.

Repair of a perineal laceration immediately after injury is usually unsuccessful because contraction of the rectal and vestibular musculature rapidly widens and lengthens the wound and because the lacerated tissue soon becomes inflamed. By 4 weeks, the wound is usually healed sufficiently to allow repair. The mare's reproduc-tive tract should be palpated per vagina and per rectum before repair, to determine whether the mare has also incurred a cervical laceration, has uterine adhesions or pyo-metra, or is pregnant. Histologic evaluation of the endometrium may be indicated if the mare has gone through more than one reproductive season. Even though the vagina is constantly contaminated with feces, the uterus is unlikely to be permanently damaged, provided that reconstruction of the perineum was not neglected beyond several reproductive seasons.

The mare's stool should be softened and its bulk decreased in preparation for surgery, but the mare's ration should allow the mare to maintain weight. Adminis-tering mineral oil (2.25–4.5 L [0.5–1 gallon] orally by stomach tube) or raw linseed oil (30–60 mL [1–2 ounces] in the feed) the day before surgery assures that the stool is soft and unformed at surgery. A stool softener often need not be administered if the mare has been grazing a lush pasture. A broad-spectrum antimicrobial drug should be administered before surgery.

The mare is restrained in a stock and sedated, and the perineal region is desensi-tized by administering epidural anesthesia. The tail is bandaged, elevated, and tied, and feces are evacuated from the rectum. Some surgeons insert a tampon cranial to the defect to prevent feces from leaking into the surgical site during repair, but inser-tion of a tampon is not necessary because epidural anesthesia prevents movement of feces into the surgical site. The vagina, vestibule, rectum, and perineal region are cleaned, and the laceration is exposed by clamping the dorsal aspect of each labium and ventral aspect of right and left sides of the anus to adjacent skin with towel clamps. Using long surgical instruments to reconstruct the rectum and vestibule is helpful.

The repair consists of 2 stages: rectovestibular reconstruction and anoperineal reconstruction. Both stages can be performed during the same operation, or the ano-perineal reconstruction can be completed 3 weeks or more after rectovestibular reconstruction. To reconstruct the rectovestibular tissue, regardless of whether or not both stages of reconstruction are to be performed during a single session, submu-cosa, between the ventral aspect of the rectum and the dorsal aspect of the vagina, at the cranial border of the laceration, is separated using scissors. The submucosa is separated for 5 to 10 cm cranial to the cranial border of the defect, and dissection is continued caudolaterally along the right and left walls of the common vault of the rectum and vestibule, using a scalpel, to the ventralmost aspect of each side of the torn anus. This incision along each wall of the rectovestibular vault is deepened ven-trolaterally, using scissors, to form the right and left flaps used to recreate the dorsal aspect of the vestibule. Dissection is continued until right and left flaps can be sutured together on midline without tension. The caudal portion of the flaps is dissected ventral to the anus to the point at which the dorsal commissure of the vulva is to be created. At this point, rectovestibular reconstruction can be completed by suturing the vestibular flaps together with a continuous horizontal mattress suture pattern using no. 1 or no. 2 absorbable or nonabsorbable suture oversewn with a simple continuous or simple interrupted suture of heavy absorbable or nonabsorbable suture (Aanes technique; **Fig. 9**). The anus and perineum can be reconstructed 3 or 4 weeks later, after the rec-tovestibular reconstruction has healed.

To reconstruct the anus and perineum at the same time as rectovestibular recon-struction, the longitudinal incision in the rectovestibular vault is deepened dorsally on each side of the vault to create flaps used to form the ventral aspect of the rectum. Using the Goetz technique of rectovestibular reconstruction, the edges of the right and left rectal and vestibular flaps are sutured together, cranially to caudally, with no. 1 or no. 2, absorbable or nonabsorbable sutures, placed 0.5 to 1 cm apart, using an inter-rupted, 6-bite suture pattern. The dorsal portion of this suture resembles a Lembert su-ture, and the ventral aspect of this suture resembles a vertical mattress suture (**Fig. 10**). This pattern causes the edges of the vestibular flaps to invert into the vestibular lumen and the edges of the rectal flaps to invert into the rectal lumen. These sutures can be alternated with no. 2-0 or no. 0 monofilament absorbable sutures inserted in the rectal submucosa in an interrupted Lembert pattern, which inverts the edges of rectal mucosa into the rectal lumen, ensuring close apposition of rectal mucosa, so that the likelihood of leakage of rectal contents between the sutured flaps is minimized.

The rectum and vestibule are reconstructed, using the 6-bite suture pattern, until the region of the perineal body is reached. To repair the perineal body, the remaining portion of the right and left flaps created to form the vestibule are sutured together with a continuous, horizontal mattress pattern using no. 1 or no. 2 monofilament, absorbable suture. The caudal aspect of the sutured flaps forms the dorsal commis-sure of the vulva. The rectal submucosa of the right rectal flap is sutured to that of the left rectal flap with 2-0 absorbable suture using a continuous Lembert pattern, so that the sutured edges are inverted into the rectal lumen. Tissue between the newly created rectum and vestibule is apposed with multiple, simple continuous rows of no. 0 or no. 2-0 absorbable suture. Nonabsorbable sutures are placed in the skin of the perineal body and, to ensure a good labial seal, the mare should receive a Caslick vulvoplasty.

Aanes Technique

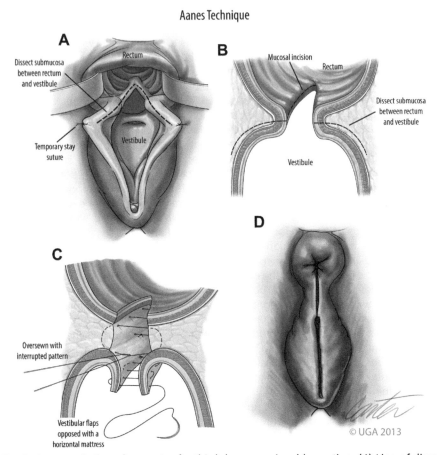

Fig. 9. Aanes technique for repair of a third-degree perineal laceration. (*A*) Line of dissection of the healed edges of the laceration. The dissection should be between the line of rectal mucosa and vestibular mucosa. (*B*) Dissection is continued ventrolaterally through the submucosa alongside the vestibule until the flaps can be apposed without tension. (*C*) The vestibular flaps are closed by everting the edges into the vestibule with a Lembert suture pattern. This suture pattern is then oversewn with a simple interrupted pattern. The rectal mucosa is not involved in the oversow. (*D*) Appearance of the perineum after completion of the Aanes technique. Anoperineal reconstruction still needs to be done but can be done in 3 to 4 weeks, after the rectovestibular reconstruction has healed.

A rectovestibular fistula should be converted into a laceration for repair only if the fistula is larger than 2 fingers in diameter or is within the caudal portion of the perineal body. A rectovestibular fistula, 2 fingers or less in diameter, can be repaired using the Forssell technique to spare the intact perineal body. Using this technique, the skin of the perineum is incised in a horizontal plane midway between the anus and the dorsal commissure of the vulva. The incision is deepened cranially beyond the fistula, separating the rectovestibular hole into a rectal hole and a vestibular hole. The rectal portion of the fistula is closed in a transverse plane because the musculature of the rectum is primarily circular, and sutures placed perpendicular to the muscle fibers are less likely to tear through tissue than are sutures placed parallel to the direction of the muscle fibers. The vestibular portion of the fistula is closed in a sagittal plane

Goetz Technique

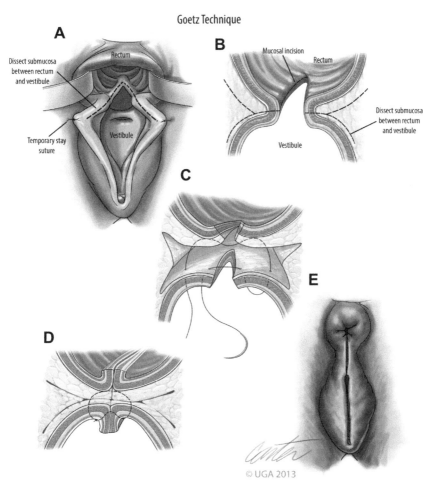

© UGA 2013

Fig. 10. Goetz technique for repair of a third-degree perineal laceration. (*A*) Line of dissection of the healed edges of the laceration. The dissection should be between the line of rectal mucosa and vestibular mucosa. (*B*) The line of dissection should be one-third of the distance from the vestibular mucosa and two-thirds of the distance from the rectal mucosa. The dissection is continued dorsolaterally and ventrolaterally to create 2 vestibular flaps and 2 rectal flaps. (*C*) A 6-bite interrupted suture pattern is used to evert the rectal mucosa into the rectum and the vestibular mucosa into the vestibule. The knot is tied within the vestibular lumen. (*D*) The apposition of tissue when the suture has been tied. (*E*) Appearance of the perineum after completion of the Goetz technique for rectovestibular reconstruction. Anoperineal reconstruction still needs to be performed.

because the musculature of the vestibule is primarily longitudinal. Both holes are closed using no. 0 or no. 2 absorbable sutures placed in an interrupted Lembert pattern. Preplacing all sutures and then tying the sutures from the center outward may allow the sutures to be placed more uniformly. The perineal dissection is difficult to close and so is usually left unsutured to heal by second intention.

Postoperative treatment of a mare after repair of a third-degree perineal injury usually includes administration of an antimicrobial drug and a nonsteroidal antiinflammatory drug for several days. The mare's stool should be kept soft and scanty for at least 8 days by feeding a pelleted feed and by administering a stool softener. The integrity of the repair can be evaluated by palpation on the eighth or ninth day. Most mares are capable of eliminating bacteria from the endometrium within 1 estrous cycle and, although natural breeding should not be allowed for 2 months, mares may be bred by artificial insemination within 2 weeks.

TREATMENTS FOR PNEUMOVAGINA

Pneumovagina, or wind sucking, is an abnormality characterized by persistent fecal contamination of the tubular portion of the reproductive tract resulting from conformational faults that cause a mare to aspirate air into the vestibule and vagina. Causes of pneumovagina include tearing or stretching of the labial seal or the vestibulovaginal sphincter. Affected mares typically have a cranially displaced anus and cranial inclination of the vulva dorsal to the brim of the pelvis. The surgical procedure used most commonly to correct pneumovagina is the Caslick vulvoplasty, a procedure in which the labia are sutured together from the dorsal commissure to slightly below the floor of the ischium after a thin strip of tissue has been excised from the mucocutaneous margin of each labium.

A Caslick vulvoplasty may be insufficient to correct pneumovagina when the vulva is deviated far cranially and dorsally, and, if so, a perineoplasty or vestibuloplasty may correct the condition. This surgery entails excising a triangle of mucosa and submucosa from the dorsum of the vestibule to expose the vestibular musculature. The right and left sides of the triangle are sutured to each other to return the vulva to a more vertical position.

TREATMENTS FOR UROVAGINA

Urovagina (ie, vesicovaginal reflux, urine pooling) is the accumulation of urine in the vagina. Urine in the vagina causes vaginitis, cervicitis, and endometritis and is associated with poor conception and early embryonic death. Urine within the vagina may decrease viability of sperm by changing the vaginal pH and may cause the corpus luteum to lyse prematurely. Urovagina occurs when the vaginal fornix is positioned ventral to the external urethral orifice and occurs most commonly in thin, aged, pluriparous mares that have poor muscular tone of the vagina and elongated ovarian ligaments, resulting from multiple pregnancies.

Before performing surgery to alleviate urine pooling, a sample of endometrium should be examined histologically. Surgery is unlikely to restore the mare's fertility if the mare has severe, widespread, periglandular, endometrial fibrosis. Surgical techniques described to alleviate urine pooling include extending the transverse fold caudally (ie, the Monin technique) and various techniques to create a tunnel from the external urethral orifice to the labia, such as the McKinnon and the Brown techniques of urethroplasty. The McKinnon technique may be superior to the Brown technique because the McKinnon technique provides a more spacious extension and is less likely to decrease the circumference of the vestibule.

To perform the McKinnon technique of urethroplasty, the mare is sedated and its perineal region is desensitized using epidural anesthesia. The tail is bandaged and tied dorsally, and the perineal region is cleaned with an antiseptic soap. The lumen of the vestibule and the urethral orifice are exposed with a self-retaining retractor fixed to the base of the tail or with hand-held tissue retractors. A U-shaped, mucosal flap is created in the vestibule that extends laterally from the floor of the vagina 2 to 4 cm cranial to the caudal border of the transverse fold, and then caudally, midway between the dorsal and ventral borders of the vestibule, to the labia. The incision is then directed ventrally toward the ventral commissure of the vulva. Using scissors, the submucosa at the transverse, cranial aspect of the incision is undermined caudally, and submucosa at the ventral margin of the right and left longitudinal portions of the incision is undermined toward the ventral aspect of the vestibule, to form a U-shaped flap. Dissection is continued until the right and left sides of the edge of the flap meet on the midline without tension.

The right and left sides of the U-shaped mucosal flap are sutured together with no. 0 monofilament, absorbable suture placed in a continuous Lembert pattern to create a mucosa-lined tunnel that extends from a point cranial to the external urethral orifice to the mucocutaneous junction of the labia. Suturing begins cranially and laterally at the juncture of the transverse and longitudinal portions of the U-shaped incision (either right or left side) apposing the edge of transverse portion of the U-shaped incision to the adjacent aspect of the edge of the longitudinal portion of the incision on the lateral wall of the vestibule. Suturing is continued caudally until half of the horizontal portion of the flap has been sutured to the caudal aspect of the longitudinal portion of the incision on the vestibule. The continuous pattern is ended with a knot. The contralateral side of the transverse portion of the U-shaped incision is sutured in a similar manner, beginning cranially and laterally at the juncture of the transverse and longitudinal portions of the U-shaped incision. Suturing is continued to the labia, past the end point of the first suture pattern, to create a Y-shaped suture line. Transposing the right and left sides of the flap to create the tunnel exposes the submucosa of the ventral half of the vestibule, and this exposed submucosa eventually epithelializes.

A Caslick vulvoplasty is performed if the mare also has pneumovagina, a condition that commonly accompanies urovagina, and many mares may also require a vestibuloplasty. The mare is administered a nonsteroidal antiinflammatory drug and a broad-spectrum antimicrobial drug for 3 to 5 days.

REMOVAL OF UTERINE CYSTS

Uterine cysts can be a cause of infertility. They are frequently diagnosed by ultrasonography or hysteroscopy. Multiple methods of removing cysts have been reported, but the most accepted technique is to ablate the cysts using a laser, such as a diode laser or an neodymium:yttrium-aluminum-garnet (Nd:YAG) laser.[4,33] The mare is sedated, and the perineum is cleaned. A sterilized, 1-m, flexible endoscope is passed into the uterus. The laser fiber is passed through the biopsy channel of the endoscope to puncture and drain the cyst and then to desiccate its lining. A power setting of 15 W is recommended.[4] The uterus should be lavaged after the procedure and for 2 to 3 days.

REMOVAL OF CYSTIC CALCULI

Cystic calculi are uncommon in mares because the urethra of mares is short. The urethra of the mare can be digitally dilated for removal of small calculi. If removal of a cystic calculus necessitates transection of the urethral sphincter, the transected sphincter must be repaired to avoid urinary incontinence. This repair can be accomplished by apposing the ends of the transected urethralis muscle.[34] The incision is sutured in 3 layers using absorbable suture placed in a simple continuous suture pattern. The first suture line apposes adventitia and the outermost portion of the ends of the urethralis muscle, the second suture line apposes the innermost portions of the ends of urethralis muscle and the tunica muscularis, and the third suture line apposes the urethral mucosa.

REFERENCES

1. Kamm JL, Hendrickson DA. Clients' perspectives on the effects of laparoscopic ovariectomy on equine behavior and medical problems. J Equine Vet Sci 2007; 27(10):435–8.
2. Tate LP Jr, Fogle CA, Bailey CS, et al. Laparoscopic-assisted colpotomy for ovariectomy in the mare. Vet Surg 2012;41(5):625–8.
3. Embertson RM. Selected urogenital surgery concerns and complications. Vet Clin North Am Equine Pract 2008;24(3):643–61, ix.
4. Auer JA, Stick JA. Equine surgery. 4th edition. St Louis (MO): Elsevier/Saunders; 2012.
5. Goodin JT, Rodgerson DH, Gomez JH. Standing hand-assisted laparoscopic ovariectomy in 65 mares. Vet Surg 2011;40(1):90–2.
6. Rocken M, Mosel G, Seyrek-Intas K, et al. Unilateral and bilateral laparoscopic ovariectomy in 157 mares: a retrospective multicenter study. Vet Surg 2011; 40(8):1009–14.
7. Rodgerson DH, Brown MP, Watt BC, et al. Hand-assisted laparoscopic technique for removal of ovarian tumors in standing mares. J Am Vet Med Assoc 2002; 220(10):1503–7, 1475.
8. Hanson CA, Galuppo LD. Bilateral laparoscopic ovariectomy in standing mares: 22 cases. Vet Surg 1999;28(2):106–12.
9. Hendrickson D. Laparoscopic cryptorchidectomy and ovariectomy in horses. Vet Clin North Am Equine Pract 2006;22(3):777–98.
10. Boure L, Marcoux M, Laverty S. Paralumbar fossa laparoscopic ovariectomy in horses with use of Endoloop ligatures. Vet Surg 1997;26(6):478–83.
11. Cokelaere SM, Martens AM, Wiemer P. Laparoscopic ovariectomy in mares using a polyamide tie-rap. Vet Surg 2005;34(6):651–6.
12. Smith LJ, Mair TS. Unilateral and bilateral laparoscopic ovariectomy of mares by electrocautery. Vet Rec 2008;163(10):297–300.
13. Alldredge JG, Hendrickson DA. Use of high-power ultrasonic shears for laparoscopic ovariectomy in mares. J Am Vet Med Assoc 2004;225(10):1578–80, 1548.
14. Hand R, Rakestraw P, Taylor T. Evaluation of a vessel-sealing device for use in laparoscopic ovariectomy in mares. Vet Surg 2002;31(3):240–4.
15. Hubert JD, Burba DJ, Moore RM. Evaluation of a vessel-sealing device for laparoscopic granulosa cell tumor removal in standing mares. Vet Surg 2006;35(4): 324–9.
16. De Bont MP, Wilderjans H, Simon O. Standing laparoscopic ovariectomy technique with intraabdominal dissection for removal of large pathologic ovaries in mares. Vet Surg 2010;39(6):737–41.
17. Van Hoogmoed LM, Galuppo LD. Laparoscopic ovariectomy using the endo-GIA stapling device and endo-catch pouches and evaluation of analgesic efficacy of epidural morphine sulfate in 10 mares. Vet Surg 2005;34(6):646–50.
18. Rodgerson DH, Belknap JK, Wilson DA. Laparoscopic ovariectomy using sequential electrocoagulation and sharp transection of the equine mesovarium. Vet Surg 2001;30(6):572–9.
19. Palmer SE. Standing laparoscopic laser technique for ovariectomy in five mares. J Am Vet Med Assoc 1993;203(2):279–83.
20. Lloyd D, Walmsley JP, Greet TR, et al. Electrosurgery as the sole means of haemostasis during the laparoscopic removal of pathologically enlarged ovaries in mares: a report of 55 cases. Equine Vet J 2007;39(3):210–4.

21. Dusterdieck KF, Pleasant RS, Lanz OI, et al. Evaluation of the harmonic scalpel for laparoscopic bilateral ovariectomy in standing horses. Vet Surg 2003;32(3):242–50.
22. Virgin J, Hendrickson D, Wallis T, et al. Comparison of intraoperative behavioral and hormonal responses to noxious stimuli between mares sedated with caudal epidural detomidine hydrochloride or a continuous intravenous infusion of detomidine hydrochloride for standing laparoscopic ovariectomy. Vet Surg 2010; 39(6):754–60.
23. Alford C, Hanson R. Evaluation of a transvaginal laparoscopic natural orifice transluminal endoscopic surgery approach to the abdomen of mares. Vet Surg 2010;39(7):873–8.
24. Pader K, Lescun TB, Freeman LJ. Standing ovariectomy in mares using a transvaginal natural orifice transluminal endoscopic surgery (NOTES®) approach. Vet Surg 2011;40(8):987–97.
25. Leblanc MM. The chronically infertile mare. Proc Am Assoc Equine Practnr 2008; 54:391–407.
26. Troedsson MH. Uterine clearance and resistance to persistent endometritis in the mare. Theriogenology 1999;52(3):461–71.
27. Brink P, Schumacher J, Schumacher J. Elevating the uterus (uteropexy) of five mares by laparoscopically imbricating the mesometrium. Equine Vet J 2010;42(8):675–9.
28. Allen WR, Wilsher S, Morris L, et al. Laparoscopic application of PGE2 to re-establish oviducal patency and fertility in infertile mares: a preliminary study. Equine Vet J 2006;38(5):454–9.
29. Weber JA, Freeman DA, Vanderwall DK, et al. Prostaglandin E2 secretion by oviductal transport-stage equine embryos. Biol Reprod 1991;45(4):540–3.
30. Weber JA, Freeman DA, Vanderwall DK, et al. Prostaglandin E2 hastens oviductal transport of equine embryos. Biol Reprod 1991;45(4):544–6.
31. Hemberg E, Lundeheim N, Einarsson S. Retrospective study on vulvar conformation in relation to endometrial cytology and fertility in thoroughbred mares. J Vet Med A Physiol Pathol Clin Med 2005;52(9):474–7.
32. Miller CD, Embertson RM. Surgical repair of cervical lacerations in thoroughbred mares: 53 cases (1986-1995). Proc Am Assoc Equine Practnr 1996;42:154–5.
33. Griffin RL, Bennett SD. Nd:YAG laser photoablation of endometrial cysts: a review of 55 cases (2000-2001). Proc Am Assoc Equine Practnr. 2002;48:58–60. Paper presented at: Proceedings AAEP 2002.
34. Schumacher J, Brink P. Repair of an incompetent urethral sphincter in a mare. Vet Surg 2011;40(1):93–6.
35. Trim C. The changing face of epidural analgesia. Equine Vet Educ 2007;19(11): 595–6.
36. Goodrich LR, Nixon AJ, Fubini SL, et al. Epidural morphine and detomidine decreases postoperative hindlimb lameness in horses after bilateral stifle arthroscopy. Vet Surg 2002;31(3):232–9.
37. DeRossi R, Maciel FB, Modolo TJ, et al. Efficacy of concurrent epidural administration of neostigmine and lidocaine for perineal analgesia in geldings. Am J Vet Res 2012;73(9):1356–62.
38. DeRossi R, Módolo TJ, Pagliosa RC, et al. Comparison of analgesic effects of caudal epidural 0.25% bupivacaine with bupivacaine plus morphine or bupivacaine plus ketamine for analgesia in conscious horses. J Equine Vet Sci 2012; 32(3):190–5.

Diagnostic and Therapeutic Arthroscopy in the Standing Horse

Janik C. Gasiorowski, VMD[a],*, Dean W. Richardson, DVM[b]

KEYWORDS

- Standing arthroscopy ● Diagnostic arthroscopy ● Fetlock ● Carpus ● Stifle

KEY POINTS

- Arthroscopy in the standing horse is most appropriate for exploration and treatment of the dorsal aspect of the metacarpophalangeal, metatarsophalangeal, middle carpal, and radiocarpal joints.
- Standing arthroscopy of the stifle joints is diagnostic only.
- Special consideration must be given to preoperative preparation, including local anesthesia, positioning of the horse, surgical equipment, and draping methodology.
- Physical and chemical restraint must be properly used to maximize the safety and efficiency of these procedures.

INTRODUCTION

The switch from arthrotomy to arthroscopic surgical technique significantly increased the success rate and decreased the incidence of complications associated with joint surgery.[1] In human medicine, complication rates have decreased further with the growing use of local or regional instead of general anesthesia.[2] Cost savings and increased hospital efficiency have also been documented.[2,3] These advances have yielded similar benefits in equine medicine.[1]

Arthroscopy in the horse is typically performed while the animal is under general anesthesia. However, some arthroscopic surgical procedures are so rapidly performed that the amount of time spent inducing, positioning, and recovering a horse from general anesthesia seems disproportionate. General anesthesia carries its own risks for the horse during the procedure and recovery from anesthesia, including myositis, neuropathy, postoperative pneumonia, and traumatic injuries during recovery, all of which may occur in young and healthy athletic horses.[4] It is important to emphasize, however, that these risks are still low and certainly do not demand an

[a] Department of Surgery, Mid-Atlantic Equine Medical Center, 40 Frontage Road, Ringoes, NJ 08551, USA; [b] Section of Surgery, New Bolton Center, University of Pennsylvania, 382 West Street Road, Kennett Square, PA 19348, USA
* Corresponding author.
E-mail address: Dr_Gasiorowski@midatlanticequine.com

Vet Clin Equine 30 (2014) 211–220
http://dx.doi.org/10.1016/j.cveq.2013.11.011
0749-0739/14/$ – see front matter © 2014 Elsevier Inc. All rights reserved.
vetequine.theclinics.com

alternative approach to surgery. An alternative such as a standing approach should not be selected unless the procedure can be performed equally well or the alternative approach affords some other specific advantage.

Surgeons must have an honest appraisal of their abilities as an arthroscopist. If one cannot consistently complete a routine chip fracture removal in less than 10 minutes without a tourniquet, standing removal should not be attempted. This technique should not be attempted without a lightweight videoendoscopic system (fetlock, carpus) or purpose-built equipment (stifle).

INDICATIONS
The Metacarpophalangeal Joint

The best indication for standing arthroscopic surgery in the horse is removal of chip fractures from the proximal dorsal aspect of the proximal phalanx, which is the single most common chip fracture in thoroughbred racehorses.[5] The arthroscopic portals are straightforward, intra-articular dissection is minimal, and the procedure can be performed easily without manipulation of the joint. In fact, the standing weight-bearing posture of the horse maximizes fetlock joint extension, making the dorsal joint pouch more readily accessible. Retrieval of dorsal proximal osteochondral fragmentation of the sagittal ridge of the third metacarpal bone and partial exploration of the proximal aspect of the palmar joint pouch are also possible in the standing horse.

The Radiocarpal Joint

Simple chip fractures of the distal dorsolateral radius and proximal intermediate carpal bone can be removed with the horse standing. The antebrachiocarpal joint has adequate space in which to maneuver the scope and the instruments along the dorsal rim with the horse bearing weight.

The Femoropatellar and Femorotibial Joints

A technique for standing arthroscopic evaluation of the equine stifle has been described.[6] The technique is intended as a diagnostic option for horses with stifle disease, as evidenced by clinical signs and diagnostic analgesia, in which radiographic and sonographic examinations have not yielded a diagnosis and whose owners are reluctant to pursue general anesthesia and/or conventional arthroscopy. This technique is strictly diagnostic. The goal is "to distinguish between horses in which training can, with appropriate management, reasonably be expected to continue and those in which arthroscopic surgery under general anesthesia is indicated."[7]

Other Synovial Structures

Other synovial structures have been endoscopically examined but are currently seen rarely enough in routine practice to warrant only brief mention.

RESTRAINT
Physical

The procedure is best performed with the horse restrained in stocks, and with its head controlled by an experienced handler. If head ties are used, they should be easily releasable. Some horses respond well to a lip-chain or twitch, whereas others do not.

Chemical

Patients are sedated with intravenous xylazine hydrochloride (0.4–0.5 mg/kg) for clipping, primary limb preparation, and local anesthesia. Intravenous or intramuscular detomidine hydrochloride (0.015–0.022 mg/kg) is administered after moving to the stocks and immediately before surgery. Additional doses are administered as needed.

EQUIPMENT
Fetlock

- Powerful fluid delivery system (Arthro-Flo, Davol, Warwick, RI, USA); hemorrhage is more significant with the horse standing
- 4-mm arthroscope
- Lightweight videoendoscopic equipment

Carpus

- Same as for the fetlock

Stifle

- Arthroscopic fluid pump or irrigation fluid in a pressure bag
- 18-gauge (1.3 mm) arthroscopic system (arthroscope, light source, camera, and monitor) (BioVision Technologies, Golden, CO, USA) (**Fig. 1**).
- 2.5-mm cannula/obturator with a 30° scope lens system

ANESTHESIA

Local anesthesia for standing arthroscopy must be comprehensive enough to ensure the safety of the patient and the surgeon. If possible, however, it should be focused enough to preserve some sensation to the limb, which might help minimize stumbling under the effects of sedation. The authors believe that it is better if the horse can feel part of its distal limb so that the limb can be more easily and safely repositioned by the surgeon or assistants during the procedure.

Fetlock

The joint is tautly distended with intra-articular 2% mepivacaine hydrochloride, and greater than 20 mL of the anesthetic is usually required. The distention clearly outlines the proximal margins of the dorsal joint pouch (**Fig. 2**). A dorsal subcutaneous half-ring block is then performed just proximal to the joint capsule to desensitize the skin. Using a 1.5-inch 22-gauge needle, this usually can be performed with 2 "sticks." This

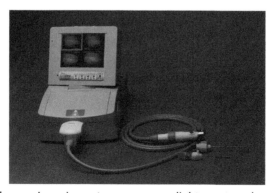

Fig. 1. Needle arthroscopic equipment: screen, xenon light source and camera cable, arthroscope and cannula/obturator combination. (*Courtesy of* BioVision, Milpitas, CA; with permission.)

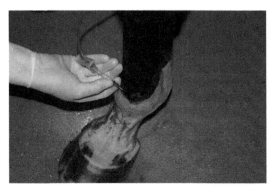

Fig. 2. Local anesthesia of the fetlock: the intra-articular block has already been performed; the distension outlines the dorsal joint pouch. A 22-gauge needle is being used to create a subcutaneous half-ring block just proximal to the proximal aspect of the dorsal joint pouch.

technique has the advantages of being technically simple, rapid to perform, and consistent in its effects, and it distends the joint pouch in preparation for placement of the arthroscope cannula.

Carpus

The same technique that is used for the fetlock is used for the radiocarpal joint.

Stifle

Each joint compartment is individually blocked using 20 to 30 mL of local anesthetic at least 20 minutes before surgery. The skin and deep tissues at each portal site are blocked with 5 to 10 mL of 2% mepivacaine hydrochloride.

PREPARATION AND POSITIONING
Patient

The horse should be carefully groomed or bathed to remove gross debris, bedding, and hair. The hooves are picked, cleansed, and dried. For fetlock arthroscopy, the hair is clipped from the coronary band to the mid metacarpus. For carpal arthroscopy, the hair is clipped from the mid metacarpus to the mid antebrachium. For the stifle, the hair is clipped from just distal to the tibial crest to the top of the patella. In horses with very short, fine hair coats, clipping is not necessary for needle stifle arthroscopy. The horse is then moved into stocks and routine aseptic preparation of the surgical site is performed while the surgeon scrubs. A nonsterile assistant who can manipulate the limb is useful when performing surgery on the carpus, and is a necessity for standing stifle arthroscopy. Custom-made positioning devices are available.[6]

Room

The arthroscopy tower is positioned according to the direction the surgeon will face. When positioned cranially, the tower should be far enough to the side to prevent crossing of the light and camera cables in front of the patient or around the handler. The instrument table is positioned on the same side as the operated limb. Because the surgeon is kneeling and cannot let go of the arthroscope, a capable surgical assistant not only simplifies the task of exchanging instruments but also decreases motion around the horse. This minimizes the surgeon's risk of breaking aseptic technique.

Draping (Fetlock)

A large paper drape (150 × 200 cm) is spread out on the floor, wrapped around the distal limb just below the fetlock, and clamped to itself (not to the horse; palmar skin is not desensitized) behind the pastern. An adhesive transparent drape (Ioban 2; 3M, St. Paul, MN, USA) is then applied circumferentially proximal to the surgical site to drape off the carpus and distal antebrachium. Finally, a plastic split sheet with adhesive edges (Split Sheet; General Econopak Inc, Philadelphia, PA, USA) is placed under the fetlock and the adhesive strips stuck to the palmar aspect of the limb and the adhesive drape proximally. The plastic drape is spread out on the floor surrounding the limb undergoing surgery (**Fig. 3**).

Draping (Carpus)

Draping protocol for the carpus is similar to that described for the fetlock. A single paper drape is wrapped around the limb just below the carpus and clamped to itself (not to the horse; palmar skin is not desensitized) behind the metacarpus. An adhesive transparent drape is then applied circumferentially proximal to the surgical site to drape off the antebrachium. Finally, a plastic split sheet with adhesive edges is placed under the carpus and the adhesive strips stuck to the caudal aspect of the carpus and the adhesive drape proximally. The plastic drape is spread out on the floor surrounding the limb undergoing surgery.

Draping (Stifle)

No drapes are used for needle stifle arthroscopy.

Surgeon

A long sterile gown is worn so that the surgeon can kneel with the sterile gown on the sterile floor drape. Carpet layer's kneepads are strongly recommended for the surgeon's comfort during fetlock arthroscopy. For needle stifle arthroscopy, only sterile gloves are worn. The surgeon performed the operation while kneeling at the lateral aspect of the limb. The nondominant hand will operate the arthroscope, which should be positioned opposite the lesion. For example, for a right-handed surgeon, if the lesion were a dorsomedial fragment in the left metacarpophalangeal joint, the surgeon would kneel to the left of the left forelimb and face cranially to view the monitor. For a

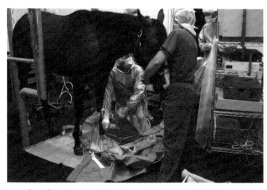

Fig. 3. Image showing the draping protocol and the organization of the room for standing arthroscopy of the fetlock.

dorsomedial fragment in the right metacarpophalangeal joint, the right-handed surgeon would kneel to the right of the right forelimb and faced caudally.

SURGICAL TECHNIQUE

Basic arthroscopic technique for the fetlock and carpus is no different from that used under general anesthesia. The surgeon must work while kneeling and pay close attention to asepsis caused by awkward positioning. Skin anesthesia must be checked with hemostats or a towel clamp (needle prick may be insufficient to induce a response in some sedated horses) before a skin incision is made. Sudden movement by the horse in response to pain is dangerous to the surgeon and handler, and creates a disturbingly large incision when the scalpel is applied.

FETLOCK

The arthroscope portal is proximally positioned so that the camera/scope system can be comfortably directed distally to view the lesion. A slightly more distal portal may be used for sagittal ridge lesions. The authors prefer to leave the fluids running at full pressure while a stab incision is made with a #11 blade and a blunt obturator is used to enter the joint. The instrument portal is made according to the location of the lesions. Medial and lateral dorsal proximal fractures of the proximal phalanx can almost always be debrided through a single instrument portal (**Fig. 4**). If both medial and lateral lesions are identified after insertion of the arthroscope, the instrument portal should be positioned more axially so that the sagittal ridge is not in the way when reaching across the joint. If the palmar aspect of the joint must be examined, an assistant can hold the distal limb in palmar flexion, but standing surgery is not recommended if anything more than a brief examination is anticipated. (*N.B.* The dorsal half ring block must be extended palmar if examination of the palmar aspect of the joint is planned. The described local anesthetic strategy does not desensitize the skin in this location.)

Carpus

The arthroscope portal is positioned opposite the lesion. The lateral portal is placed between the extensor carpi radialis and common digital extensor tendons. The medial portal is placed just medial to the extensor carpi radialis tendon. Insertion of the arthroscope and examination of the joint is performed as described for the metacarpophalangeal joint. Complete examination of the joint, especially the articular surface, is difficult and requires limb manipulation by an assistant.

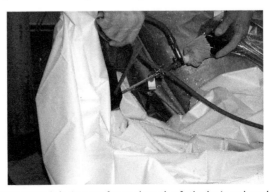

Fig. 4. Arthroscopic surgery is being performed on the fetlock via a dorsolateral arthroscope portal and a dorsomedial instrument portal.

Stifle

The preferred limb positioning is flexed. The joints can be entered with the horse bearing weight, but the soft tissue anatomy will appear markedly different. The sharp trocar and cannula are inserted through a small stab incision made through the skin. Prior distension of the joint is unnecessary (**Fig. 5**). The cranial compartment of the medial femorotibial joint is assessed using both cranial and lateral approaches.[5] The caudal aspect of the medial femorotibial joint is entered as described by Trumble and colleagues,[8] and the lateral femorotibial joint is entered as described by Moustafa and colleagues.[9] The caudal compartment of the lateral femorotibial joint is entered 2.5 cm proximal to the tibial plateau and 3 cm caudal to the lateral collateral ligament, in the flexed position.[6] The femoropatellar joint is entered through the craniolateral approach with the limb extended.[5] The image produced is not as clear as with conventional arthroscopic equipment but is certainly of diagnostic quality (**Fig. 6**).

OTHER LOCATIONS

The authors have performed standing arthroscopic procedures in the palmar metacarpophalangeal, middle carpal, tarsocrural, and distal interphalangeal joints. Standing arthroscopy will likely never be the preferred technique for these locations, although in certain situations it is possible and can be successful.

PERIOPERATIVE CARE

The authors do not administer antimicrobials of any sort for standing arthroscopic procedures. All horses are given intravenous phenylbutazone (2.2 mg/kg) at the time of surgery. A bandage is applied after closure of the arthroscopic portals in the fetlock and carpus. Bandaging is continued for 1 week after suture removal, with the dressing changed every 2 to 3 days or as necessary. No bandages are used after stifle arthroscopy, but cyanoacrylate skin glue can be used in cases of persistent bleeding.

REHABILITATION AND RECOVERY

As with arthroscopic surgery of any kind, the rehabilitation program is determined by the lesion and the state of the joint. Because most articular lesions treated with a standing approach are simple, rehabilitation periods are often short. Horses undergoing diagnostic needle arthroscopy of the stifle joints return to exercise in 3 to 5 days.

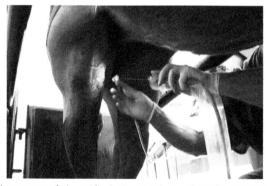

Fig. 5. Needle arthroscopy of the stifle being performed in the standing, weight-bearing position.

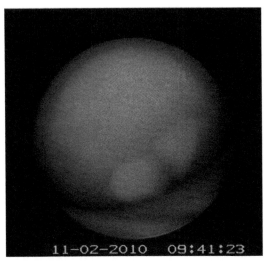
11-02-2010   09:41:23

Fig. 6. A subchondral bone cyst is visible in the medial femoral condyle. The stifle is being held in passive flexion to expose the lesion.

Rehabilitation after standing arthroscopic removal of a simple dorsoproximal chip fracture of the proximal phalanx may include:

- Exercise: the horse should be receive stall rest with hand grazing only for 2 weeks, followed by gradually increased hand-walking exercise for another 6 weeks. The horse may then be allowed turnout in a small paddock. The horse should be tranquilized before the first several times being turned out.
- Medication: the horse should be given 1 g of phenylbutazone orally twice daily for 3 days, then once daily for another 4 days.
- Bandage: a distal limb bandage should be maintained for 2 weeks, and changed every 2 to 3 days or sooner if it slips or become soiled.
- Sutures: the skin sutures should be removed in 10 to 12 days using aseptic technique.
- Follow-up care: the affected joint should be injected with sodium hyaluronate in 2 weeks.
- Monitoring: the horse should be monitored for any swelling, discharge, fever, or lameness.

CLINICAL RESULTS IN THE LITERATURE

A retrospective evaluation of arthroscopic removal of dorsoproximal chip fractures of the proximal phalanx from standing horses ($n = 104$) found that no major operative or postoperative complications occurred. A total of 91% of racehorses raced after surgery, with 78% returning to race at the same or higher level.[10]

Proof of the concept of needle stifle arthroscopy was recently published.[6] In clinical cases in which the authors of that study followed standing needle arthroscopy with conventional arthroscopic surgery, no further lesions were identified.

SUMMARY

The principles of standing arthroscopy have been discussed. Detailed in **Box 1** is an example of the chronologic order of events used by the authors when performing standing arthroscopic surgery in the fetlock joint.

Box 1
Technique for performing standing arthroscopic surgery in the fetlock joint

- Equipment positioned in the surgical suite
  - Instrument table ready but unopened
- Initial preparation of the horse (recovery stall)
  - Groom horse
  - Pick and clean feet
  - Primary sedation: intravenous xylazine hydrochloride, 0.5 mg/kg
  - Clip hair
  - Initial skin preparation
    - Full 5-minute aseptic preparation for intra-articular block
  - Local anesthesia
    - Intra-articular: ≥25 mL mepivacaine hydrochloride
    - Subcutaneous: dorsal half-ring block just proximal to capsular distension
  - Move horse into the stocks
  - Final aseptic preparation of the skin (surgeon scrubs at the same time)
  - Prepare instrument table/open instruments
- Draping
  - Apply single paper drape around the pastern
  - Place adhesive transparent drape proximal to the surgical site
  - Apply plastic split sheet
    - Spread distal plastic drape on the floor around the hoof
- Surgery
  - Secondary sedation: intravenous detomidine hydrochloride (0.02 mg/kg)
  - Test skin anesthesia
  - Create arthroscopic portal
    - Proximal stab incision (#11 blade)
    - Blunt obturator
    - Evaluate joint, document lesions and state of articular cartilage
  - Create the instrument portal
    - Plan proposed portal site with an 18-gauge needle
    - Stab incision (#11 blade)
    - Debride lesion
    - Thoroughly lavage joint
    - Document removal/debridement
  - Complete surgery
    - Close skin portals
    - Remove drapes
    - Bandage limb

REFERENCES

1. McIlwraith CW. Experiences in diagnostic and surgical arthroscopy in the horse. Equine Vet J 1984;16(1):11–9.
2. Lintner S, Shawen S, Lohnes J, et al. Local anesthesia in outpatient knee arthroscopy: a comparison of efficacy and cost. Arthroscopy 1996;12(4):482–8.
3. Jacobson E, Forssblad M, Rosenberg J, et al. Can local anesthesia be recommended for routine use in elective knee arthroscopy? A comparison between local, spinal, and general anesthesia. Arthroscopy 2000;16(2):183–90.
4. Klein L. Anesthetic complications in the horse. Vet Clin North Am Equine Pract 1990;6(3):665–92.
5. McIlwraith CW, Nixon AJ, Wright IM, et al, editors. Diagnostic and surgical arthroscopy in the horse. 3rd edition. Elsevier-Mosby Limited; 2005.
6. Frisbie D, Barrett M, McIlwraith C, et al. Diagnostic arthroscopy of the stifle joint using a needle arthroscope in standing horses: a novel procedure. Vet Surg, in press.
7. McIlwraith CW, Nixon AJ, Wright IM, et al, editors. Diagnostic and surgical arthroscopy in the horse. 4th edition. Elsevier-Mosby Limited; 2014.
8. Trumble TN, Stick JA, Arnoczky SP, et al. Consideration of anatomic and radiographic features of the caudal pouches of the femorotibial joints of horses for the purpose of arthroscopy. Am J Vet Res 1994;55(12):1682–9.
9. Moustafa MA, Boero MJ, Baker GJ. Arthroscopic examination of the femorotibial joints of horses. Vet Surg 1987;16(5):352–7.
10. Elce YA, Richardson DW. Arthroscopic removal of dorsoproximal chip fractures of the proximal phalanx in standing horses. Vet Surg 2002;31(3):195–200.

Recent Advances in Standing Equine Orthopedic Surgery

Thomas O'Brien, MVB[a],*, Robert J. Hunt, DVM, MS[b]

KEYWORDS

- Equine • Fracture • Transphyseal screw • Dorsal spinous process
- Sequestrectomy

KEY POINTS

- Appropriate case selection is essential when an orthopedic procedure is to be performed with the patient standing.
- Surgical repair of select fractures with the patient standing and sedated and through the use of regional/local anesthesia can be performed successfully.
- Catastrophic failure of a surgically repaired fracture or implant failure may occur during recovery from anesthesia. This situation may be avoided by repairing the fracture with the patient standing and sedated.
- Hemostasis, soft tissue dissection, surgical exposure, and operator orientation may be superior in surgeries performed with the patient standing, such as implant removal, dorsal spinous process resection/desmotomy, or sequestrectomy.
- The safety of the personnel and animal involved should not be compromised and neither the principles nor outcomes of the surgical procedure jeopardized by performing a surgery with the horse standing and sedated.

INTRODUCTION

The range of orthopedic procedures regularly performed in the standing equine patient is ever increasing. Although current textbooks on equine surgery and previous editions of *Veterinary Clinics of North America* offer information on many of these standing orthopedic procedures, the purpose of this article is to review those more recently described and, if appropriate, to present the authors' techniques and experiences in performing them.[1,2] If possible, clinical data substantiating the rationale for performing the standing surgical procedure rather than with the patient under general anesthesia are provided. Orthopedic procedures performed with the patient standing have clear benefits in avoiding the risks and increased costs associated with general

[a] Fethard Equine Hospital, Fethard, Tipperary, Ireland; [b] Davidson Surgery Center, Hagyard Equine Medical Institute, 4250 Iron Works Pike, Lexington, KY 40511, USA
* Corresponding author.
E-mail address: tom@obyrneandhalley.ie

Vet Clin Equine 30 (2014) 221–237
http://dx.doi.org/10.1016/j.cveq.2013.11.006
0749-0739/14/$ – see front matter © 2014 Elsevier Inc. All rights reserved.

anesthesia. In addition, hemostasis, soft tissue dissection, surgical exposure, and operator orientation may be improved.

FRACTURE REPAIR

Parasagittal fracture of the third metacarpal or metatarsal condyles (MC3/MT3 condylar fracture) and sagittal fracture of the first phalanx (P1) are common long bone fractures in racehorses. In longitudinal fractures of MC3/MT3 that propagate proximally (spiral), the risk for catastrophic failure during recovery from general anesthesia or in the early postoperative period is possible, regardless of treatment method.[3–6] Recently, screw fixation in lag fashion of proximally propagating MC3/MT3 condylar fractures with the horse standing and sedated has been described in an effort to minimize the risk of catastrophic failure of the repair during recovery from anesthesia.[7,8] In both case series, screw fixation in lag fashion was performed on the epiphyseal and distal metaphyseal portions of the fracture. Although nondisplaced incomplete or complete condylar fractures and incomplete P1 fractures do not carry the same risk of catastrophic failure as do proximally propagating condylar fractures, the same technique for standing repair of propagating condylar fractures has been successfully adapted for their repair.[9,10] The results of the case series by O'Brien and colleagues[10] are highlighted in **Table 1**. In addition to reducing the risks associated with general anesthesia, in particular the risks of catastrophic failure during recovery, the ability to repair fractures with the patient standing offers a clear economic advantage. Furthermore, correct positioning of the implants may be easier with the patient standing. **Fig. 1** give an overview and comparison of the reported outcomes in numerous studies after MC3/MT3 condylar and P1 fracture repair in both anesthetized and standing horses.[4,7,9–15] From the figures, it is clear that standing repair of appropriately selected fracture configurations is a suitable technique, with good postoperative outcomes, which are comparable with those achieved after repair of similar fractures under general anesthesia.

More recently, the successful repair of a fracture of the greater tubercle of the humerus in a standing horse, using bone screws, has been reported.[16] This is another fracture configuration, in which implant failure and catastrophic failure of the humerus during recovery from anesthesia have been reported.[17] The aforementioned case report[16] detailing standing repair of a fracture of the greater tubercle of the humerus warrants consideration when surgical repair of a similar fracture is performed.

In addition, the first author has recently placed a 6.3-mm centrally threaded positive profile pin in the distal cannon bone of a standing horse, which was subsequently

Table 1						
Postoperative outcomes after standing repair of 37 nondisplaced condylar fractures in thoroughbred racehorses						
Variables	Incomplete	Complete	Propagating	Female	Male	Total
Number of returns to athletic performance (%)	6/6 (100)	17/22 (77)	5/9 (56)	12/19 (63)	16/18 (89)	28/37 (76)
Days to start	270	303	362	323	306	320
Number of postoperative starts	11.5	7.4	3.2	6	8.3	7.1

Data from O'Brien T, Gomez J, Hunt RJ, et al. Standing surgical repair of non-displaced metacarpal and metatarsal condylar fractures in thoroughbred racehorses. In: Proceedings of Annual Scientific Meeting of the American College of Veterinary Surgeons–ACVS. Chicago, IL. November 3rd, 2011.

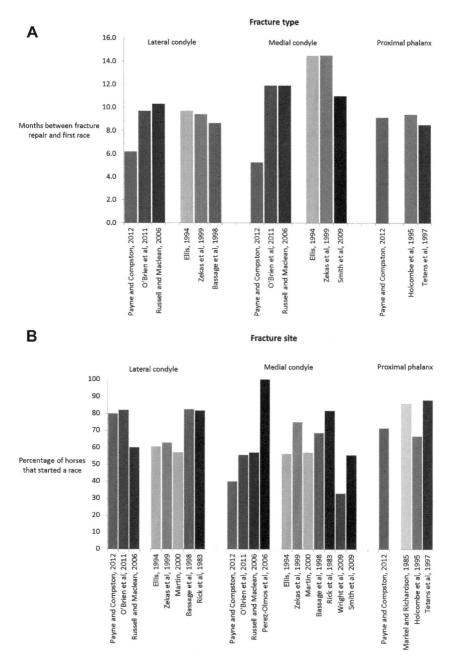

Fig. 1. (*A*) Comparison of reported number of days from repair to return to racing after repair of nondisplaced condylar and P1 fractures in studies on fractures repaired standing (*red bars*) as well as under general anesthesia (*blue bars*). (*B*). Comparison of reported percentage of horses to start a race after repair of nondisplaced condylar and P1 fractures in studies on fractures repaired standing (*red bars*) as well as under general anesthesia (*blue bars*). (*Courtesy of* Polly Compston, BVM&S, MSc, MRCVS. Rossdales Equine Hospital & Diagnostic Centre, Newmarket, Suffolk.)

incorporated into a fiberglass cast in the treatment of a comminuted fracture of the proximal phalanx (Thomas O'Brien, personal communication, 2013). Regional anesthesia, as outlined for standing repair of condylar fractures, was used, and the procedure was well tolerated by the animal.

The following is a description of our technique in performing repair of a standard nondisplaced condylar fracture. The limb is approached from the lateral aspect when possible (**Fig. 2**).

- Broad-spectrum antibiotics and antiinflammatories are administered.
- The patient is positioned in a quiet room with a firm rubber floor (stocks optional).
- The horse is sedated. Our preference is a combination of detomidine hydrochloride and butorphanol tartrate administered intravenously as a bolus and topped up as required.
- The hair is clipped, and aseptic preparation of the entire lower limb is performed.
- Regional anesthesia of the distal limb is achieved with either a high 4-point (forelimbs; medial and lateral branches of palmar and palmar metacarpal nerves) or high 6-point block (hind limbs; medial and lateral branches of plantar, plantar metatarsal, and dorsal metatarsal nerves). A subcarpal/tarsal subcutaneous ring block is also performed.
- After further aseptic preparation of the surgical site, the limb is minimally draped.
- Needles (18 G × 8.89 cm [3.5 in], 20 G × 2.54 cm [1 in]) and skin staples are placed as radiographic markers. Correct positioning of the epicondylar screw hole, in the center of the epicondylar fossa, is determined using digital radiography. Placing a needle in the fetlock joint slightly palmar/plantar to the central area of the epicondylar fossa is a good radiographic reference point for determining the correct positioning of the distalmost screw.

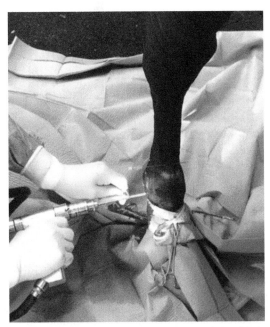

Fig. 2. Standing repair of a nondisplaced condylar fracture of the third metatarsal. Skin staples and a spinal needle are used as radiographic markers to determine correct positioning for placement of screws in lag fashion.

- It may be beneficial to remember that the trajectory required to obtain a true standing lateral radiographic projection of the fetlock joint is the same trajectory necessary for correct placement of the epicondylar screw.
- Standard technique for placement of a 4.5-mm (preferably self-tapping) cortical screw in lag fashion follows.
- Final tightening of the screw is performed with the horse momentarily non–weight bearing on that limb, facilitating compression of the fracture. Multiple orthogonal radiographs ensure correct screw positioning.
- Additional screws are placed in a similar manner at intervals of 1.5 to 2 cm proximal to the epicondylar screw. All screws should be tightened again, if possible, after placement of each additional screw.
- The skin incisions are sutured, and a sterile dressing and half limb bandage are applied.

In most nondisplaced fractures, which do not propagate proximally, 2 screws are usually sufficient to achieve complete radiographic reduction after repair. Proximally propagating fractures may require a greater number of screws (3–4), but screw placement should not be performed beyond a clearly visible fracture line on radiographs. For fractures involving the palmar or plantar cortex only, a single epicondylar screw is usually sufficient. Because these fractures are typically more chronic at presentation, complete radiographic reduction may not be achieved after repair. We use battery-powered hardware drills for this procedure, and the process may be expedited by using 2 drills, one for the 4.5-mm drill bit and the other for the 3.2-mm drill bit. In addition, self-tapping cortical bone screws can also be used to reduce the surgical time.

Postoperative care, including exercise restrictions, antibiotic and antiinflammatory administration, and bandaging, as well as radiographic follow-up, is as for similar fractures repaired under general anesthesia. Nondisplaced fractures that do not propagate/spiral proximally can be repaired on an outpatient basis. The first author recommends hospitalizing horses with proximally propagating fractures for 24 to 48 hours, because marked postoperative discomfort has been observed in 2 patients within 12 hours of repairing a proximally propagating fracture. In both these horses, further radiographic evaluation of MT3 revealed fracture lines proximal to the repair. Further screws were placed as previously described (1 and 2 screws, respectively), and comfort levels markedly improved within 24 hours of the second surgical procedure.

Alternatively, a standard half limb fiberglass cast may be applied in those horses with severe lameness after repair of a proximally propagating fracture, which is maintained upwards of 4 weeks. Application of a standard half-limb or bandage cast is easily performed with the horse standing and sedated. The horse is positioned squarely on all 4 limbs. The pair of limbs involved (front or hind) is placed on individual wooden blocks approximately 5 cm (2 in) thick. The limb to be casted is placed so that the palmar/plantar one-third of the foot is overhanging the back of the wooden block. The dressings and padding underneath the cast are applied in routine manner. The horse should be equally weight bearing on the pair of limbs being worked on. Fiberglass casting tape (4–6 layers) is applied from the level of proximal MC3/MT3 to the foot, including the foot overhanging the back of the block. Once this portion of the cast has sufficiently cured, the foot is then incorporated in a similar manner, with the affected limb elevated. When incorporating the foot in a hind limb cast, the limb should be brought forward underneath the horse to prevent flexing of the lower portion of the limb. Once the foot is incorporated, the foot should be replaced on the block and weight bearing resumed to allow final curing of the cast. Once the cast has cured fully, a hoof acrylic or thermoplastic is applied to the weight-bearing surface of the foot to prevent wearing through of the cast.

Diaphyseal screws should be removed before commencement of training, which can be performed with the horse standing under chemical restraint. Between the first and second authors' practices, approximately 100 horses have been treated in this manner, 25% of which were proximally propagating fractures. Postoperative catastrophic failure, implant failure, or surgical site infection has not been reported in any of these cases.

TRANSPHYSEAL SCREW IMPLANTATION AND REMOVAL

The surgical correction of angular limb deformities is performed primarily for cosmetic appeal and as a means of altering a conformation believed to be associated with musculoskeletal injuries incurred during an athletic career.[18] Retardation or temporary arrest of growth on 1 side of a physis by mechanical restriction is a commonly used technique in the surgical correction of angular limb deformities.[19] The use of a single cortical screw, to traverse and temporarily close the physis on the convex side of the limb, has been well documented in recent years.[20–23] Single cortical screws, placed so as to traverse the lateral distal radial physis for correction of carpal varus angular limb deformity, can be placed and removed in the standing patient.[24] Transphyseal implants placed at other locations can also be removed in the standing patient depending on location, surgeon preference, and temperament of the patient.

The following is a description of a documented technique in placing a single cortical screw across the lateral aspect of the distal radial physis (**Fig. 3**).[24]

- Routine broad-spectrum perioperative antimicrobials and antiinflammatories are administered.
- The horses are sedated with a combination of detomidine hydrochloride and butorphanol tartrate administered as a bolus intravenously.
- The hair is clipped from the skin, extending from midradius to proximal metacarpus, which is then aseptically prepared in routine fashion.
- Local anesthetic solution (3–5 mL of 2% mepivicaine hydrochloride) is injected subcutaneously proximal to the proposed incision site (2–3 cm proximal to the distal radial physis).
- After further aseptic preparation of the surgical site, the limb is draped surgically.
- A small 1-cm to 2-cm skin incision, which is continued all the way through the periosteum, is made approximately 1.5 cm proximal to the distal radial physis (the widest point of the distal radius) in between the lateral digital extensor tendon and the ulnaris lateralis muscle.
- A 4.5-mm drill bit is placed though this incision and is used to make a 3-mm to 5-mm deep shelf, perpendicular to the long axis of the bone.
- A 3.2-mm drill bit is then placed on this shelf at approximately 20° to the long axis of the radius and a hole drilled from the metaphysis, across the physis, and extending approximately 10 to 20 mm into the epiphysis. In general, aiming to place the screw as close as possible to parallel to the long axis of the bone is recommended. This strategy ensures that only the most abaxial portions of the physis are engaged, which may allow for an increased speed of correction of the angular limb deformity, desirable for when little growth potential of the physis remains.
- Appropriate positioning and hole depth are confirmed with intraoperative radiography.

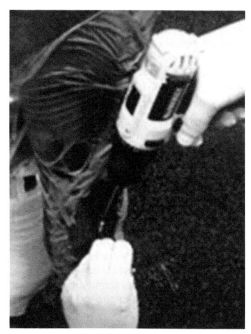

Fig. 3. A single transphyseal screw is being placed for correction of carpal varus angular deformity in a thoroughbred yearling. A 4.5-mm self-tapping cortical bone screw is placed at approximately 20° to the long axis of the leg. (*Courtesy of* Dwayne Rodgerson, DVM, Hagyard Equine Medical Institute, Davidson Surgery, Lexington, Kentucky.)

- The hole is measured and a 4.5-mm self-tapping cortical bone screw is placed (typically 56–60 mm in length), which is lightly tightened by hand. The screw, after tightening, should be backed out one-half of a revolution, because this facilitates ease of removal.
- Skin incisions are closed routinely, and the limb bandaged.

Postoperative care is routine, with perioperative antimicrobials continued for 5 to 7 days, and perioperative antiinflammatories continued for 3 to 5 days. Horses are on stall rest for 5 to 7 days, followed by limited turnout (4–6 hours per day) for a further 14 days. Exercise is progressively increased after this period. The bandages are maintained for 10 to 14 days after the surgery, and the implants are removed once correction has occurred.

IMPLANT REMOVAL

Implants that traverse or bridge an open physis must be removed promptly when the required degree of correction has been achieved, because failure to do so may result in overcorrection and deformity in the opposite direction. In addition, implants placed across the diaphysis of long bones and infected or broken implants may also require removal. After placement of transphyseal screws for correction of angular limb deformities, appropriate postoperative bandaging may help limit the local tissue reaction and production of fibrous tissue, which impedes implant removal. However, during the healing process, granulation tissue and periosteal callus may encompass the screw head and fill out the recess in the screw head, the screw drive. This situation can result in difficulty locating and properly seating the end of the screwdriver in the screw drive. Inadequate seating can then lead to stripping of the screw drive or breaking of the screw head. To avoid either of these complications, it is imperative that encroaching bone and soft tissue in and around the head of the screw is removed before any attempt at screw loosening and removal. Implants are removed when the deformity has been corrected.

The following is a description of our technique in removing a single cortical screw placed across the lateral aspect of the distal radial physis in the standing patient.

- Please follow the initial steps for placement of a transphyseal screw in the standing patient with regard to patient and surgery site preparation and anesthesia.
- The screw head is located by palpation, and the overlying skin incised. Should difficulty in locating the implant occur, the use of intraoperative radiographic control and radiopaque markers is beneficial.
- Having located the screw head, a stab incision is made, and any fibrous tissue or periosteal callus occupying the screw drive or surrounding the screw head removed, using the tip of a hypodermic needle, mosquito forceps, or a bone curette.
- The hexagonal head of the screwdriver is then firmly seated in the screw drive. Light tapping of the screwdriver with a mallet may help to seat the screwdriver in the screw drive and also help to disrupt any callus that is impeding removal.
- The screw is removed, the skin incisions may be sutured or left open to heal by second intention, and the limb is bandaged in routine fashion.

Postoperative care is routine, with perioperative antimicrobials continued for 3 to 7 days, and perioperative antiinflammatories continued for 3 to 5 days. Horses are on stall rest for 5 to 7 days, followed by limited turnout (4–6 hours per day) for a further 14 days. Exercise is progressively increased after this period. The bandages are maintained for 10 to 14 days after implant removal.

Standing removal of other orthopedic implants can also be performed in a similar manner to removal of single transphyseal screws. Implants are typically removed 60 to 90 days after fracture repair, unless indications for earlier removal (eg, infection, implant failure) are present. The distal portion of the limb is amenable to regional anesthesia, facilitating patient compliance in removing both bone screws and plates. Otherwise, direct infiltration with local anesthetic over the implant may be sufficient to provide adequate anesthesia to facilitate implant removal. Digital radiography aids in implant localization where callus and fibrous tissue have been laid down. Again, it is important to remove all fibrous tissue or periosteal callus occupying the screw drive or surrounding the screw head. The head of the screwdriver should be firmly seated in the screw drive to prevent stripping of the screw head. Again, light tapping of the screwdriver with a mallet may help to seat the screwdriver and may also help to loosen the implant. In some instances, in which a screw is difficult to loosen, taking the limb out of weight bearing may be advantageous. When an orthopedic bone plate is to be removed, the most proximal screw is located and partially removed through a stab incision. Using a similar sized bone plate as a template, placed on the skin over the site of the implants, the remaining location of the screws can then be determined, and the screws removed through stab incisions (**Fig. 4**).[25] Once all screws have been loosened and removed, the plate is then removed. The plate can be elevated with an osteotome and secured with sterile vise grips and extracted.[25]

DORSAL SPINOUS PROCESS IMPINGEMENT, FRACTURE, AND OSTEOMYELITIS

Surgical access to the dorsal spinous processes (DSP) may be desirable for treatment of impinging DSP or in the treatment of fistulous withers complicated by osteomyelitis.

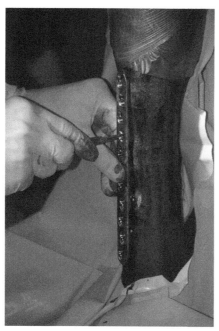

Fig. 4. Using a similar sized bone plate as a template, placed on the skin over the site of the implants, the remaining location of the screws can then be determined, and the screws removed through stab incisions. (*Courtesy of* Dean Richardson, DVM, University of Pennsylvania.)

Subtotal ostectomy of DSP with the horse standing has been reported, with the primary benefits of less hemorrhage in the surgical field, an easier soft tissue dissection, and better exposure of the diseased bone when subjectively compared with the same procedure performed under general anesthesia.[26,27] This factor is advantageous when resecting DSP for the treatment of osteomyelitis, because severe hemorrhage obscures the surgical field and recognition and removal of all the diseased bone may not be performed. In addition, duration of hospitalization and the incidence of postoperative wound complications are less after standing DSP resection than when compared with the same procedure performed under general anesthesia.[27] Obviously, any postoperative complication results in increased veterinary interventions and increased costs for the horse owner. Furthermore, the recuperation period is prolonged. Reported outcomes after standing DSP resection are favorable (77%) and comparable with the outcomes after the same procedure performed under general anesthesia (72%).[26–30]

The following is a description of a documented technique in subtotal ostectomy of the DSP in standing horses (**Fig. 5**).[26]

- Routine broad-spectrum perioperative antimicrobials and antiinflammatories are administered.
- The horse is sedated with a combination of detomidine hydrochloride and butorphanol tartrate and restrained in stocks.
- The hair is clipped from the skin over the proposed surgery site (determined radiographically using radiopaque markers), which is then aseptically prepared in routine fashion.

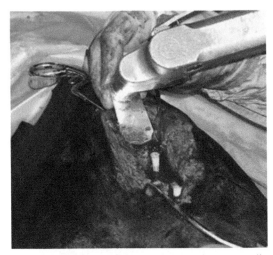

Fig. 5. Resection of the DSP using an oscillating saw. Hypodermic needles have been used as radiographic markers to determine the portions of the spinous processes to be removed. (*Courtesy of* Jim Schumacher, DVM, Department of Large Animal Clinical Sciences, College of Veterinary Medicine, The University of Tennessee, Knoxville.)

- Local anesthetic solution (40–60 mL of 2% mepivicaine hydrochloride) is injected in the soft tissues adjacent to the DSP to be removed to a depth of approximately 10 cm and subcutaneously along the proposed incision site.
- The skin over the affected DSP is incised longitudinally on dorsal midline, and the incision extended sharply through the supraspinous ligament.
- Using both sharp and blunt dissection, the affected portion of the DSP was separated from the supraspinous and interspinous ligaments and surrounding muscle and fascia.
- The dorsal aspect of the affected DSP is resected using an oscillating saw. Each DSP is severed obliquely, craniodorsal to caudoventral and then caudodorsal to cranioventral.
- Any abnormal soft tissues in cases of infected DSP are sharply excised, and the wound lavaged.
- In horses with impinging DSP, the incision is closed in 3 layers (supraspinous ligament, subcutaneous tissues, and skin) and a stent is applied for 48 to 72 hours.
- In horses with infected DSP, the incision is closed similarly with the addition of a closed suction drain placed through a stab incision placed at the most dependent aspect of the surgical site.

Postoperatively, the horses receive antibiotics and antiinflammatories on a case-by-case basis after DSP resection for treatment of osteomyelitis and for 5 to 7 days after DSP resection for treatment of impinging DSP. Box rest is observed for 8 weeks, with hand walking commencing after 8 weeks.

More recently, interspinous ligament desmotomy with the horse standing has been reported in the treatment of impinging DSP.[31] In this study, comparisons were made between a group of horses treated medically and a group of horses treated surgically. Initial responses to treatment were similar between groups. However, complete resolution was seen in 100% of the horses treated surgically and in only 50% of the horses treated medically. Furthermore, wound healing is not a significant concern with interspinous ligament desmotomy when compared with DSP resection, and horses return to exercise immediately after desmotomy.

Desmotomy of the interspinous ligaments for treatment of impinging DSP is performed in a similar manner in the initial stages as that for DSP resection, including patient and surgical site preparation and anesthesia (**Fig. 6**). The remainder of the described technique is as follows.[31]

- After imaging conformation of the center of the surgery site, each affected interspinous space, a 1-cm-long paramedian skin incision is made 3 cm from the left of midline.
- Through this incision, a pair of Mayo scissors is passed axially beneath the supraspinous ligament.
- The interspinous ligament is then severed for a depth of up to 6 cm using Mayo scissors.
- Conformation of complete severance of the interspinous ligament is confirmed using a probe.
- The portals are closed routinely.

Postoperative care includes antimicrobial and antiinflammatory therapy for 5 and 10 days after surgery, respectively. Hand walking exercise commences immediately and continues for 3 weeks. Lunging exercise follows this stage and is performed for 6 weeks. A gradual return to regular exercise follows, with owners being advised to recheck saddle fit.

PEDAL OSTEITIS/SEQUESTRATION

Septic pedal osteitis can occur secondary to penetrating injuries, laminitis, or most commonly, to extension of soft tissue infection in the foot (eg, subsolar abscess). Septic pedal osteitis involves the distal phalanx, the laminae and hoof wall, and the soft tissues of the sole. The disease process is characterized by purulent exudate draining from the sole and radiographic evidence of osteolysis. Sequestrum formation may develop secondary to the osteitis, because the infection disrupts the blood supply to a portion of the pedal bone. The avascular bone separates from the pedal bone, forming a sequestrum.[2] In cases of septic pedal osteitis (with or without a sequestrum

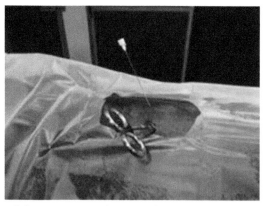

Fig. 6. Desmotomy of the interspinous ligament for the treatment of impinging DSP in a horse. (*Courtesy of* Richard Coomer, MA Vet MB, MRCVS. Cotts Farm Equine Hospital Ltd., Cotts Farm, Narberth, Pembrokeshire.)

formation), surgical debridement is the treatment of choice. In horses, the surgical treatment of pedal osteitis/sequestration with the patient standing and appropriately restrained may be advantageous for several reasons. In addition to avoiding the costs and risks of general anesthesia, appropriate homeostasis and exposure of the affected tissues are easily achieved with the patient standing. Either a solar (if a defect already exists and with the limb elevated and flexed) or a hoof wall approach (foot on the ground) may be used to gain access to the lesion. In gaining access to the lesion, through either approach, radiographic control is frequently used, and correct surgical orientation may be easier in the standing patient. A hoof wall approach may offer benefits in increasing postoperative comfort, but in cases in which an extensive solar hoof defect already exists (as often is the case before referral for surgery), it may offer little benefit over a solar approach. In addition, a solar approach may allow the required exposure to remove all contaminated and infected tissues of the hoof and not only the radiographically apparent necrotic pedal bone, as well as allowing postoperative drainage. Reported outcomes after surgical treatment are favorable, with approximately 73% of horses returning to previous or expected levels of performance.[32–34] Factors that affected outcomes in these reports include the amount of bone to be removed and the involvement of adjacent synovial structures.

The following is a description of our technique in performing standing surgical debridement/sequestrectomy of pedal bone osteitis (**Fig. 7**).

- After radiographic conformation of the lesion, the hoof wall is lightly debrided with a Dremel tool or hoof rasp, and the foot wrapped in an antiseptic and soaked for several hours.
- With the animal sedated, anesthesia of the medial and lateral palmar/plantar nerves is performed using 2% mepivicaine hydrochloride at the level of the abaxial sesamoids.
- A tourniquet is applied from the level of the proximal sesamoids to just below the carpus.
- An intravenous regional limb perfusion containing a combination of an antibiotic and a local anesthetic is then performed. Typically, 1 g of amikacin sulfate or ceftiofur sodium and 10 mL of 2% mepivicaine hydrochloride are diluted with 0.9% NaCl to a volume of 30 to 60 mL and injected into one of the digital veins below the tourniquet. The injection site is covered with a pressure bandage to prevent extravasation.
- The limb above the coronary band is wrapped in an adhesive bandage to the level of the proximal metacarpus/metatarsus, and the foot is aseptically prepared for surgery.

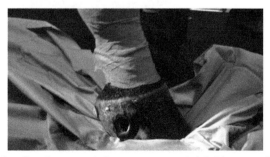

Fig. 7. A standing hoof wall approach for curettage and debridement of septic pedal osteitis of the plantar process of the distal phalanx in a broodmare.

- The lower portion of the limb is wrapped in a sterile adhesive bandage from the level of the coronary band to the level of the proximal metacarpus/metatarsus, and the foot is placed on a sterile impervious drape on the ground.
- Radiographic markers (typically needles) are placed in the hoof wall and radiographs (lateromedial, dorsopalmar/plantar, and dorsal-65° proximal-distal) are obtained to determine the landmarks to ensure access to the bony lesion.
- If a solar approach is used, an assistant has to hold the affected limb in flexion, allowing access to the sole. With a hoof wall approach, the horny tissue is removed with a Dremel tool or trephine, whereas in a solar approach, a sterile hoof knife can be used to remove any remaining horny tissue covering the lesion (a selection of sterile hoof knives is recommended, including a loop knife).
- After removal of the horn, the soft tissues (sensitive lamina, subcutis, and periosteum) and necrotic bone are easily removed with surgical blades, rongeurs, and curettes.
- In cases in which a distinct pedal bone sequestrum is present, it is now exposed and can be removed. In cases in which ill-defined necrotic bone is present, its complete removal may be appreciated only when normal surrounding pedal bone is accessed. Normal surrounding bone is hard and not discolored.
- Repeat radiographic examination confirms that all necrotic or sequestered bone has been removed.
- The soft tissues surrounding the defect in the pedal bone should be fully debrided to remove any remaining necrotic material.
- The defect in the foot is packed with a sterile dressing, and a heavily padded foot bandage and standard half-limb bandage are placed.

Postoperative care is continued in routine manner. The foot dressing is changed the following day, and the packing removed from the defect. After this process, the defect is only loosely packed with a sterile dressing, and this typically improves postoperative comfort levels. The foot bandage is replaced at 4-day to 5-day intervals for 6 to 8 weeks until the defect has cornified. Antibiotic administration should continue until healthy granulation tissue has covered the surgically exposed pedal bone (7–10 days). Additional intravenous regional limb perfusions with antibiotics may be performed in the 2 to 3 days after surgery. Application of a hospital treatment plate after surgery may make postoperative care easier, in addition to increasing patient comfort. The use of a hospital plate reduces the amount of bandage material required and also protects the sole and prevents any bandage material from becoming compressed in to the surgery site, which may result in patient discomfort. Bandaging is required for 6 to 8 weeks until the defect has cornified, although soundness at a walk usually takes 2 to 4 weeks to return. Once the defect has cornified, the affected foot and contralateral limb should be shod. If necessary, the sole can be protected with a pad.

There should be little to no drainage apparent at the surgery site after surgical debridement at successive bandage changes. Persistent drainage typically indicates the continued presence of necrotic material and the foot should be radiographed. A second surgical procedure may be required to remove any remaining necrotic or sequestered bone.

HARVESTING BONE MARROW–DERIVED MESENCHYMAL STEM CELLS

The use of mesenchymal stem cells or progenitor cells is advocated in the treatment of tendonitis, desmitis, and joint disease.[35] Bone marrow–derived mesenchymal stem cells show superiority to fat-derived progenitor cells in comparative studies in their ability to heal the various target tissues of the musculoskeletal system.[36,37] Bone marrow can be easily harvested from either the ilium or sternum in the standing sedated patient.[38,39] It is our preference to harvest bone marrow from the sternum, which is performed as follows (**Fig. 8**)

- The horse is sedated with a combination of detomidine hydrochloride and butorphanol tartrate and restrained in stocks.
- The hair is clipped from the skin from between the forelimbs, 2 cm either side of midline and extending caudally for 8 to 10 cm. The clipped area is then aseptically prepared in routine fashion.
- Bone marrow may be aspirated from the fourth, fifth, or conjoined sixth/seventh sternebrae, with the fifth being the sternebra of choice.
- The sternebrae can be identified using ultrasound guidance using a 7.5-MHz to 14-MHz linear transducer. Starting caudally at the xiphisternum and moving cranially, the intersternebral space between the fifth and sixth sternebrae can be imaged. Further cranially, the space between the fourth and fifth sternebra can be identified.
- The cranial and caudal boundaries of the fifth sternebra can be marked using skin staples.
- An area on midline (skin, subcutis, deep muscle, and periosteum) over the fifth sternebra is desensitized using 5 mL of 2% mepivacaine hydrochloride.
- A stab incision is made on midline over the central portions of the fifth sternebra through the skin to the periosteum, a depth of approximately 2 cm.
- A Jamshidi needle is inserted through the skin portal until contact is made with the ventral aspect of the fifth sternebra.
- With the Jamshidi needle in contact with the sternum, it should be advanced a further 2 cm into the fifth sternebra through gentle rotation.

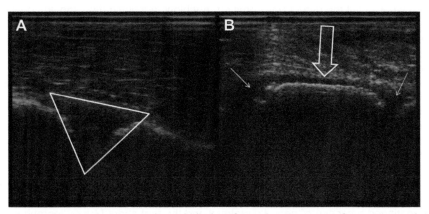

Fig. 8. Ultrasonographic images (*A* and *B*) identifying the correct site for puncture of the sternebra. (*A*) Longitudinal ultrasonographic image of the intersternebral space between the fifth and sixth sternebrae. Note the characteristic V-shaped (*white triangle*) indentation representing the cartilaginous space between sternebrae. (*B*) Longitudinal ultrasonographic image of the fifth sternebrae, with the center and site for puncture identified with the large white arrow. The cartilage separating the sternebra from adjacent sternebrae are identified with the thin white arrows at either end. By appreciating the limits of the fifth sternebra and identifying the central portion using ultrasonographic guidance, bone marrow aspirate can be obtained safely.

- The obturator is removed and the heparinized (0.5 mL of 5000 IU/mL of heparin) 10-mL syringe is connected to the needle and 9.5 mL of bone marrow aspirate collected.
- After collection of appropriate quantities of bone marrow, the Jamshidi needle is withdrawn, and a skin staple may be placed to close the stab incision.
- Bone marrow may be aspirated from the sixth sternebra in a similar manner, if necessary.

The syringes of bone marrow are packaged and shipped as outlined by the company performing the expansion.

SUMMARY

Certain orthopedic issues are amenable to successful surgical treatment in the standing patient, and treatment in this manner may be favored in an effort to reduce complications and costs. In all surgeries to be performed with the patient standing under chemical and physical restraint, patient compliance is of the utmost importance in an effort to ensure the safety of both the personnel and the animal. Appropriate case selection is essential for a successful outcome to be achieved, because all MC3/MT3 condylar or P1 fractures are not amenable to internal fixation with the horse standing, and young unhandled horses may not have a suitable disposition for standing surgical treatment of septic pedal osteitis, or implantation and removal of transphyseal screws. Previous operator experience in performing the procedure or technique under general anesthesia, which is now to be performed with the patient standing, is beneficial in performing the surgery correctly and expeditiously. Furthermore, appreciation of appropriate topographic anatomic landmarks is important, and intraoperative radiographic control is useful. It is important that proper surgical principals are adhered to and that the patient's well-being and the principles and outcomes of the surgical procedure are not jeopardized by performing an orthopedic surgical procedure with the animal standing and sedated rather than under general anesthesia.[40]

ACKNOWLEDGMENTS

The authors would like to acknowledge the contributions of Ms Polly Compston, Mr Richard Coomer, Mr Gerard Kelly, Mr Richard Payne, Dr Dwayne Rodgerson, and Dr Michael Spirito in the development of the outlined procedures, and in the provision of case information, graphs, and images.

REFERENCES

1. Sullins KE. Standing musculoskeletal surgery. Vet Clin North Am Equine Pract 1991;7(3):685–94.
2. Honnas CM. Standing surgical procedures of the foot. Vet Clin North Am Equine Pract 1991;7(3):695–722.
3. Richardson DW. Medial condylar fractures of the third metatarsal bone in horses. J Am Vet Med Assoc 1984;185:761–5.
4. Bassage LH II, Richardson DW. Longitudinal fractures of the condyles of the third metacarpal and metatarsal bones in racehorses: 224 cases (1986–1995). J Am Vet Med Assoc 1998;212:1757–64.
5. James FM, Richardson DW. Minimally invasive plate fixation of lower limb injury in horses: 32 cases (1999–2003). Equine Vet J 2006;38(3):246–51.

6. Levine D, Richardson DW. Clinical use of the locking compression plate (LCP) in horses: a retrospective study of 31 cases (2004–2006). Equine Vet J 2007;39: 401–6.

7. Russell TM, Maclean AA. Standing surgical repair of propagating metacarpal and metatarsal condylar fractures in racehorses. Equine Vet J 2006;38:423–7.

8. Perez-Olmos JF, Schofield WL, McGovern F, et al. Standing surgical treatment of spiral longitudinal metacarpal and metatarsal condylar fractures in 4 horses. Equine Vet Educ 2006;18:309–13.

9. Payne RJ, Compston PC. Short- and long-term results following standing fracture repair in 34 horses. Equine Vet J 2012;44:721–5.

10. O'Brien T, Gomez J, Hunt RJ, et al. Standing surgical repair of non-displaced metacarpal and metatarsal condylar fractures in thoroughbred racehorses. In: Proceedings of Annual Scientific Meeting of the American College of Veterinary Surgeons–ACVS. Chicago, IL. November 3rd, 2011.

11. Ellis DR. Some observations on condylar fractures of the third metacarpus and third metatarsus in young thoroughbreds. Equine Vet J 1994;26:178–83.

12. Zekas LJ, Bramlage LR, Embertson RM, et al. Characterization of the type and location of fractures of the third metacarpal/metatarsal condyles in 135 horses in central Kentucky (1986–1994). Equine Vet J 1999;31:304–8.

13. Smith LC, Greet TR, Bathe AP. A lateral approach for screw repair in lag fashion of spiral metacarpal and metatarsal medial condylar fractures in horses. Vet Surg 2009;38:681–8.

14. Holcombe SJ, Schneider RK, Bramlage LR, et al. Lag screw fixation of noncomminuted sagittal fractures of the proximal phalanx in racehorses: 59 cases (1973-1991). J Am Vet Med Assoc 1995;206:1195–9.

15. Tetens J, Ross MW, Lloyd JW. Comparison of racing performance before and after treatment of incomplete, mid sagittal fractures of the proximal phalanx in standardbreds: 49 cases (1986-1992). J Am Vet Med Assoc 1997;210: 82–6.

16. Madron M, Caston S, Kersh K. Placement of bone screws in a standing horse for treatment of a fracture of the greater tubercle of the humerus. Equine Vet Educ 2013;25:381–5.

17. Mez JC, Dabareiner RM, Cole RC, et al. Fractures of the greater tubercle of the humerus in horses: 15 cases (1986–2004). J Am Vet Med Assoc 2007;230: 1350–5.

18. Auer JA. Angular limb deformities. In: Auer JA, Stick JA, editors. Equine surgery. 4th edition. St Louis (MO): Saunders Elsevier; 2012. p. 1201–20.

19. Bramlage LR. The science and art of angular limb deformity correction. Equine Vet J 1999;31:182–3.

20. Witte S, Thorpe PE, Hunt RJ, et al. A lag-screw technique for bridging of the medial aspect of the distal tibial physis in horses. J Am Vet Med Assoc 2004; 225:1581–3.

21. Kay AT, Hunt RJ, Thorpe PE, et al. Single screw transphyseal bridging for correction of forelimb angular limb deviation. In: 51 Annual Convention of the American Association of Equine Practitioners–AAEP. Seattle, WA. December 7th, 2005.

22. Baker WT, Slone DE, Lynch TM, et al. Racing and sales performance after unilateral or bilateral single transphyseal screw insertion for varus angular limb deformities of the carpus in 53 thoroughbreds. Vet Surg 2011;40:124–8.

23. Carlson ER, Bramlage LR, Stewart AA, et al. Complications after two transphyseal bridging techniques for treatment of angular limb deformities of the distal radius in 568 thoroughbred yearlings. Equine Vet J 2012;44:416–9.

24. Modesto RB, Rodgerson DH, Masciarelli AE, et al. How to place distal lateral radial transphyseal screws in a standing horse. In: 57 Annual Convention of the American Association of Equine Practitioners–AAEP. San Antonio, TX. November 18th, 2011.
25. Richardson DW. Third metacarpal and metatarsal bones. In: Auer JA, Stick JA, editors. Equine surgery. 3rd edition. St Louis (MO): Saunders Elsevier; 2012. p. 1325–38.
26. Perkins JD, Schumacher J, Kelly G, et al. Subtotal ostectomy of dorsal spinous processes performed in nine standing horses. Vet Surg 2005;34(6):625–9.
27. Owen KR, Milner PI, Talbot A, et al. A comparison of partial ostectomy of the dorsal spinous processes in the horse; standing sedation versus general anaesthesia (28 cases). In: Annual Scientific Meeting of the European College of Veterinary Surgeons–ECVS. Barcelona, Spain. July 6th, 2012.
28. Brink P. Subtotal ostectomy of impinging dorsal spinous processes in 23 standing horses. In: Annual Scientific Meeting of the European College of Veterinary Surgeons–ECVS. Barcelona, Spain. July 6th, 2012.
29. Compston PC, Gapp JI, Payne RJ. Dorsal spinous process resection in 18 standing horses. In: Annual Scientific Meeting of the European College of Veterinary Surgeons–ECVS. Barcelona, Spain. July 6th, 2012.
30. Walmsley JP, Pettersson H, Winberg F, et al. Impingement of the dorsal spinous processes in two hundred and fifteen horses: case selection, surgical technique and results. Equine Vet J 2002;34:23–8.
31. Coomer RP, McKane SA, Smith N, et al. A controlled study evaluating a novel surgical treatment for kissing spines in standing sedated horses. Vet Surg 2012;41: 890–7.
32. Gaughan EM, Rendano VT, Ducharme NG. Surgical treatment of septic pedal osteitis in horses: nine cases (1980-1987). J Am Vet Med Assoc 1989;195(8): 1131–4.
33. Cauvin ER, Munroe GA. Septic osteitis of the distal phalanx: findings and surgical treatment in 18 cases. Equine Vet J 1998;30:512–9.
34. Neil KM, Axon JE, Todhunter PG, et al. Septic osteitis of the distal phalanx in foals: 22 cases (1995–2002). J Am Vet Med Assoc 2007;230(11):1683–90.
35. Fortier LA, Smith RK. Regenerative medicine for tendinous and ligamentous injuries of sport horses. Vet Clin North Am 2008;24:191–201.
36. Hayashi O, Katsube Y, Hirose M, et al. Comparison of osteogenic ability of rat mesenchymal stem cells from bone marrow, periosteum, and adipose tissue. Calcif Tissue Int 2008;82:238–47.
37. Kisiday JD, Kopesky PW, Evans CH, et al. Evaluation of adult equine bone marrow- and adipose-derived progenitor cell chondrogenesis in hydrogel cultures. J Orthop Res 2008;26:322–31.
38. Goodrich LR, Frisbie DD, Kisiday JD. How to harvest bone marrow derived mesenchymal stem cells for expansion and injection. In: 54th Annual Convention of the American Association of Equine Practitioners - AAEP. San Diego, CA. December 10th, 2008.
39. Kasashima Y, Ueno T, Tomita A, et al. Optimisation of bone marrow aspiration from the equine sternum for the safe recovery of mesenchymal stem cells. Equine Vet J 2011;43:288–94.
40. Compston PC, Payne RJ. Standing fracture repair–a new chapter. Equine Vet Educ 2013;25:386–8.

New Concepts in Standing Advanced Diagnostic Equine Imaging

Erin G. Porter, DVM*, Natasha M. Werpy, DVM

KEYWORDS

- Standing computed tomography • Standing low-field magnetic resonance imaging
- Equine

KEY POINTS

- Standing magnetic resonance imaging (MRI) and computed tomography (CT) eliminate the need for general anesthesia, reducing risk to the patient and cost to the client.
- Standing MRI of the carpus and tarsus distally is well described; diagnostic MR images are often comparable with high-field MR images.
- Standing CT of the equine head and distal limb has been successfully performed at a limited number of institutions where CT scanners are modified to accommodate the standing horse.
- Standing CT and high-field standing MRI will possibly become more available for horses in the near future.

INTRODUCTION

This article addresses the clinical application of magnetic resonance imaging (MRI) and computed tomography (CT) as applied to the standing equine patient. This discussion includes the logistics, advantages, disadvantages, and limitations of imaging a standing horse. In addition, a brief review is given of the physics of these modalities as applied in clinical practice, as well as the currently available hardware and software required by these techniques for image acquisition and artifact reduction. Finally, the appropriate selection of clinical cases for standing MRI and CT is reviewed, focusing on cases that are capable of undergoing standing surgeries following lesion diagnosis.

BENEFITS OF ADVANCED DIAGNOSTIC IMAGING IN THE STANDING HORSE

The benefits of imaging the standing equine patient include elimination of general anesthesia, increased availability of standing magnets, and, in most cases, reduced

The authors have no funding sources or conflicts of interest to disclose.
Diagnostic Imaging, Department of Small Animal Clinical Sciences, University of Florida, PO Box 100126, Gainesville, FL 32610, USA
* Corresponding author.
E-mail address: Gordone@ufl.edu

cost to the client. Arguably the most important benefit of standing diagnostic imaging is that it negates the need for general anesthesia and eliminates the associated risk to the patient. Anesthetic complications in horses are well described. The most common perioperative (and perianesthetic) complications include cardiac arrest, fractures in recovery, and myopathy. One study performed to evaluate the risk of general anesthesia in horses undergoing MRI found the mortality rate to be 0.6%,[1] which is similar to that of healthy horses undergoing nonabdominal surgeries.[1–3] Interestingly a greater proportion of horses suffered myopathy after MRI (2.3%) than after surgery (0.8%).[1] In this study, horses in the MRI group were heavier, whereas horses that underwent surgery had longer anesthetic duration. The increase in myopathy in horses undergoing MRI was not statistically significant, which the investigators attributed to the limited power of the study. Nonetheless, it was concluded that the 8 cases of myopathy seen in the MRI group versus 2 in the surgical group may represent a clinical difference. In a multi-institutional study assessing the risk of general anesthesia in horses, it was shown that the likelihood of patient death increases if the duration of anesthesia exceeds 61 minutes.[3,4] Anesthesia time for an equine patient to undergo a recumbent MR examination of bilateral distal forelimbs in a 1.5-T magnet is approximately 1 to 2 hours. Although sedation is required to perform an MRI or CT examination on a standing horse to limit patient motion and protect the patient and equipment from damage, the need for general anesthesia is eliminated, thus making standing imaging a lower-risk procedure than recumbent MR or CT imaging.

In general, high-field (recumbent) MR examinations are often more costly than their low-field counterparts. High-field magnets are built to produce a stronger magnetic field than low-field magnets, thus providing higher-resolution images. However, this benefit comes at a price. High-field magnets are more expensive than low-field magnets to purchase and maintain. Because of the increased strength of their magnetic field, high-field magnets require a large room with conductive material built into the walls, termed a Faraday cage, the purpose of which is to protect the surrounding areas from the stray magnetic field produced by the magnet and to prevent stray radiofrequencies, such as radio waves, from interfering with the function of the magnet and quality of the images produced. The need for the large room to accommodate the size of the magnetic field, and the Faraday cage, adds to the expense of high-field MRI. By eliminating the need for general anesthesia with standing diagnostic imaging, the overall cost of the procedure is inherently reduced.

STANDING MRI IN THE HORSE
Magnetic Field Strength and Magnet Configuration

MR scanners can be in either an open or closed configuration (**Fig. 1**). Until recently, high-field magnets required a closed (tube-shaped) configuration to produce a stronger magnetic field than low-field magnets. This closed configuration limits the size of the patient that can be imaged. Closed magnets with a wider-bore diameter (71 cm) and magnets with shorter bore lengths (125 cm long) and flared ends have been developed to accommodate larger human patients and claustrophobics. These developments have helped to improve the ease of positioning and to accommodate the larger and more proximally located anatomy of equine patients. However, regardless of bore length or size, general anesthesia is required to position a horse in the closed bore of a high-field magnet. Open magnets have a C-shaped configuration whereby the anatomy to be imaged is only partially enclosed (**Fig. 2**). It is this open configuration that allows for an MR examination to be performed on horses in the standing position. The open magnets that can be used to image standing horses are of low field strength at present.

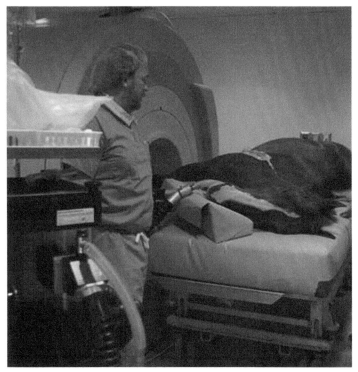

Fig. 1. Positioning of an anesthetized horse in a closed magnet.

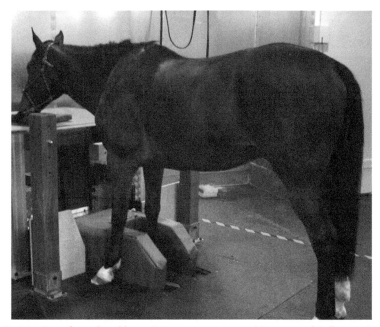

Fig. 2. Positioning of a sedated horse in an open magnet. (*Courtesy of* Hallmarq Veterinary Imaging, Ltd; with permission.)

Magnetic field strength, rated in units of Tesla (T), is the major determinant of image contrast and resolution.[5] The principal method of increasing MR image quality is through increased signal-to-noise ratio, which is fundamentally achieved by increasing the strength of the main magnetic field.[5–7] Magnets in current clinical use range from 0.5 to 3 T, with even higher field strengths being used for research purposes. Field strength can be broken down into low (0.1–0.5 T), medium (0.5–1.0 T), high (1.5 T), or ultrahigh (3.0 T or greater) (**Fig. 3**).[5,8] For the purposes of this article, magnets with field strengths of less than 0.5 T are referred to as low field

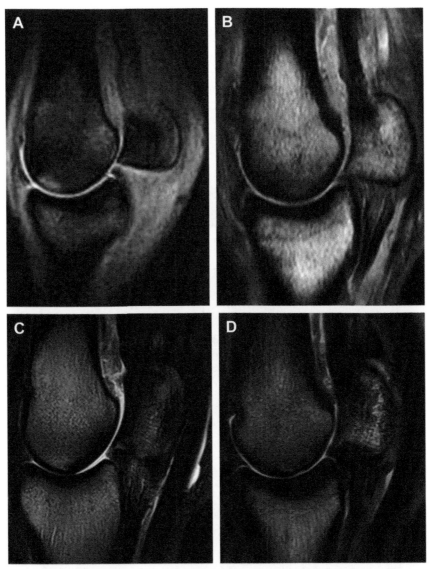

Fig. 3. Sagittal plane magnetic resonance (MR) images of the equine fetlock joint obtained at 0.27 T (*A*), 1 T (*B*), 1.5 T (*C*), and 3 T (*D*). The image resolution increases as magnetic field strength increases.

strength, and those with field strengths of greater than 1 T are referred to as high field strength.

The disadvantages of low strength of magnetic field include decreased signal-to-noise ratio, longer scan times, thicker image slices, and increased patient motion, all of which result in decreased image resolution and image quality in comparison with high-field images.[9–11] Recently in human medicine, there has been a drive toward improving the image quality of open magnets to better accommodate claustrophobic and bariatric patients and to allow quicker access and ease of patient positioning for orthopedic imaging. With recent advances, the image quality produced by these magnets has significantly improved in order for them to become more competitive with their closed, high-field counterparts. Magnets of high field strength with an open configuration are now becoming available for clinical use in humans, and will likely be available for veterinary patients in the near future. This technology will offer the best of both worlds: high-resolution imaging without the risks associated with general anesthesia.

Procedure

Regardless of the type of magnet used, lesion localization before MRI examination or study is performed is crucial. Lesion localization should consist of thorough passive and active lameness examinations as well as regional perineural, intrathecal, and/or intra-articular diagnostic analgesia. Imaging techniques such as radiography, ultrasonography, and nuclear scintigraphy are often performed before or after MRI, ruling out apparent disease processes that can be diagnosed with these methods and further localizing the source of the lameness. MR examinations are time consuming, and should not be used as screening examinations. Ideally the MR examination is limited to 1 or 2 joints or portions of a limb. However, even with thorough lesion localization, MRI findings do not always correlate with the degree of lameness or suspected lesion location. In such cases, one benefit of standing MRI is the ability to repeat the MR examination on another anatomic site, proximal or distal to the initial site, on the following day. Such a repeat examination becomes more expensive, time consuming, and risky when general anesthesia is required.

Once the region of interest has been localized, the horse shoes are removed from the limb to be imaged as well as from the contralateral forelimb or hindlimb, to avoid magnetic attraction of the shoe to the walls of the magnet and avoid susceptibility artifact, which is caused by interference of metal with the magnetic field.[12] With standing MRI the patient is lightly sedated, and more sedative is administered as needed to maintain an adequate plane of sedation. The region of interest is carefully aligned in the magnet, and images of the affected limb and, often, the contralateral limb are acquired. In routine examinations, a standardized protocol is used to acquire the necessary images in the correct imaging planes. In complicated cases, images can be evaluated as they are acquired by a veterinary radiologist experienced in MR image interpretation. This evaluation can be done by remote access, so the interpreting radiologist does not have to be on site at the time of the MR examination. The procedure usually takes anywhere from 1 to 3 hours. Scan times should be kept as short as possible for each sequence acquired so as to limit artifact associated with patient motion. After images are acquired the patient is allowed to wake up from sedation, and little further monitoring is necessary. Although this is often an outpatient procedure, temporarily holding the patient at the clinic while the images are evaluated is beneficial, as further imaging may be indicated. Once the study is completed, Digital Imaging and Communication in Medicine (DICOM) images can be transferred to a Picture Archiving and Communication System (PACS) workstation and/or burned onto a CD for image interpretation. After thorough evaluation of the study, an MRI report is created by a radiologist or the interpreting veterinarian.

Clinical Applications

Our ability to image certain anatomic regions of the horse, such as the carpus and stifle joint, is limited by the length of the patient's limbs and width of the shoulder or pelvic regions. Using a closed (high-field) magnet with the largest bore size available or a low-field open magnet with general anesthesia, it is sometimes possible to image as far proximal as the stifle joint in the hindlimb and the distal radius in the forelimb. The region of interest has to be positioned as close to the center (termed isocenter) of the magnet to optimize image quality. With an open magnet, images can be obtained from foot distally to as far proximal as the carpus and tarsus. In the open magnet, the ability to image more proximal anatomic regions is limited by magnet size. Larger anatomic regions require longer scanning times, which increases the likelihood of motion and associated artifacts in the nonanesthetized patient. In addition, the more proximal aspects of the extremities are more severely affected by the swaying motion of a sedated horse.

Since MRI of the standing horse was first described, numerous articles have described normal anatomy of the equine limb as well as numerous soft-tissue and osseous lesions as observed on standing MR images. In one article comparing 0.27-T, 1.5-T, and 3-T MR images of normal equine cadaver distal limbs, the investigators found all 3 examinations to be of diagnostic value with the exception of evaluation of the hoof capsule, whereby artifacts, distortion, and signal loss limited the assessment of the dorsodistal aspect of the hoof on low-field images.[13] In addition, the investigators found high-field MR images to be significantly better than low-field images for the evaluation of anatomic structures.[13] It must be noted that because this study was performed on cadaver limbs, patient motion was not a factor. However, in a clinical situation patient motion has the most significant detrimental effect on the quality of a standing MR image. This factor should be considered when evaluating literature that compares standing and recumbent MRI performed on cadaver limbs.

The low-field MR appearance of soft-tissue structures in the foot,[14–16] metacarpophalangeal region,[17] carpus and proximal metacarpus,[18,19] and tarsus and proximal metatarsus[20,21] have been described. Subtle soft-tissue abnormalities are more easily recognized with MRI than with other imaging modalities, such as ultrasonography, radiography, nuclear scintigraphy, and CT, because of the superior soft-tissue resolution it provides. MRI allows evaluation of the intricate ligaments and tendons contained within the hoof capsule, an area in which even ultrasonographic evaluation of soft tissues is limited at best. Furthermore, MRI allows for thorough evaluation of joints, periarticular structures, and bursas, which are difficult to thoroughly evaluate with other modalities. Another advantage of MRI is that it is the only modality that allows detection of fluid accumulation in bone caused by inflammation, neoplasia, infection, contusions, osteonecrosis, or edema,[22] or stress at points of ligamentous attachments.[23] The following sections describe some common abnormalities that can be identified with MRI, with a focus on those disorders that can be surgically treated in the standing horse.

Tendons and ligaments

After lameness is localized to a specific anatomic region in the horse, radiographs are often the first test performed to rule out osseous abnormalities. When musculoskeletal soft-tissue injury is suspected, ultrasonography of the affected region is often the next step in the diagnostic workup. In the hands of an experienced sonographer, ultrasonography can be very sensitive for evaluation of soft-tissue injury, such as ten-dinopathy and desmopathy. However, ultrasonography has limited sensitivity to certain types of lesions and in certain anatomic regions where the window for trans-ducer placement is limited, such as within the hoof capsule, or in regions with complex osseous anatomy such as the carpus and tarsus.

MRI is extremely useful for evaluation of the complex soft-tissue structures encased within the hoof capsule. Deep digital flexor tendinopathy is a common cause of lame-ness localized to the equine foot (21%–54%).[16,24,25] Deep digital flexor tendon (DDFT) lesions in the equine foot have been described as having an appearance on low-field MR images similar to that on high-field MR images of the same locations.[26] Although a direct comparison has not been made between low-field and high-field images to assess relative sensitivity and specificity,[24,26] standing, low-field MRI is generally considered to be a sufficient method for evaluating certain lesions of the DDFT (**Fig. 4**). Other soft-tissue structures of the foot that are frequently affected in lame horses include the navicular bursa, the collateral sesamoidean ligament, the distal sesamoidean impar ligament, and the collateral ligaments of the distal interphalangeal joint.[16,27–32] Injury to these tendinous and ligamentous structures of the foot, including the soft tissues of the podotrochlear apparatus[16] and the navicular bone as well as the supporting structures of the metacarpophalangeal joint, can be adequately evaluated using low-field MRI in the standing horse.[17]

Navicular syndrome is the most common indication for palmar digital neurectomy.[33] With MRI the specific structures involved in navicular syndrome and other causes of chronic foot lameness can be determined, and prognosis more accurately assessed. If deemed appropriate, medial and lateral palmar digital neurectomies can subse-quently be performed in those horses with chronic lameness that resolves with a palmar digital nerve block. This procedure is routinely performed in the standing horse under local analgesia.

Low-field MRI can also be used to evaluate the anatomy of the proximal meta-carpus/metatarsus, including the proximal suspensory ligament (third interosseous muscle). Several structures in the proximal metacarpus/metatarsus can be evaluated

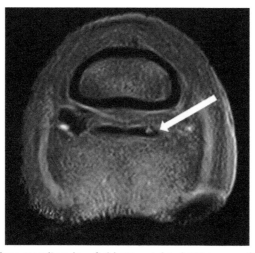

Fig. 4. Transverse plane standing, low-field, T1-weighted MR image of a core lesion in the lateral lobe of the deep digital flexor tendon (DDFT) (*arrow*). Lateral is to the left and the injury is in the lateral lobe that is on the right.

on both high-field and low-field MR images that cannot easily be imaged using other modalities such as radiography, ultrasonography or nuclear scintigraphy (**Fig. 5**). These structures include the interosseous ligaments between the metacarpal bones, the abaxial margins of the suspensory ligament, and the carpometacarpal ligaments.[19] When evaluating this region with a low-field MR examination, the interpreting veterinarian should keep in mind that low-field MR images have decreased resolution in comparison with their high-field counterparts. This decreased resolution makes differentiation between smaller anatomic structures more difficult on low-field images. Evaluation of the complicated anatomy of the proximal metacarpal/metatarsal region on low-field images should be viewed in light of the appearance of this anatomy on higher-resolution MR images.[19] One study evaluating the use of both high-field and low-field MRI for proximal metacarpal pain found decreased signal intensity on T1-weighted and T2-weighted images in the carpal bones and the proximal carpal region to be the most common abnormality, with a lower proportion of horses having desmopathy of the accessory ligament of the DDFT and proximal suspensory ligament.[18]

Synovial structures

Distal interphalangeal arthritis and synovitis, and navicular bursitis are other common findings in horses with lameness localized to the foot, and have been described on low-field MR images of the standing horse (**Fig. 6**).[16] Evaluation of the thin articular cartilage layers in the joints of the equine limb continues to present a challenge. Resolution and motion artifact are limiting factors when imaging the standing horse. In cadaver limbs, where motion artifact is not a factor for consideration, the articular cartilage of the distal interphalangeal joint can be evaluated on low-field MR images with moderate to good sensitivity and accuracy when appropriate sequence selection is used.[34] In the standing horse, on the contrary, mild amounts of motion, joint space asymmetry, and decreased synovial fluid resulting from weight bearing complicate the evaluation of articular cartilage. In addition, assessment of superficial erosions and

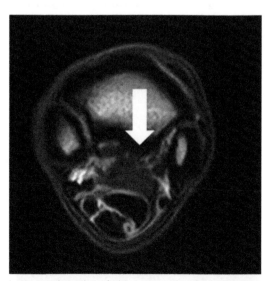

Fig. 5. Transverse plane standing, low-field, proton-density MR image at the level of the proximal metacarpus. The proximal suspensory ligament (*arrow*) is enlarged with loss of the normal fiber pattern. There is bone loss of the adjacent palmar aspect of the proximal metacarpus. Lateral is to the left of the image.

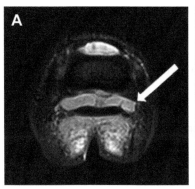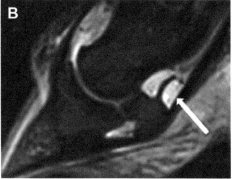

Fig. 6. Transverse (*A*) and sagittal plane (*B*) standing, low-field, T2-weighted MR images of a horse with navicular bursitis. Moderate to severe effusion and synovial proliferation is seen in the podotrochlear bursa on both planes (*arrows*). Lateral is to the left on the transverse plane image.

fibrillations in the articular cartilage of the distal interphalangeal and metacarpophalangeal joints has been found to be unreliable on low-field images.[34,35] Abnormalities such as osteophyte formation and subchondral bone sclerosis add supporting evidence in the evaluation of osteoarthrosis. Likewise, increased synovial fluid, synovial proliferation, and joint-capsule thickening can be identified with low-field MR images in the standing horse, and help to support a diagnosis of synovitis. Similar findings including synovial proliferation, effusion, and thickening of the synovial membrane are seen with podotrochlear bursitis and tenosynovitis. If adhesions between the podotrochlear bursa and adjacent soft-tissue structures such as the collateral sesamoidean ligament, the distal sesamoidean impar ligament, and/or the DDFT are suspected, MRI can be performed after distending the proximal recess of the podotrochlear bursa with saline (MR bursography) in the anesthetized horse.[36] In addition to better delineating adhesions, MR bursography can help to more accurately evaluate the fibrocartilage of the navicular bone.[37] Unfortunately, separation of the DDFT from the navicular bone cannot be achieved in weight-bearing horses even after navicular bursal distension.

MRI can also be used in horses to support a diagnosis of septic arthritis. Septic arthritis can have career-ending and life-threatening consequences in horses. Diagnosis of septic arthritis should be made and treatment initiated as early as possible to achieve the most successful outcome. MRI is considered the gold standard for diagnosing septic arthritis in humans,[38–42] and high-field MRI findings of septic arthritis and osteomyelitis have been described to a limited extent in horses.[43,44] MRI features of septic arthritis in horses include increased signal intensity in bone and periarticular tissues on fat-suppressed images, joint effusion, synovial proliferation, and thickening of the joint capsule.[44] In one study, osseous lesions with increased signal intensity and a peripheral, low-signal rim were described as the most common abnormality in foals with septic arthritis.[43] Of importance is that radiographic lesions were not detected in many of these foals, making MRI one of the earliest imaging indicators of septic changes. In addition, on MR images the joint effusion from septic joints has been described to have decreased or heterogeneous signal intensity, likely as a result of increased cells and protein content.[43,44] Nonseptic inflammatory changes are often difficult to distinguish from septic arthritis in the absence of osteolysis or osseous proliferation. Intravenous gadolinium contrast medium increases the conspicuity of hyperemic tissue and increased vascular permeability.[45] Gadolinium has been investigated as a method to increase the diagnostic accuracy of MRI for infection.[45] Some human studies have shown that administration of intravenous gadolinium contrast medium during the MR examination can increase specificity for osteomyelitis[46] while others report an inability to distinguish the enhancement of septic from nonseptic inflammatory change.[47] It must be noted that these findings have been described on high-field images, which is a limiting factor when evaluating for the possibility of septic arthritis in the standing horse. Although MRI alone does not provide a definitive diagnosis of septic arthritis, it may help to provide additional information when arthrocentesis is unsuccessful, when cytology and/or culture results are inconclusive, or when looking for a source of a persistent infection.

Penetrating wounds

The structures most commonly affected by penetrating wounds to the sole include the DDFT, the distal sesamoidean impar ligament, the distal interphalangeal joint, the podotrochlear bursa, the navicular bone, and the distal phalanx.[48] Timely determination of the anatomic structures involved and prompt, aggressive treatment are considered paramount to obtaining a successful outcome.[49] Radiographic fistulography using iodinated contrast media or with a lead probe inserted into the wound tract can be helpful for determining the depth of penetration. Likewise, transcuneal ultrasonography may be helpful to determine involvement or extent of injury to the adjacent soft-tissue structures.[22] Unfortunately, it is not possible to evaluate the soft-tissue structures within the hoof capsule using radiography alone; moreover, transcuneal ultrasonography requires the examiner to be skilled in this technique, and the information provided is limited. Other modalities including CT, MRI, and nuclear scintigraphy can also be used to evaluate these types of injuries. Low-field MR images have been shown to afford easy evaluation of the structures commonly injured by penetrating wounds, and allow the examiner to assess the extent of injury of the affected structures. Although the appearance of more chronic penetrating wounds has been described, the wound tract is most easily identified when the injury is less than 1 week old.[48] Wound tracts appear as low signal intensity or a heterogeneous tract extending through the soft tissues, and foreign material such as metallic fragments, debris, and/or hemorrhage may be identified within the tract (**Fig. 7**). The presence of low-signal osseous lesions on MRI of penetrating injuries may be due to hemorrhage degradation products and mineralization,[50] and may persist for years after the inciting incident.

MRI is also helpful for treatment planning and prognosis for horses with penetrating wounds to the sole, with prognosis being most dependent on the anatomic region affected by the penetrating wound.[48,50,51] Treatment of penetrating wounds to the sole depends on identification of the structures involved as well as severity of the injury to these structures. Some treatment options, including intravenous regional limb perfusion with antibiotics, synovial or intrathecal lavage, or local debridement, may be performed on the standing horse with the use of local anesthesia. In these cases a diagnosis can be made, prognosis can be determined, and treatment can be initiated while avoiding the use of general anesthesia altogether. In more severe cases; however, aggressive treatment including surgical debridement under general anesthesia may be required.

Osseous structures

Bone marrow edema (also called bone bruise or bone contusion) was first described by Yao and Lee[52] in 1988, and has since become a common MRI finding in humans,

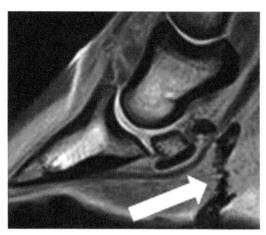

Fig. 7. Sagittal plane standing, low-field, T1-weighted MR image of a horse with a penetrating wound to the sole. A low-signal (*black*) fistulous tract (*arrow*) is seen extending from the sole to the level of the DDFT.

dogs, and horses. Histologically it may consist of trabecular bone microfractures with associated edema and hemorrhages,[52] fibrosis, and/or necrosis.[53] Bone marrow edema may be associated with direct trauma on subchondral bone, strain from ligamentous structures, or chronic degenerative processes leading to necrosis. Bone marrow edema is a nonspecific finding characterized by regions of low signal intensity on T1-weighted images and intermediate to high signal intensity on T2-weighted and fat-suppressed images[53,54] (**Fig. 8**). In horses, bone marrow edema is easily identified by standing MRI and has been clinically associated with lameness.

Both high-field and low-field MRI have proved to be effective for early fracture evaluation (**Fig. 9**). In the authors' opinion, certain types of osseous abnormalities are much less susceptible to motion artifact on MR images in comparison with

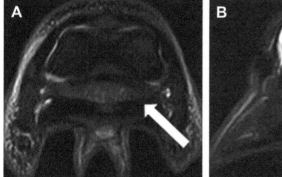
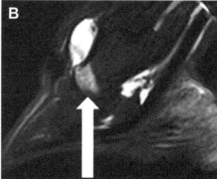

Fig. 8. Transverse plane standing, low-field, short-tau inversion recovery (STIR) MR image of a horse with increased signal, representing fluid in the navicular bone (*arrow*) (*A*), and sagittal plane standing, low-field, STIR MR image of a horse with fluid in the distal aspect of the middle phalanx (*arrow*) (*B*). Moderate to severe effusion is also seen in the distal interphalangeal joint. Lateral is to the left on the transverse plane image.

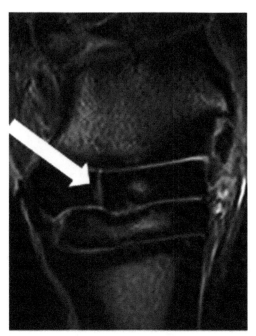

Fig. 9. Dorsal plane standing, low-field T1-weighted MR image of a horse with a proximo-distally oriented slab fracture of the central tarsal bone (*arrow*). The surrounding low signal intensity represents sclerosis. Lateral is to the left of the image.

soft-tissue structures. This aspect is important in standing MRI whereby motion arti-fact is a common cause of decreased image quality. In racing horses, a high incidence of stress fractures occurs at the level of the fetlock joint involving the distal third meta-carpal/metatarsal condyles and proximal phalanx. Standing MRI can detect a wide range of disease processes within equine fetlock joints, including bone contusions, condylar and proximal phalangeal fractures, palmar/plantar osteochondral disease, and arthritis.[55] Both condylar and incomplete sagittal P1 fractures have a character-istic linear hyperintensity on multiple sequences, with fluid signal in the surrounding bone. In condylar fractures, this hyperintensity extends proximally from the parasagit-tal groove, and surrounding subchondral bone sclerosis may be present. In many of these cases, including early, incomplete fractures, radiographic findings are often inconclusive.[55] It is essential to obtain a definitive diagnosis of the pathologic change involved in a timely manner, so as to instill appropriate treatment and prevent cata-strophic injury. With standing MRI, horses can be imaged early in the disease process and progression of pathologic change can be followed over time. In some instances, fractures of the third metacarpal/metatarsal condyles and proximal phalanx can be addressed in the standing horse, without ever risking catastrophic injury during anes-thetic recovery.[56,57] MRI findings of the distal phalanx and ossified ungual cartilage fractures have also been characterized. These fractures tend to be simple, nonarticu-lar, and nondisplaced, and extend from the base of the ossified ungual cartilage into the distal phalanx. The intricate ligamentous structures associated with the ungual cartilages are often affected in these cases, with enlargement and altered signal inten-sity, and are thought to contribute to the lameness. Evaluation of these subtle findings is limited with radiography and near impossible with ultrasonography.[58] Nondisplaced fractures of the middle phalanx have also been described on MRI of 2 horses. In both cases, radiographs were unremarkable with the exception of smooth periosteal new bone production on the dorsal aspect of the middle phalanx.[59]

Treatment and Recheck Examinations

Once injury to a soft tissue, bursa, or joint is diagnosed with MRI, treatment can be initiated. The clinician can perform image-guided intralesional injections, intravenous regional limb perfusions, or intra-articular or intrathecal injections with therapeutic or regenerative agents. For more permanent injuries, neurectomy can be decided upon at the clinician's discretion. With the use of standing magnets, all of the injuries already mentioned can be diagnosed, prognosis determined, and treatment initiated without ever having to incur the risks of general anesthesia.

It is important that the patient's response to therapy and progression of healing are followed once treatment is instituted. Complications should be evaluated with the most appropriate imaging modality, which may include sequential MR examinations.[60] Recheck MR examinations can be used to evaluate disease progression after a neurectomy is performed, to prevent catastrophic injury or to evaluate fracture healing or resolution of inflammation or infection. In addition, recheck MR examinations are often indicated to monitor healing or evaluate complications after surgery. The increased availability, decreased cost, and lower risk of standing MRI make this modality advantageous for these types of targeted examinations. Time frames for reevaluation with MRI vary based on the nature and extent of the initial injury, and may range from weeks to years. The possibility of recheck MR examination(s) should be discussed with the owner before the initial examination, as this may present a financial limitation.

MR Artifacts

This section briefly discusses common artifacts that can occur with standing MRI of the horse and affect the diagnostic quality of MR images. This review of artifacts, though not exhaustive, is intended to familiarize the practitioner with the more commonly occurring artifacts so that misinterpretation of these artifacts as lesions might be prevented. A brief review of how to prevent, avoid, or decrease the severity of each artifact is included.

Motion

Motion artifact appears as ghosting (the appearance of multiple images) or blurring of the image, and can drastically decrease the ability of the examiner to resolve fine details (**Fig. 10**). In severe cases, motion artifact can render the study nondiagnostic. Any motion greater than one-half the pixel resolution of the MR image, which corresponds to submillimeter movements, can degrade image quality.[61] In the standing horse, the distal limb is the least likely to have associated motion artifact. As one images further proximally on the limb, even the subtle swaying motion of a sedated horse becomes a more severe issue. As discussed earlier, the signal-to-noise ratio is decreased in the low magnetic field strengths used for standing MRI. Decreased signal-to-noise ratio, which translates to degraded image quality, can be improved by increasing the length of time over which the image is acquired. Unfortunately, the prolonged scan times needed to improve image quality will increase the opportunity for motion artifact to occur.

Motion-correction techniques have been developed over recent years, and can improve MR image quality in the face of mild to moderate swaying motion. Such methods include faster scanning sequences and retrospective motion-correction techniques.[12,61] Some of these techniques have been shown at least to be effective

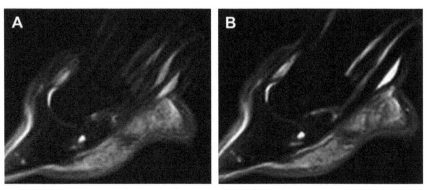

Fig. 10. Sagittal plane standing, low-field, STIR MR image of a foot with motion artifact (*A*), and a repeat image without motion artifact (*B*). Note the appearance of multiple superimposed images created by motion artifact.

on high-field MR images of cadaveric equine limbs with motion mimicking that of a standing horse.[61] Dedicated motion-correction software and supportive hardware are necessary to provide motion-correction techniques.

Motion can also be limited by providing an adequate plane of sedation while avoiding heavier sedation protocols, which may cause more severe swaying or wobbling. In addition, if the patient is in pain when bearing weight on the limb to be imaged, local analgesia can be provided to promote weight bearing on the affected limb.

Magic angle

An artifactual increase in signal intensity will occur in structures oriented at angles of 55° ± 10° relative to the main magnetic field when imaged with sequences that have a short echo time.[62,63] This increase is termed magic-angle artifact, and has been described at similar anatomic locations in the equine limb on high-field MR images.[64,65] With the patient in a standing position, the conformation and position of the foot will affect the signal intensity of structures including the DDFT and the collateral ligaments of the distal interphalangeal joint, and can mimic lesions.[66] Collateral ligaments of the distal interphalangeal joint are specifically affected by magic-angle artifact in standing magnets. In limbs positioned adequately in the magnet, the base wide stance needed to position the patient within the bore and the resulting medial joint compression causes the collateral ligaments to be affected asymmetrically. For clinical MRI, the collateral ligaments have a heterogeneous signal pattern with low signal center and increased signal peripherally, owing to their orientation and fiber configuration (**Fig. 11**).[67] If images are not interpreted with knowledge of how different anatomic structures are affected by magic-angle artifact, the regions of increased signal can be confused with pathologic change.

To prevent magic-angle artifact the limb should be carefully positioned in the magnetic field, attempting to avoid placing structures of interest at 55° to the main magnetic field. Furthermore, magic-angle artifact can be reduced by choosing pulse sequences with a longer echo time. A T2-weighted fast spin-echo sequence with an echo time of 120 milliseconds has been shown to maintain image quality while minimizing the magic-angle effect in the collateral ligaments of the distal interphalangeal joint.[68] When the artifact cannot be prevented, the examiner should evaluate the study based on knowledge of the common structures where the artifact occurs and should have the ability to recognize this artifact, thus avoiding misinterpretation.

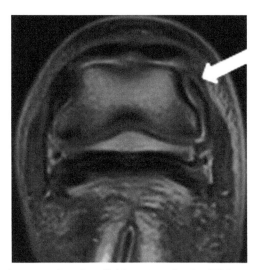

Fig. 11. Transverse plane standing, low-field, proton-density MR image at the level of the collateral ligaments of the distal interphalangeal joint. Increased signal intensity is present in the periphery of the lateral collateral ligament because of magic-angle artifact (*arrow*). The medial collateral ligament has normal, low signal intensity, as it is not affected by magic-angle artifact in the image. Lateral is to the right of the image.

Magnetic susceptibility

Magnetic susceptibility artifacts are manifested as regions of signal void (black regions), with a peripheral rim of increased signal intensity and distortion of the MR image (**Fig. 12**).[12,69] Although magnetic susceptibility artifacts decrease with field strength, making them less severe in low-field magnets, they still exist and often obscure the quality of low-field images. These artifacts are often associated with metallic fragments, and are especially common when imaging the equine foot. Metallic debris is commonly found in the hoof even after the shoe and nails have been removed. For many common MR sequences used in low-field MRI, there is a linear relationship between the size of the metallic debris and the size of the artifact created.[70]

It is imperative that all shoes and shoeing nails are removed from the hoof before imaging the distal limb. Magnetic susceptibility can be further prevented by radiographically screening for metal, and removing any metallic fragments from the hoof wall before performing the MR examination. If metallic fragments cannot be removed, fast spin-echo sequences, which are less prone to magnetic susceptibility artifacts, will more accurately represent the tissues in this region, whereas gradient-echo sequences will exacerbate these artifacts.

STANDING CT IN THE HORSE
Basic CT Technology

CT allows acquisition of 2-dimensional, cross-sectional images obtained by rapid rotation of an x-ray generator and detectors around the patient. X-ray detectors are positioned across the gantry from the x-ray generator, and detect radiation transmitted through the patient. The resultant CT image is generated by a computer, allowing the internal structure of the object imaged to be reconstructed from the collective information obtained from multiple x-ray beams. The original CT scanners acquired CT

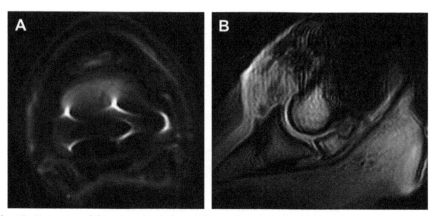

Fig. 12. Transverse (*A*) and sagittal plane (*B*) standing, low-field spin-echo MR images at the level of the proximal interphalangeal joint. Large signal voids, caused by metallic implants associated with a prior proximal interphalangeal arthrodesis, obscure the anatomy.

images one slice at a time. To increase the amount of anatomy imaged, the patient was moved a determined distance between the acquisition of each slice. Technological advances have led to the development of spiral (also known as helical) CT scanners, which are in common use today. These scanners allow the patient to move slowly through the path of a continuously emitted x-ray beam. The radiation transmitted is in the form of a spiral. Spiral CT enables very efficient anatomic coverage during the CT scan, making the studies much more time effective than MRI.

Arguably the largest disadvantage of CT is exposure to ionizing radiation. To prevent radiation exposure to personnel, proper safety precautions are necessary and include limiting the amount of exposure time, maximizing distance from the primary beam and scattered radiation, and x-ray shielding. The technician performing the scan is positioned behind a leaded wall while the scan is in progress.

Procedure

To prevent gross motion artifact, animals are routinely placed under general anesthesia for the duration of the CT scan (**Fig. 13**). In small animals, heavy sedation is often adequate for motion reduction during the scan, limiting the use of general anesthesia. If properly restrained, even unsedated small animals can be imaged. However, in nonanesthetized animals, respiratory motion creates a challenge when performing thoracic imaging, whereas breath-holding can help limit respiratory motion in intubated patients under general anesthesia. Until very recently, general anesthesia was considered mandatory for equine patients undergoing a CT examination. In a few locations across the world today, modifications have been made to allow for CT imaging to be performed on the standing horse. To scan the head of the sedated horse, the CT gantry must be elevated to the level of the horse's neck (**Fig. 14**), which can be achieved by elevating the CT scanner or positioning the horse within a trench to have the head level with the gantry. In 2002, a peripheral quantitative CT scanner was specifically designed to image the distal equine limb in either the standing or recumbent position (Equine XCT 3000; Norland-Stratec Medical Systems, Fort Atkinson, WI).[71] Images from this CT scanner were considered diagnostic in 89% of cases reported in a retrospective study. With this standing CT, several people may be needed to accompany the horse during the scan to restrain the animal, creating radiation exposure to personnel that would be unnecessary in an anesthetized horse. As

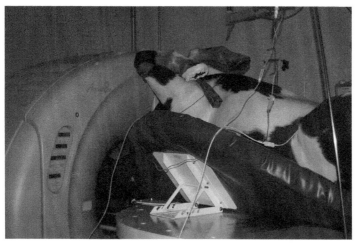

Fig. 13. Positioning of an anesthetized horse with its head in the computed tomography (CT) gantry.

with MRI, the horse shoe and nails must be removed before CT imaging to avoid artifact created by having metal within the field of view.

As with MRI, the size of the CT gantry limits the ability to image certain anatomic regions. Currently available CT scanners have gantry sizes of up to 85 cm in diameter. The gantry of CT scanners consists of a closed construct, thus limiting the ability to position larger equine anatomy within the gantry. However, whereas most MR

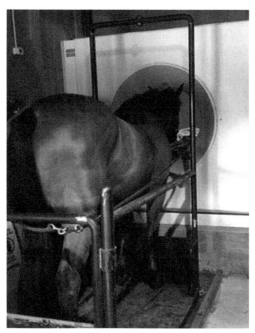

Fig. 14. Positioning of a sedated horse with its head in a CT gantry, modified for a standing horse. (*Courtesy of* Dr Kurt Selberg, Animal Imaging, Irving, TX.)

scanners have a longer, more tubular shape; CT scanners have more of a simple ring or circular construct, making the positioning of anatomy within the center of the gantry less complicated with CT in comparison with MRI scanners.

Similar to that described with standing MRI, the ideal plane of sedation maximally limits patient motion while limiting the swaying or wobbling motions of a heavily sedated patient. Because CT image acquisition is rapid, and reformatted images are made by the computer after the data set is obtained from the patient, scan time is significantly quicker with CT than with MRI. The length of sedation needed for a patient is relatively short, with a typical CT scan of a single anatomic region taking approximately 20 minutes. Sedation duration is lengthened by the time needed to adequately position the standing, sedated patient before initiating the scan.

In addition to being time efficient, CT is much more cost efficient than MRI. The lower initial setup and maintenance costs of CT scanners makes them more appealing to practice owners, thus increasing their availability. As mentioned earlier, however, the availability of CT scanners modified for the standing equine patient is still extremely limited. As with MRI, once the study is completed, DICOM images can be transferred to a PACS workstation and/or burned onto a CD for image interpretation. After thorough evaluation of the study, a CT report is created by a radiologist or the interpreting veterinarian.

Clinical Applications

Because of its relative technical simplicity, better availability, and lower cost, a radiographic examination is often performed before advanced imaging to rule out gross disease. However, the sensitivity of radiography relative to 3-dimensional imaging, such as CT, is low. This factor is even more significant with regard to the complicated anatomy of the equine skull. CT allows for evaluation of the skull without anatomic superimposition, and provides excellent contrast and spatial resolution. For these reasons, CT allows for a more accurate assessment of the extent and physical features of diseases of the skull than conventional radiographs.[72] Both soft tissues and bone can be imaged with CT; however, the soft-tissue contrast resolution of MRI is superior to that of CT. In the standing horse, CT imaging of the equine head and the distal limbs has been described to a limited extent. The following sections discuss the use of CT imaging in the standing horse as applied to specific, commonly encountered disease processes that can be surgically addressed in the standing horse.

Dental structures

Dental disease is the third most common medical problem in large animal practice in the United States, and the most common oral disorder encountered in equine practice.[73,74] Radiographic evaluation of small structures in the equine skull, such as the teeth and alveolar bone, is limited by superimposition of anatomic structures. Three-dimensional imaging, specifically CT, has become routine for evaluation of dental disease in the horse. In one study comparing dental radiography with CT for nonneoplastic mandibular disease, it was concluded that some findings of dental disease, including tooth pulp involvement, lamina dura destruction, presence of bone fragments, mandibular bone periosteal reaction, and cortical bone destruction, are more conspicuous with CT.[75] If the CT scanner is modified to accommodate the standing horse, the head is easily positioned in the gantry for evaluation of the maxillary and mandibular arcades as well as the paranasal sinuses.

Common equine dental disorders include apical abscesses, fractured teeth or tooth roots, retained deciduous teeth, abnormalities of wear, supernumerary teeth, congenital anomalies, and periodontal disease.[74] CT imaging is helpful in evaluating features of dental disease such as diastema widening, alveolar bone sclerosis and/or osteolysis, blunting of the tooth root, gas within the tooth root, and fragmented teeth.[76] Although infundibular gas can be seen in both normal and diseased teeth, it may lead to tooth decay with subsequent tooth root infection and fracture within the maxillary teeth.[76] The roots of the maxillary fourth premolar through second molar teeth are intimately associated with the maxillary sinuses. Infection of these tooth roots can lead to sinusitis, with the first molar, fourth premolar, and third premolar tooth roots being most commonly involved.[77] The CT findings of sinusitis are further discussed in the next section.

Oral and endoscopic dental evaluation, tooth extraction, and other dental surgeries are routinely performed in the standing horse. It is imperative that the appropriate diagnosis be obtained before performing dental surgery. Long-term complications including development of oronasal, orosinus, or orocutaneous fistulas can result from performing dental surgeries without an accurate diagnosis.[76] With the use of CT in the standing horse a thorough evaluation can be performed, an accurate diagnosis made, and surgical treatment initiated without the need for general anesthesia.

Sinonasal region

Common sinonasal disorders encountered with CT include sinusitis, paranasal sinus cysts, aggressive and nonaggressive sinonasal neoplasia (**Fig. 15**), and ethmoid hematomas.

Sinusitis can be primary or secondary. Primary sinusitis is caused by an upper respiratory tract infection involving the paranasal sinuses, whereas secondary sinusitis is

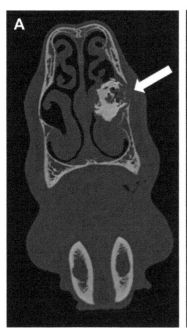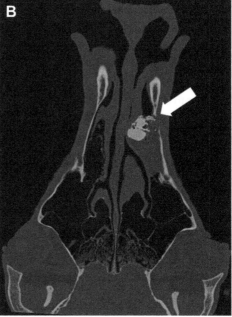

Fig. 15. Transverse (A) and dorsal plane (B) CT images of an equine head acquired in a standing horse and processed in a bone algorithm. Soft tissue–attenuating material and a well-defined, mineral-attenuating mass (*arrow*) is seen in the left middle nasal meatus, with associated, complete disruption of the left maxillary bone. Left is to the left of the images. (*Courtesy of* Dr Mads Kristofferson, Regional Veterinary Clinic of Helsingborg, Sweden.)

usually caused by tooth-root infections. Characteristics of sinusitis on CT may include nasal mucosal thickening, accumulation of fluid, mucus, or purulent material in the sinus, with a decreased volume of air in the sinus, thickening and sclerosis of the maxilla, and expansion and/or regional osteolysis of the sinus.[78] The rostral and caudal maxillary and ventral conchal sinuses are most commonly affected by sinusitis; however, any of the sinuses can be involved.[76] Sinusitis may be treated with lavage or surgical debridement via an osteotomy in the standing horse.[77]

Paranasal sinus cysts may be single or loculated fluid-filled structures with a thin epithelial lining, which develop in the maxillary sinuses or ventral conchae and can extend into the frontal sinus.[77] Clinically they may cause mucopurulent nasal discharge, facial swelling, or partial airway obstruction, and can occur in horses of any age.[79] On CT examination they are well-defined, fluid-attenuating structures with a thin, soft tissue–attenuating wall. Paranasal sinus cysts can be removed in the standing horse with very successful outcomes.[80]

Both benign and malignant sinonasal neoplasia have been reported in the horse. Multiple tumor types have been reported; including neuroendocrine tumors, undifferentiated carcinomas, myxosarcomas, adenocarcinoma, hemangiosarcoma, chondroblastic osteosarcoma, anaplastic sarcoma, squamous cell carcinoma, histiocytic sarcoma, cementoma, myxoma, and ossifying fibroma.[80–82] Neoplasia may involve the nasal cavities and one or multiple sinuses, and may extend into the retrobulbar space. On CT, a homogeneous mass with poorly defined margins and moderate to severe regional osteolysis has been described, and osteolysis of the cribriform plate with intracalvarial extension may be seen as well.[81] Radiographs, although useful as a screening tool for identification of masses, may underestimate features of malignancy, such as severity of osteolysis or osseous proliferation. CT can be more informative than radiography with regard to mass extent, features of malignancy, and important prognostic indicators, and may be helpful in differentiating neoplasia from nonneoplastic sinonasal disorders.[81] Although reports are limited, neoplasia has been reported to enhance after administration of intravenous contrast, so contrast-enhanced CT may help to further differentiate neoplastic processes.[81] This observation has also been noted in the authors' experience. If neoplasia is suspected the diagnosis should be confirmed with histopathology, and tumor staging should be performed.

Ethmoid hematomas are slow-growing, locally invasive masses that can originate from the ethmoid labyrinth or the maxillary sinuses, and rarely involve the nasal passages.[77,83,84] Clinically, ethmoid hematomas most commonly cause mild, unilateral epistaxis. CT is specifically helpful for diagnosing ethmoid hematomas when the hematoma cannot be seen endoscopically, if there is involvement of the paranasal sinuses, and/or when multifocal disease is present. With CT imaging, ethmoid hematomas appear as well-defined, homogeneous or heterogeneous, soft tissue–attenuating masses adjacent to the ethmoturbinates or within the paranasal sinuses. These hematomas may contain swirling hyperattenuating regions resulting from recent hemorrhage, and may be characterized by mild regional osseous destruction.[85] In a recent study, CT was shown to better define the location and extent of disease than a combination of clinical examination, endoscopy, and radiography. In addition, CT findings affected treatment decisions in most horses.[85] Treatment options for ethmoid hematomas include intralesional injection of 10% formalin, laser ablation, or surgical removal through a frontonasal osteotomy, all of which may be performed in the standing horse.[77,86]

For many of these disease processes, CT can help to form a differential diagnosis list and raise the index of suspicion for one disease process over another; however, imaging diagnoses are often not definitive. After a differential diagnosis list is generated with CT imaging, endoscopy or surgery can be performed on the standing horse to obtain biopsies for histopathology. Often sinonasal disease can subsequently be surgically managed in the standing horse. With the use of standing CT imaging, many common sinonasal diseases can be diagnosed and the prognosis determined, and the lesion can be surgically treated, all without the need for general anesthesia.

Calvarium

CT is often recognized for its superior ability to image osseous structures. One study evaluated the diagnostic utility of CT for evaluation of different intracranial lesions.[87] In this study, CT was not only determined to be excellent for identifying multiple skull fractures but also for evaluation of space-occupying lesions such as neoplasia and ventriculomegaly, and acute hemorrhage, similar to what has been observed in human medicine. CT was also considered helpful for ruling in intracranial disorders. The sensitivity of CT for identifying inflammatory disorders, such as meningoencephalitis, and small parenchymal lesions of the brain was limited in this study. Intravenous contrast administration helped to elucidate an inflammatory lesion in one case. The use of intravenous contrast-enhanced CT has also been described in a standing horse to evaluate a cholesterol granuloma.[88]

If inflammatory or infectious causes are suspected, cerebrospinal fluid can be collected in the standing horse with ultrasound guidance after the CT scan.[89] Although MRI is commonly known to be more sensitive for evaluation of subtle lesions of the brain because of its superior soft-tissue contrast, the possibility of obtaining a CT diagnosis in a neurologic horse without the risks of anesthetic recovery is a huge benefit of standing CT.

Guttural pouch and hyoid apparatus

Temporohyoid osteopathy (THO) is a disorder characterized by osseous proliferation of the temporohyoid joint, and can result in cranial nerve deficits and/or other behavior such as head shaking, ear rubbing, or resentment of the bit. Historically, THO has been diagnosed with radiography and endoscopy. More recently, however, findings of THO have been described with CT.[90–92] Osseous proliferation of the stylohyoid bone and temporohyoid articulation was found to be a consistent CT finding, while ceratohyoid bone thickening and osseous proliferation of the articulation of the ceratohyoid and stylohyoid bones was also commonly seen. CT has been shown to allow identification of abnormalities not diagnosed with endoscopy or radiography in some horses, such as middle and external ear disease, ceratohyoid bone thickening, and fracture of the petrous temporal and stylohyoid bones.[90] Subclinical, bilateral disease has also been seen on CT images of horses thought to be unilaterally affected based on clinical examination.[90] The ability to make this diagnosis in the standing horse is advantageous, as recovering a neurologic horse from anesthesia poses increased risk to the patient.

The guttural pouches are extensions of the Eustachian tube that connect the pharynx to the middle ear bilaterally. Diseases of the guttural pouches, although uncommon, include guttural pouch empyema, guttural pouch tympany, and guttural pouch mycosis. CT anatomy of the guttural pouches has been described.[93] Medical management of these diseases may include aggressive guttural pouch lavage, decompensation of guttural pouch tympany, and endoscopic removal of chondroids, and can often be addressed in the standing horse.[94] In some cases surgical management can also be performed in the standing horse.[95,96]

Orthopedic

CT has been shown to be effective for evaluating anatomic structures and abnormalities of the distal limb in lame horses.[14,15,97,98] As mentioned earlier, CT of the limbs of standing horses has been performed to a very limited extent.[71] A case series of CT scans on 47 clinically abnormal horses and 4 normal horses has been reported. Of the 47 abnormal scans, the majority (26) were evaluated for foot pain, 7 were assessed for bone cysts, 5 for fracture of the distal phalanx, 4 for foot abscesses, 2 for keratoma assessment, 1 for chronic lameness evaluation secondary to a previous distal phalanx fracture, 1 for internal fixation of a distal phalanx fracture, and 1 to confirm navicular bone fragmentation.[71] In these cases, standing CT allowed good evaluation of the osseous structures of the distal limb; including the distal aspect of the middle phalanx, the distal phalanx, and the navicular bone. Evaluation of the surrounding soft tissues was inadequate. Of the 26 evaluations for foot pain, CT was considered to be more clinically useful than radiography in only 5 cases. The investigators considered it likely that pathologic change of the soft tissues, which could not be assessed on CT, may have contributed to the lameness in many of these cases. The limited ability of recumbent CT with and without contrast enhancement, and low-field MRI, to delineate the margins of many of the soft-tissue structures of the distal limb has been previously described.[14] However, CT is more diagnostic than low-field MRI for soft-tissue mineralization.[15] Because the ability to perform standing CT is so new, further studies comparing standing CT findings with recumbent CT findings, as well as other imaging modalities, are necessary before more conclusions can be drawn about this technology.

Fractures of the middle and distal phalanx may be difficult to detect radiographically. Middle phalangeal fractures are often comminuted, which complicates interpretation. CT evaluation of comminuted middle phalanx fractures has been described, and this modality has been advocated for more complete evaluation of the fracture configurations.[98] Radiographic examination of the distal phalanx often requires multiple oblique projections to follow the fractures and determine whether an articular component exists. In one study evaluating fractures of the distal phalanx, more fractures were identified, and small fissure fractures were identified to be associated with a larger fracture with CT more commonly than with radiography.[99] In another case report an oblique, nonarticular fracture of the palmar process of the distal phalanx could only be identified with radiography after CT was used to find the fracture and then used as a guide to obtain the appropriate radiographic projection.[100] For evaluation of fractures of the distal limb, CT has been shown to better determine fracture configuration, provide surgical planning, and help determine prognosis.

Keratomas are benign hyperplastic keratin masses that can originate from the coronary band, hoof wall, or sole, and are an infrequent cause of lameness in horses.[101,102] Keratomas have been adequately evaluated with both CT and low-field MRI (**Fig. 16**).[103] On CT they appear as a mass originating from the hoof wall, which is isoattenuating to the hoof wall on CT, and causes a semicircular region of osteolysis in the adjacent distal phalanx.[103] Cross-sectional imaging allows the exact location of the keratoma to be determined. Treatment most often consists of surgical debridement with resection of hoof wall. Using cross-sectional imaging as a guide, the keratoma can be completely surgically resected while minimizing the hoof-wall defect that must be made.[103] Keratomas can often be removed while the horse is standing.[104,105]

The early stages of navicular disease may present with soft-tissue abnormalities and subtle osseous changes. Both CT and MRI have been shown to better define the size, shape, and location of synovial invaginations in the distal border of the navicular bone when compared with radiography.[97,106] Furthermore, radiography is known to underestimate the number and size of distal border synovial invaginations in the navicular bone.[106] CT may be best for identifying contour changes on the flexor surface of the navicular bone, whereas MRI is more effective for evaluation of navicular bone

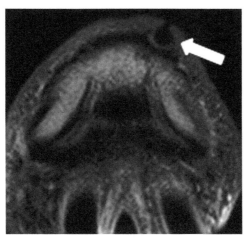

Fig. 16. Transverse plane, standing, low-field, proton-density MR images at the level of the distal phalanx. A round, hypointense (*dark*) keratoma (*arrow*) is seen in the hoof wall, causing lysis of the adjacent solar margin of the distal phalanx.

fibrocartilage and the adjacent soft tissues.[97] However, the addition of intra-arterial contrast before CT can improve evaluation of the soft tissues within the hoof capsule.[107] With CT imaging of the distal limb, one may be able to diagnose lesions associated with navicular disease earlier, and thus initiate therapeutic interventions in hopes of slowing the progression of disease.

Many of the lesions evaluated with standing CT can subsequently be surgically addressed in the standing horse. Intravenous limb perfusions of antibiotics and/or intra-articular lavage can be initiated for septic processes; some fractures can be repaired or stabilized,[56,57] in some cases CT can be used to guide implant placement for fracture repair,[108] and image-guided hoof-wall resections can be performed. The risk of catastrophic outcomes in anesthetic recovery of a horse with a fracture can be prevented in these cases.

CT Artifacts

This section briefly discusses artifacts that commonly occur with standing CT imaging of the horse, which can affect the diagnostic quality of CT images. As in the section on MR artifacts, this is not intended to be an exhaustive review. The goal is to familiarize the practitioner with more commonly occurring artifacts so as to prevent misinterpretation of these artifacts as lesions. A brief review of how to prevent, avoid, or decrease the severity of each artifact is included.

Motion

In the standing horse, patient motion is probably the artifact most detrimental to image quality. Patient motion during the CT scan can result in artifacts severe enough to render the reconstructed image nondiagnostic. Motion artifacts on CT images usually appear as shading or streaking of the image. Some motion, such as cardiac motion, cannot be avoided; however, voluntary motions are typically limited by anesthetizing or heavily sedating veterinary patients.

In the standing horse, motion is limited by maintaining an adequate plane of sedation while avoiding sedation so heavy that the patient becomes wobbly. In addition, positioning aids can be used to help stabilize the area of interest within the gantry. Motion-correction techniques such as overscan and underscan modes, which are built into the CT scanner, and software correction can also help to limit motion arti-fact.[109] Unfortunately, the standing CT modalities currently in use do not use motion-correction techniques.[71]

Photon starvation

Photon starvation occurs in anatomic regions that greatly attenuate the x-ray beams. The classic example of this is the shoulder region in humans, when the x-ray beam is oriented horizontally (from one shoulder to the other). Photon starvation appears as a streaking of the image. This artifact (in addition to gantry width) limits the capability of CT scanners to obtain a diagnostic image of the larger anatomic regions in equine patients.[109]

This artifact can be mitigated to an extent by increasing the tube current when scan-ning larger structures. In some CT scanners, the tube current is automatically modu-lated to provide higher current to thicker anatomic regions and to reduce excess current in regions where it is not necessary. In addition, adaptive filtration software correction techniques can be used to smooth out the streaky appearance of this arti-fact before the image is reconstructed.[109]

Metal

The density of metal is beyond the normal range of attenuation values that can be managed by the computer. When metallic structures are present within the scanning field of view, severe streaking artifacts can occur.[109] The best way to avoid this artifact is to remove any metallic objects from the field of view. As with MRI, any metallic frag-ments should be removed from the hoof wall before performing a CT scan of the distal limbs.

Limitations of Standing CT

At present, the limited availability of CT scanners modified to accommodate the stand-ing horse is the most prevalent limitation. Anatomic sites that can be evaluated are limited by gantry diameter and artifact. The swaying motion of the standing horse can limit the image quality of both CT and MRI, and motion artifact becomes more sig-nificant as the scanner is moved proximally along the extremities. In addition, radiation exposure to personnel needed to restrain a sedated horse during a CT examination is another concern that must be addressed.

The Future of Standing CT

The concept of standing CT is currently in its infancy. However, the benefits of limiting general anesthesia and recumbency are clinically significant. As standing surgical pro-cedures become more available, the option to limit general anesthesia altogether with the use of standing advanced imaging becomes even more desirable. Continued development of standing CT scanners is on the horizon. As more standing CT technol-ogy is developed, better motion correction/artifact reduction software will likely become more available in the future, thus improving image quality.

SUMMARY

Both MRI and CT can be performed in the standing horse. The greatest benefit of per-forming cross-sectional imaging in the standing patient is that it eliminates the risks associated with general anesthesia. With both modalities, careful case selection is paramount to ensuring that the maximum information is obtained from these studies. Limitations of the use of both modalities in the standing horse are addressed. In stand-ing MRI, decreased image quality resulting from the low field strength of most available open magnets and motion artifact are the most significant limitations. The low availability of facilities equipped to perform CT examinations in the standing horse is the most significant limitation of this modality. With the rapid progression of MRI technology and continued demand for availability of these modalities, it is likely that high-quality standing MR and CT imaging will become available for equine patients in the near future.

REFERENCES

1. Franci R, Leece EA, Brearley JC. Post anaesthetic myopathy/neuropathy in horses undergoing magnetic resonance imaging compared to horses undergoing surgery. Equine Vet J 2006;38:497–501.
2. Johnston GM, Eastment JK, Taylor PM, et al. Is isoflurane safer than halothane in equine anaesthesia? Results from a prospective multicentre randomised controlled trial. Equine Vet J 2004;36:64–71.
3. Johnston GM, Eastment JK, Wood JL, et al. The confidential enquiry into perioperative equine fatalities (CEPEF): mortality results of phases 1 and 2. Vet Anaesth Analg 2002;29:159–70.
4. Johnston GM, Steffey E. Confidential enquiry into perioperative equine fatalities (CEPEF). Vet Surg 1995;24:518–9.
5. Jacobs MA, Ibrahim TS, Ouwerkerk R. AAPM/RSNA physics tutorial for residents - MR imaging: brief overview and emerging applications. Radiographics 2007;27:1213–29.
6. Hoult DI, Lauterbur PC. Sensitivity of the zeugmatographic experiment involving human samples. J Magn Reson 1979;34:425–33.
7. Hoult DI, Richards RE. The signal-to-noise ratio of the nuclear magnetic resonance experiment. 1976. J Magn Reson 2011;213:329–43.
8. Bottomley PA, Foster TH, Argersinger RE, et al. A review of normal tissue hydrogen NMR relaxation-times and relaxation mechanisms from 1-100 MHz—dependence on tissue-type, NMR frequency, temperature, species, excision, and age. Med Phys 1984;11:425–48.
9. Patton JA. The AAPM RSNA physics tutorial for residents—MR-imaging instrumentation and image artifacts. Radiographics 1994;14:1083–96.
10. Tucker RL, Sande RD. Computed tomography and magnetic resonance imaging in equine musculoskeletal conditions. Vet Clin North Am Equine Pract 2001;17:145–57, vii.
11. Rutt BK, Lee DH. The impact of field strength on image quality in MRI. J Magn Reson Imaging 1996;6:57–62.
12. Zhuo JC, Gullapalli RP. AAPM/RSNA physics tutorial for residents—MR artifacts, safety, and quality control. Radiographics 2006;26:275–97.
13. Bolen G, Audigié F, Spriet M, et al. Qualitative comparison of 0.27T, 1.5T, and 3T magnetic resonance images of the normal equine foot. J Equine Vet Sci 2010; 30:9–20.
14. Vallance SA, Bell RJ, Spriet M, et al. Comparisons of computed tomography, contrast enhanced computed tomography and standing low-field magnetic resonance imaging in horses with lameness localised to the foot. Part 1: anatomic visualisation scores. Equine Vet J 2012;44:51–6.
15. Vallance SA, Bell RJ, Spriet M, et al. Comparisons of computed tomography, contrast-enhanced computed tomography and standing low-field magnetic resonance imaging in horses with lameness localised to the foot. Part 2: lesion identification. Equine Vet J 2012;44:149–56.

16. Gutierrez-Nibeyro S, Werpy N, White Ii N. Standing low-field magnetic resonance imaging in horses with chronic foot pain. Aust Vet J 2012;90:75–83.

17. Smith MA, Dyson SJ, Murray RC. The appearance of the equine metacarpophalangeal region on high-field vs. standing low-field magnetic resonance imaging. Vet Radiol Ultrasound 2011;52:61–70.

18. Nagy A, Dyson S. Magnetic resonance imaging findings in the carpus and proximal metacarpal region of 50 lame horses. Equine Vet J 2012;44:163–8.

19. Nagy A, Dyson S. Magnetic resonance anatomy of the proximal metacarpal region of the horse described from images acquired from low- and high-field magnets. Vet Radiol Ultrasound 2009;50:595–605.

20. Lempe-Troillet A, Ludewig E, Brehm W, et al. Magnetic resonance imaging of plantar soft tissue structures of the tarsus and proximal metatarsus in foals and adult horses. Vet Comp Orthop Traumatol 2013;26:192–7.

21. Blaik MA, Hanson RR, Kincaid SA, et al. Low-field magnetic resonance imaging of the equine tarsus: normal anatomy. Vet Radiol Ultrasound 2000;41:131–41.

22. Balassy C, Hormann M. Role of MRI in paediatric musculoskeletal conditions. Eur J Radiol 2008;68:245–58.

23. Powell SE, Ramzan PH, Head MJ, et al. Standing magnetic resonance imaging detection of bone marrow oedema-type signal pattern associated with subcarpal pain in 8 racehorses: a prospective study. Equine Vet J 2010;42:10–7.

24. Mair TS, Kinns J. Deep digital flexor tendonitis in the equine foot diagnosed by low-field magnetic resonance imaging in the standing patient: 18 cases. Vet Radiol Ultrasound 2005;46:458–66.

25. Dyson S, Murray R, Schramme M, et al. Lameness in 46 horses associated with deep digital flexor tendonitis in the digit: diagnosis confirmed with magnetic resonance imaging. Equine Vet J 2003;35:681–90.

26. Zubrod CJ, Schneider RK, Tucker RL. Use of magnetic resonance imaging to identify suspensory desmitis and adhesions between exostoses of the second metacarpal bone and the suspensory ligament in four horses. J Am Vet Med Assoc 2004;224:1815–20.

27. Dyson SJ, Murray R, Schramme MC. Lameness associated with foot pain: results of magnetic resonance imaging in 199 horses (January 2001-December 2003) and response to treatment. Equine Vet J 2005;37:113–21.

28. Gutierrez-Nibeyro SD, White NA 2nd, Werpy NM, et al. Magnetic resonance imaging findings of desmopathy of the collateral ligaments of the equine distal interphalangeal joint. Vet Radiol Ultrasound 2009;50:21–31.

29. Dyson S, Murray R. Magnetic resonance imaging evaluation of 264 horses with foot pain: the podotrochlear apparatus, deep digital flexor tendon and collateral ligaments of the distal interphalangeal joint. Equine Vet J 2007;39:340–3.

30. Sampson SN, Schneider RK, Gavin PR, et al. Magnetic resonance imaging findings in horses with recent onset navicular syndrome but without radiographic abnormalities. Vet Radiol Ultrasound 2009;50:339–46.

31. Zubrod CJ, Farnsworth KD, Tucker RL, et al. Injury of the collateral ligaments of the distal interphalangeal joint diagnosed by magnetic resonance. Vet Radiol Ultrasound 2005;46:11–6.

32. Dyson SJ, Murray R, Schramme M, et al. Collateral desmitis of the distal interphalangeal joint in 18 horses (2001-2002). Equine Vet J 2004;36:160–6.

33. Jackman BR, Baxter GM, Doran RE, et al. Palmar digital neurectomy in horses. 57 cases (1984-1990). Vet Surg 1993;22:285–8.

34. Olive J. Distal interphalangeal articular cartilage assessment using low-field magnetic resonance imaging. Vet Radiol Ultrasound 2010;51:259–66.

35. Werpy NM, Ho CP, Pease AP, et al. The effect of sequence selection and field strength on detection of osteochondral defects in the metacarpophalangeal joint. Vet Radiol Ultrasound 2011;52:154–60.
36. Maher MC, Werpy NM, Goodrich LR, et al. Positive contrast magnetic resonance bursography for assessment of the navicular bursa and surrounding soft tissues. Vet Radiol Ultrasound 2011;52:385–93.
37. Schramme M, Kerekes Z, Hunter S, et al. Improved identification of the palmar fibrocartilage of the navicular bone with saline magnetic resonance bursography. Vet Radiol Ultrasound 2009;50:606–14.
38. Yang WJ, Im SA, Lim GY, et al. MR imaging of transient synovitis: differentiation from septic arthritis. Pediatr Radiol 2006;36:1154–8.
39. Learch TJ, Farooki S. Magnetic resonance imaging of septic arthritis. Clin Imaging 2000;24:236–42.
40. Lalam RK, Cassar-Pullicino VN, Tins BJ. Magnetic resonance imaging of appendicular musculoskeletal infection. Top Magn Reson Imaging 2007;18:177–91.
41. Jbara M, Patnana M, Kazmi F, et al. MR imaging: arthropathies and infectious conditions of the elbow, wrist, and hand. Radiol Clin North Am 2006;44:625–42, ix.
42. Graif M, Schweitzer ME, Deely D, et al. The septic versus nonseptic inflamed joint: MRI characteristics. Skeletal Radiol 1999;28:616–20.
43. Gaschen L, LeRoux A, Trichel J, et al. Magnetic resonance imaging in foals with infectious arthritis. Vet Radiol Ultrasound 2011;52:627–33.
44. Easley JT, Brokken MT, Zubrod CJ, et al. Magnetic resonance imaging findings in horses with septic arthritis. Vet Radiol Ultrasound 2011;52:402–8.
45. Miller TT, Randolph DA Jr, Staron RB, et al. Fat-suppressed MRI of musculoskeletal infection: fast T2-weighted techniques versus gadolinium-enhanced T1-weighted images. Skeletal Radiol 1997;26:654–8.
46. Malcius D, Jonkus M, Kuprionis G, et al. The accuracy of different imaging techniques in diagnosis of acute hematogenous osteomyelitis. Medicina (Kaunas) 2009;45:624–31.
47. Hopkins KL, Li KC, Bergman G. Gadolinium-DTPA-enhanced magnetic resonance imaging of musculoskeletal infectious processes. Skeletal Radiol 1995; 24:325–30.
48. del Junco CI, Mair TS, Powell SE, et al. Magnetic resonance imaging findings of equine solar penetration wounds. Vet Radiol Ultrasound 2012;53:71–5.
49. Furst A, Lischer C. Musculoskeletal system: foot. In: Stick JA, Auer J, editors. Equine surgery. 4th edition. 2011. p. 1274–5.
50. Boado A, Kristoffersen M, Dyson S, et al. Use of nuclear scintigraphy and magnetic resonance imaging to diagnose chronic penetrating wounds in the equine foot. Equine Vet Educ 2005;17:62–8.
51. Kinns J, Mair TS. Use of magnetic resonance imaging to assess soft tissue damage in the foot following penetrating injury in 3 horses. Equine Vet Educ 2005;17: 69–73.
52. Yao L, Lee JK. Occult intraosseous fracture: detection with MR imaging. Radiology 1988;167:749–51.
53. Zanetti M, Bruder E, Romero J, et al. Bone marrow edema pattern in osteoarthritic knees: correlation between MR imaging and histologic findings. Radiology 2000;215:835–40.
54. Lecouvet FE, van de Berg BC, Maldague BE, et al. Early irreversible osteonecrosis versus transient lesions of the femoral condyles: prognostic value of subchondral bone and marrow changes on MR imaging. AJR Am J Roentgenol 1998;170:71–7.

55. Powell SE. Low-field standing magnetic resonance imaging findings of the metacarpo/metatarsophalangeal joint of racing Thoroughbreds with lameness localised to the region: a retrospective study of 131 horses. Equine Vet J 2012;44:169–77.

56. Payne RJ, Compston PC. Short- and long-term results following standing fracture repair in 34 horses. Equine Vet J 2012;44:721–5.

57. Russell TM, Maclean AA. Standing surgical repair of propagating metacarpal and metatarsal condylar fractures in racehorses. Equine Vet J 2006;38:423–7.

58. Selberg K, Werpy N. Fractures of the distal phalanx and associated soft tissue and osseous abnormalities in 22 horses with ossified sclerotic ungual cartilages diagnosed with magnetic resonance imaging. Vet Radiol Ultrasound 2011;52: 394–401.

59. Podadera JM, Bell RJ, Dart AJ. Using magnetic resonance imaging to diagnose nondisplaced fractures of the second phalanx in horses. Aust Vet J 2010;88: 439–42.

60. Werpy NM. Recheck magnetic resonance imaging examinations for evaluation of musculoskeletal injury. Vet Clin North Am Equine Pract 2012;28:659–80.

61. McKnight AL, Manduca A, Felmlee JP, et al. Motion-correction techniques for standing equine MRI. Vet Radiol Ultrasound 2004;45:513–9.

62. Hayes CW, Parellada JA. The magic angle effect in musculoskeletal MR imaging. Top Magn Reson Imaging 1996;8:51–6.

63. Erickson SJ, Cox IH, Hyde JS, et al. Effect of tendon orientation on MR imaging signal intensity: a manifestation of the "magic angle" phenomenon. Radiology 1991;181:389–92.

64. Busoni V, Snaps F. Effect of deep digital flexor tendon orientation on magnetic resonance imaging signal intensity in isolated equine limbs-the magic angle effect. Vet Radiol Ultrasound 2002;43:428–30.

65. Werpy NM, Ho CP, Kawcak CE. Magic angle effect in normal collateral ligaments of the distal interphalangeal joint in horses imaged with a high-field magnetic resonance imaging system. Vet Radiol Ultrasound 2010;51:2–10.

66. Spriet M, Zwingenberger A. Influence of the position of the foot on MRI signal in the deep digital flexor tendon and collateral ligaments of the distal interphalangeal joint in the standing horse. Equine Vet J 2009;41:498–503.

67. Gutierrez-Nibeyro SD, Werpy NM, White NA 2nd, et al. Standing low-field magnetic resonance imaging appearance of normal collateral ligaments of the equine distal interphalangeal joint. Vet Radiol Ultrasound 2011;52:521–33.

68. Werpy NM, Ho CP, Garcia EB, et al. The effect of varying echo time using T2-weighted FSE sequences on the magic angle effect in the collateral ligaments of the distal interphalangeal joint in horses. Vet Radiol Ultrasound 2013;54:31–5.

69. Czervionke LF, Daniels DL, Wehrli FW, et al. Magnetic susceptibility artifacts in gradient-recalled echo MR imaging. AJNR Am J Neuroradiol 1988;9:1149–55.

70. Urraca del Junco CI, Shaw DJ, Weaver MP, et al. The value of radiographic screening for metallic particles in the equine foot and size of related artifacts on low-field MRI. Vet Radiol Ultrasound 2011;52:634–9.

71. Desbrosse F, Vandeweerd JM, Perrin R, et al. A technique for computed tomography (CT) of the foot in the standing horse. Equine Vet Educ 2008;20:93–8.

72. Tietje S, Becker M, Bockenhoff G. Computed tomographic evaluation of head diseases in the horse: 15 cases. Equine Vet J 1996;28:98–105.

73. Traub-Dargatz JL, Salman MD, Voss JL. Medical problems of adult horses, as ranked by equine practitioners. J Am Vet Med Assoc 1991;198:1745–7.

74. Dixon PM, Dacre I. A review of equine dental disorders. Vet J 2005;169:165–87.

75. Huggons NA, Bell RJ, Puchalski SM. Radiography and computed tomography in the diagnosis of nonneoplastic equine mandibular disease. Vet Radiol Ultrasound 2011;52:53–60.

76. Selberg K, Easley JT. Advanced imaging in equine dental disease. Vet Clin North Am Equine Pract 2013;29:397–409.

77. Freeman DE. Sinus disease. Vet Clin North Am Equine Pract 2003;19:209–43, viii.

78. Henninger W, Frame EM, Willmann M, et al. CT features of alveolitis and sinusitis in horses. Vet Radiol Ultrasound 2003;44:269–76.

79. Woodford NS, Lane JG. Long-term retrospective study of 52 horses with sinonasal cysts. Equine Vet J 2006;38:198–202.

80. Dixon PM, Parkin TD, Collins N, et al. Equine paranasal sinus disease: a long-term study of 200 cases (1997-2009): ancillary diagnostic findings and involvement of the various sinus compartments. Equine Vet J 2012;44:267–71.

81. Cissell DD, Wisner ER, Textor J, et al. Computed tomographic appearance of equine sinonasal neoplasia. Vet Radiol Ultrasound 2012;53:245–51.

82. Paciello O, Passantino G, Costagliola A, et al. Histiocytic sarcoma of the nasal cavity in a horse. Res Vet Sci 2013;94:648–50.

83. Colbourne CM, Rosenstein DS, Steficek BA, et al. Surgical treatment of progressive ethmoidal hematoma aided by computed tomography in a foal. J Am Vet Med Assoc 1997;211:335–8.

84. Sullivan M, Burrell MH, McCandlish IA. Progressive haematoma of the maxillary sinus in a horse. Vet Rec 1984;114:191–2.

85. Textor JA, Puchalski SM, Affolter VK, et al. Results of computed tomography in horses with ethmoid hematoma: 16 cases (1993-2005). J Am Vet Med Assoc 2012;240:1338–44.

86. Freeman DE, Orsini PG, Ross MW, et al. A large frontonasal bone flap for sinus surgery in the horse. Vet Surg 1990;19:122–30.

87. Lacombe VA, Sogaro-Robinson C, Reed SM. Diagnostic utility of computed tomography imaging in equine intracranial conditions. Equine Vet J 2010;42:393–9.

88. Finding E, Fletcher N, Avella C, et al. Standing CT and clinical progression of equine cholesterol granulomata. Vet Rec 2012;170:289.

89. Pease A, Behan A, Bohart G. Ultrasound-guided cervical centesis to obtain cerebrospinal fluid in the standing horse. Vet Radiol Ultrasound 2012;53:92–5.

90. Hilton H, Puchalski SM, Aleman M. The computed tomographic appearance of equine temporohyoid osteoarthropathy. Vet Radiol Ultrasound 2009;50:151–6.

91. Naylor RJ, Perkins JD, Allen S, et al. Histopathology and computed tomography of age-associated degeneration of the equine temporohyoid joint. Equine Vet J 2010;42:425–30.

92. Pownder S, Scrivani PV, Bezuidenhout A, et al. Computed tomography of temporal bone fractures and temporal region anatomy in horses. J Vet Intern Med 2010;24:398–406.

93. Tucker RL, Farrell E. Computed tomography and magnetic resonance imaging of the equine head. Vet Clin North Am Equine Pract 2001;17:131–44, vii.

94. Freeman DE, Hardy J. Guttural pouch. In: Auer JA, Stick JA, editors. Equine surgery. St Louis (MO): Saunders Elsevier; 2006. p. 591–607.

95. Munoz JA, Stephen J, Baptiste KE, et al. A surgical approach to the lateral compartment of the equine guttural pouch in the standing horse: modification of the forgotten "Garm technique". Vet J 2008;177:260–5.

96. Perkins JD, Schumacher J, Kelly G, et al. Standing surgical removal of inspissated guttural pouch exudate (chondroids) in ten horses. Vet Surg 2006;35:658–62.

97. Whitton RC, Buckley C, Donovan T, et al. The diagnosis of lameness associated with distal limb pathology in a horse: a comparison of radiography, computed tomography and magnetic resonance imaging. Vet J 1998;155:223–9.

98. Rose PL, Seeherman H, O'Callaghan M. Computed tomographic evaluation of comminuted middle phalangeal fractures in the horse. Vet Radiol Ultrasound 1997;38:424–9.

99. Crijns CP, Martens A, Bergman HJ, et al. Intramodality and intermodality agreement in radiography and computed tomography of equine distal limb fractures. Equine Vet J 2013. [Epub ahead of print].

100. Martens P, Ihler CF, Rennesund J. Detection of a radiographically occult fracture of the lateral palmar process of the distal phalanx in a horse using computed tomography. Vet Radiol Ultrasound 1999;40:346–9.

101. Lloyd KC, Peterson PR, Wheat JD, et al. Keratomas in horses: seven cases (1975-1986). J Am Vet Med Assoc 1988;193:967–70.

102. Reeves MJ, Yovich JV, Turner AS. Miscellaneous conditions of the equine foot. Vet Clin North Am Equine Pract 1989;5:221–42.

103. Getman LM, Davidson EJ, Ross MW, et al. Computed tomography or magnetic resonance imaging-assisted partial hoof wall resection for keratoma removal. Vet Surg 2011;40:708–14.

104. Honnas CM, Dabareiner RM, McCauley BH. Hoof wall surgery in the horse: approaches to and underlying disorders. Vet Clin North Am Equine Pract 2003;19:479–99.

105. Honnas CM. Standing surgical procedures of the foot. Vet Clin North Am Equine Pract 1991;7:695–722.

106. Claerhoudt S, Bergman HJ, Van Der Veen H, et al. Differences in the morphology of distal border synovial invaginations of the distal sesamoid bone in the horse as evaluated by computed tomography compared with radiography. Equine Vet J 2012;44:679–83.

107. Puchalski SM, Galuppo LD, Hornof WJ, et al. Intraarterial contrast-enhanced computed tomography of the equine distal extremity. Vet Radiol Ultrasound 2007;48:21–9.

108. Vandeweerd JM, Perrin R, Launois T, et al. Use of computed tomography in standing position to identify guidelines for screw insertion in the distal phalanx of horses: an ex vivo study. Vet Surg 2009;38:373–9.

109. Barrett JF, Keat N. Artifacts in CT: recognition and avoidance. Radiographics 2004;24:1679–91.

Index

Note: Page numbers of article titles are in **boldface** type.

A

Abdominal surgery
  diagnostic and therapeutic
    in standing horse, **143–168**
      biopsy techniques, 147
      cystic calculi removal, 163–164
      flank laparoscopy, 146–147
      flank laparotomy, 143–146
      laparoscopic nephrectomy, 156–158
      laparoscopic procedures, 156–159
      NSS closure, 152–156
      rectal prolapse, 149–150
      rectal tears, 147–149
      ureteroliths removal
        flank approach to, 159–163
      uterine torsion, 150–152
Access and trocar instruments
  in laparoscopic surgery in standing horse, 22–24
Acepromazine
  in anesthesia/analgesia for surgery in standing horse, 4
Advanced diagnostic imaging
  in standing horse
    benefits of, 239–240
    CT, 253–262. *See also* Computed tomography (CT), in standing horse
    introduction, 239
    MRI, 240–253. *See also* Magnetic resonance imaging (MRI), in standing horse
    new concepts in, **239–268**
α2-Agonists
  in anesthesia/analgesia for surgery in standing horse, 4–7
Analgesia
  for ophthalmic surgeries in standing horse, 92–96
  for surgery in standing horse, **1–17**. *See also* Anesthesia/analgesia, for surgery in
    standing horse
Anesthesia/analgesia
  in diagnostic and therapeutic arthroscopy
    in standing horse, 213–214
  for surgery in standing horse, **1–17**
    epidural, 10–13
    introduction, 1–2
    patient assessment and preparation for, 2–4
    pharmacology in, 4–10
      α2-agonists, 4–7

Vet Clin Equine 30 (2014) 269–281
http://dx.doi.org/10.1016/S0749-0739(14)00009-1
0749-0739/14/$ – see front matter © 2014 Elsevier Inc. All rights reserved.

vetequine.theclinics.com

Printed and bound by CPI Group (UK) Ltd, Croydon, CR0 4YY

03/10/2024

01040487-0012